Percutaneous Laser
Disc Decompression

Springer
New York
Berlin
Heidelberg
Hong Kong
London
Milan
Paris
Tokyo

Daniel S.J. Choy, MD
Assistant Clinical Professor of Medicine, Columbia University College of Physicians & Surgeons, New York, New York; and Director of Laser Spine Center, New York, New York

Editor

Percutaneous Laser Disc Decompression

A Practical Guide

With 149 Illustrations, 6 in Full Color

Springer

Daniel S.J. Choy, MD
Assistant Clinical Professor of Medicine
Columbia University College of
Physicians & Surgeons
New York, NY 10032
and
Director of Laser Spine Center
New York, NY 10021
USA
dchoy@nyc.rr.com

Cover illustration: Figure 2.1. Array of 24 UV lasers aimed at a suspended deuterium pellet for a fusion experiment. (Courtesy of Institute of Optics, University of Rochester, Rochester, NY.)

Library of Congress Cataloging-in-Publication Data
Percutaneous laser disc decompression : a practical guide / editor, Daniel S.J. Choy.
p. cm.
Includes bibliographical references and index.
ISBN 0-387-00260-X (alk. paper)
1. Intervertebral disk—Diseases. 2. Intervertebral disk—Surgery. 3. Intervertebral disk—Hernia. 4. Intervertebral disk displacement. 5. Lasers in surgery. 6. Lasers in medicine. I. Choy, Daniel S.J.

RD771.I6P469 2003
617.5′6—dc21 2003042428

ISBN 0-387-00260-X Printed on acid-free paper.

Printed in the United States.

9 8 7 6 5 4 3 2 1 SPIN 10904770

www.springer-ny.com

Springer-Verlag New York Berlin Heidelberg
A member of BertelsmannSpringer Science+Business Media GmbH

This book is dedicated to

Dr. Peter Wolf Ascher, former professor of neurosurgery at the University of Graz, Graz, Austria, and presently Professor and Chairman of the Department of Neurosurgery at the University of Rostock, Rostock, Germany

Professor Robert B. Case, professor of medicine at the Columbia University College of Physicians & Surgeons, New York, New York

my patients, without whose help this book would not have been possible.

Preface

Percutaneous laser disc decompression (PLDD) is an entirely new approach to the treatment of herniated intervertebral disc disease. The traditional laminectomy and discectomy procedure was first performed at the Massachusetts General Hospital in 1934. In the intervening 69 years, science has moved forward with magnetic resonance imaging, sequencing of the human genome, ion propulsion, landing men on the moon and robots on Mars, the laptop computer, global positioning system navigation, black hole theory, string theory, and the successful cloning of animals. And yet, the same soft tissue–destroying, scar-inducing, posterior wall–weakening, and spinal instability–inducing cutting operation is still being taught and performed. Advances in orthopedics and neurosurgery occur slowly.

Percutaneous laser disc decompression is minimally invasive; it can be performed as an outpatient procedure, requires no general anesthesia, and has a high success rate, a low recurrence rate, and a low complication rate. By the middle of 2002, some 35,000 PLDD procedures had been performed worldwide.

This book covers the history of the development of PLDD, laser physics, anatomy and pathophysiology of the herniated disc, the physics and mechanical principles that form the basis of PLDD, patient selection, radiographic considerations, the neurologic examination, a step-by-step description of the PLDD procedure, the complications of PLDD and their treatments, special cases amenable to PLDD, postoperative care, and rehabilitation procedures. In short, this is a compendium of PLDD from A to Z.

The author hopes the publication of this volume will persuade a new generation of orthopedic and neurologic surgeons to open their minds and hearts to a twenty-first-century innovation in the treatment of herniated intervertebral disc disease.

Daniel S.J. Choy, MD

Contents

Contributors

William Black, MD
Director of Neurosurgery (Retired), Community Medical Center, Scranton, PA 18510, USA.

John A. Botsford, MD
Director of Radiology, The Deaconness Hospital, Cincinnati, OH 45243, USA.

Daniel S.J. Choy, MD
Assistant Clinical Professor of Medicine, Columbia University College of Physicians & Surgeons, New York, NY 10032, USA; Director of Laser Spine Center, New York, NY 10021, USA; Attending Physician, Lenox Hill Hospital, New York, NY 10021, USA; Former Director, Laser Laboratory, St Luke's–Roosevelt Hospital Center, New York, NY 10027, USA; Executive Editor, *Journal of Clinical Laser Medicine & Surgery.*

Arpad S. Fejos, MD
Staff, Columbia University College of Physicians & Surgeons, New York, NY 10032, USA; Lenox Hill Hospital, New York, NY 10021, USA; Laser Spine Center, New York, NY 10021, USA.

A.K.D. Goswami, MS Mch (Orth), FRCS (Orth), DNB, DHA,
Honorary Lecturer, University of Central Lancashire, Rochdale, Lancaster OL11 4LZ, UK.

M.T.N. Knight, FRCS
Consultant Spinal Surgeon, Honorary Senior Lecturer, University of Central Lancashire, Rochdale OL11 4LZ, UK; Honorary Research Fellow, University of Manchester, Manchester M13 9PL, UK; The Spinal Centre, Rochdale, Lancaster OL11 4LZ, UK.

Sohail K. Mirza, MD
Associate Professor of Orthopedics, Department of Orthopedics & Sports Medicine and Department of Neurological Surgery, University of Washington, Seattle, WA 98195, USA; Harborview Medical Center, Seattle, WA 98104, USA.

1

Introduction: Percutaneous Laser Disc Decompression

Daniel S.J. Choy

Background

This book is devoted to a new approach in the treatment of herniated disc disease. Traditional open surgery, with its many disadvantages, has been in existence since 1934 when it was introduced at the Massachusetts General Hospital. In the intervening 69 years, science has achieved spectacular advances elsewhere: black holes, supersonic flight, the sequencing of the human genome, landing men on the moon, quarks, global position navigation, cloning. Yet spine surgeons are still making incisions, spreading and damaging muscle fibers, cutting out pieces of lamina, making holes in the annulus and removing nucleus pulposus, and leaving behind the detritus of scar tissue. These severe disturbances of normal anatomy sometimes make fusion necessary. Fusion then leads to the *adjacent disc syndrome* caused by the additional stress placed on the disc superior or inferior and adjacent to the level of fusion. This in turn has led to the development in the past few years of the various forms of artificial metal/plastic disc prostheses at great expense and effort in the new field of *vertebroplasty.* In May 2002, the author attended the "Spine Arthroplasty 2" symposium held in Montpellier, France, where numerous manufacturers displayed at least seven models of these devices. None of these would be necessary if a treatment of herniated disc disturbed the anatomy and geometry of the offending disc only minimally. Most of the panelists were of the opinion that discogenic pain arises from chemical mediators—cytokines, pH modifiers, and tumor necrosis factors—and that these arise from disc material. Hence the anatomic structure producing these offending agents must be removed as completely as possible. Sometimes an experiment in nature is more informative than a well-designed, double-blind, prospective study with crossover. The author reported on a stunt pilot with a herniated lumbar disc and sciatica whose pain was sharply aggravated by a 6 *G* pull out from a dive; independently, the pilot discovered that his pain could be almost immediately relieved by climbing to 10,000 feet and performing an outside loop, producing minus 3 *G*s. In a 6 *G* pull-out, centrifugal force increases body weight by six times gravity; in a minus 3 *G* outside loop, when the aircraft flies in a curve with the apex pointed up, the body weight is decreased threefold. The time parameters of these two maneuvers are more consistent with a pressure/mechanical mechanism of discogenic pain than a chemical one.[1]

In the healing arts there are other examples of complications of one therapy that produce the need for another therapy. Witness the early total gastrectomies causing the dumping syndrome, the early intestinal bypass operations for obesity leading to severe malabsorption syndromes and hepatic damage, the necessary immunosuppression of organ transplant recipients, which increases susceptibility to infection and lymphoma, and the implantation of metallic left ventricular assist devices, resulting in almost universal mediastinitis.

The history of interventional therapeutic modalities for back pain and sciatica due to intervertebral disc protrusion is seen in Table 1.1. When offered open surgery, many patients demur, some out of fear of having their backs "cut open," some because of a justifiable fear of general anesthesia, and some because they have heard horror stories of complications and bad results. Despite this, some 500,000 back operations are performed annually in the United States, a resident of the northwest having three times the likelihood of being operated upon than a resident of the northeast. These invasive procedures include laminectomy,

Table 1.1 Interventional Treatments for Herniated Disc Disease

History of open surgical methods	
1934	Laminectomy and discectomy, Massachusetts General Hospital, Boston, followed by microdiscectomy in the 1980s
History of percutaneous methods	
1975	Hijikata, percutaneous discectomy
1983	Kambin, trephine, rongeur, suction
1984	Onik, nucleotome
1986	Choy/Ascher, percutaneous laser disc decompression
2000	Saal, IDET (intradiscal electrothermal annuloplasty)

discectomy, microdiscectomy, fusion, and automated percutaneous nucleotomy. Chemonucleolysis with chymopapain is losing favor because of reports of neurologic complications from chymopapain leakage, with myelitis, allergic and anaphylactic reactions, and even some deaths. The latest is intradiscal electrothermal (IDET) annuloplasty, a radiofrequency method that heats up and destroys the pain fibers in the outer layers of the annulus without retracting the disc herniation.

In 1984, to address these problems, the author conceived the idea of introducing laser energy into a herniated/protruded disc to vaporize a small volume of nucleus pulposus and thus lower intradiscal pressure. The pressure reduction would create a pressure gradient, leading to migration of the herniated portion away from an involved nerve root. This approach is based on the physical principle that in an intact, enclosed hydraulic space, since water is noncompressible, a small change in volume will result in a disproportionately large change in pressure. It is well known that the water content of nucleus pulposus ranges from 50 to 89% and is age dependent, decreasing with advancing years. That was the entire concept. If it worked, it would lead to a major advance in the treatment of herniated disc disease.

Two physicians, to whom this book is dedicated, made it possible for me to test this hypothesis in the laboratory and to test it in the clinical setting. These were first, Professor Robert B. Case, Director of the Investigative Cardiology Laboratory at St. Luke's–Roosevelt Hospital, Columbia University College of Physicians & Surgeons in New York City, and second, Professor Peter Ascher at the Neurosurgical Institute of the University of Graz, Graz, Austria.

My connection with Dr. Case came about through my invention of the laser catheter for the intraoperative recanalization of obstructed coronary arteries with a laser beam. This was developed first in a basement laboratory at the Lenox Hill Hospital in New York, and when bureaucratic obstacles arose, Dr. Robert Roven persuaded his colleague to invite me to join the Investigative Cardiology Laboratory at St. Luke's. This was a completely equipped laboratory with a tinkerer's (me) dream of instrumentation, reminding me of the Aero Medical Laboratory at Wright Patterson Air Force Base, where I had spent time in the early 1950s performing the early rocketry experiments. From 1981 to 1983 the laboratory experiments validating the concept of laser angioplasty were completed,[2] and on September 17, 1983, our group performed the first five intraoperative laser coronary angioplasties successfully at the University of Toulouse in France, followed by three others in January 1984.[3]

On my return to New York, the *New York Times* report and presentations at the Texas Heart Institute and the American College of Cardiology led to inquiries from several major industrial firms producing the Gruntzig angioplasty catheters. In short order, my laser catheter patent was circumvented, leaving our laboratory with four lasers occupying space, unused.

Unwilling to allow laser equipment worth a half-million dollars to sit idle, I then drew on my 12-year experience as a part-time surgeon for the New York City Police Department. As such I regularly rode around town in police cars with flashing lights and siren, and carried a Walther PPK 9 mm automatic in a shoulder holster. With the rank of deputy inspector, I had 1500 men under me. In that capacity I saw hundreds of cases of back pain, many caused by herniated discs. An officer could retire at three-quarters pay, tax free, for life, if he could prove to the retirement board that he had had a back injury "on the job" causing total disability. It was important for me to learn all I could about bad backs and herniated disc disease. I suddenly had an insight. The intervertebral disc, I knew, was a contained hydraulic space. The nucleus pulposus is mostly water. Water is not compressible. If the volume of a noncompressible medium is reduced by a small amount, there should be a sharp decrease in pressure. The idea for using a laser to treat herniated disc disease was born.

First, the hypothesis that a small volume change in the disc would be associated with a disproportionate pressure change had to be proved.[4] Research funding and a Messerschmitt Bolkow and Blohm (MBB) Medilase Nd:YAG laser were generously provided by Walter Solomon of Endolase. Technical assistance came from Lucy Eron, chief technician of Endolase, and Peter Altman, a brilliant young bioengineer from Columbia. Always present was the eminence gris of Professor Robert B. Case, ready with advice and hands-on participation. Fresh (less than 24 hours old) cadaver lumbar spine segments were obtained. A simple pressure recording device was made from a 20-gauge needle with the tip soldered shut. A half-moon window was filed in the shaft near the tip and covered with condom rubber sheet glued on with rubber cement (Fig. 1.1). Total cost: about 24 cents. A year later,

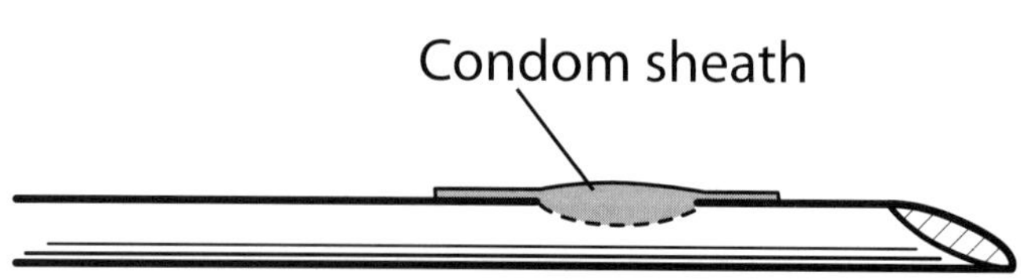

Figure 1.1. A 20-gauge needle modified with a window cut into the distal end and covered with a condom sheath glued onto the needle with rubber cement. The needle tip has been soldered shut. The modified needle is the sensor for intradiscal pressure.

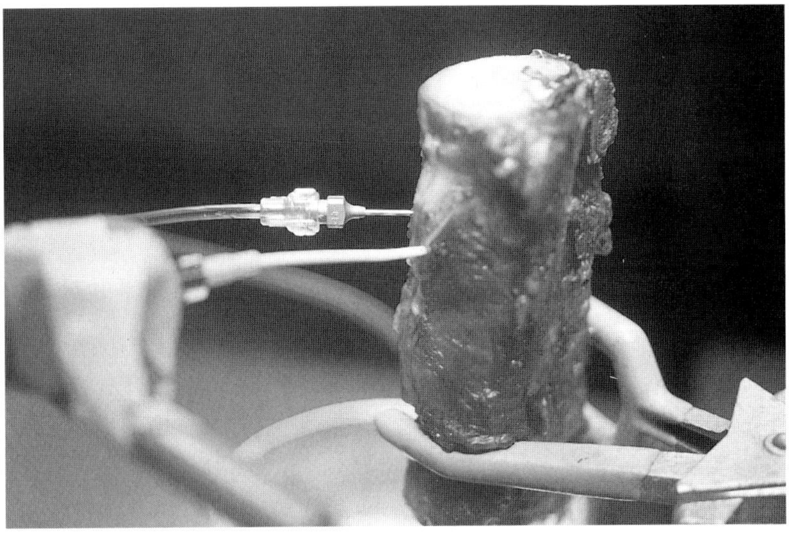

Figure 1.2. Two needles inserted into an intervertebral disc: one for pressure measurement, and one for infusion of saline with a Harvard pump.

in a telephone conversation, I mentioned this cost to Dr. Alf Nachemson, the pioneer of intradiscal pressure measurements. There was a moment of silence, then the great man remarked that the Japanese firm that made his recording needles had charged him something like U.S. $1500 each. He did not sound happy.

By filling our modified needle with saline and connecting it to a water manometer, we could obtain accurate pressure readings. The lumbar spine was immobilized with clamps to a ring stand. The pressure needle and a second 20-gauge needle were inserted into the disc at 90 degrees apart. Connected to the second needle was a Harvard pump (Fig. 1.2). Saline was pumped into the disc while pressures were recorded. The results are seen in Figure 1.3. One mL of volume change produced a pressure change of 312 kPa (= 2340 mmHg).

Next, laser dosage had to be established in terms of pressure fall induced, laser tract size, and histologic changes determined with an appropriate energy delivered. For reasons to be discussed later, it was decided to use a Neodymium:YAG (Nd:YAG) laser emitting at 1064 nm. An aluminum frame was designed and constructed by Dr. Khan of the Columbia School of Engineering to hold the lumbar spine segment upright and to exert static load pressure duplicating in some measure the weight of the upper two-thirds of the body on the lumbar spine (Fig. 1.4). Load on the spine specimen was by the addition of 20-pound lead bricks on the platform. The pressure needle was inserted, as was an 18-

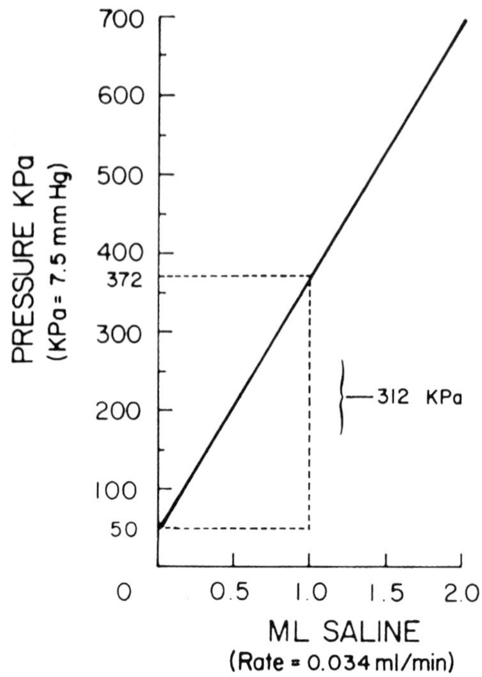

Figure 1.3. Graph plotting intradiscal pressure versus volume of saline infused. This is 312 kPa per milliliter of saline infused. (Reprinted with permission from Case RB, Choy DSJ, Altman P. Change of intradiscal pressure versus volume change. *J Clin Laser Med Surg* 1995;13:125–126.)

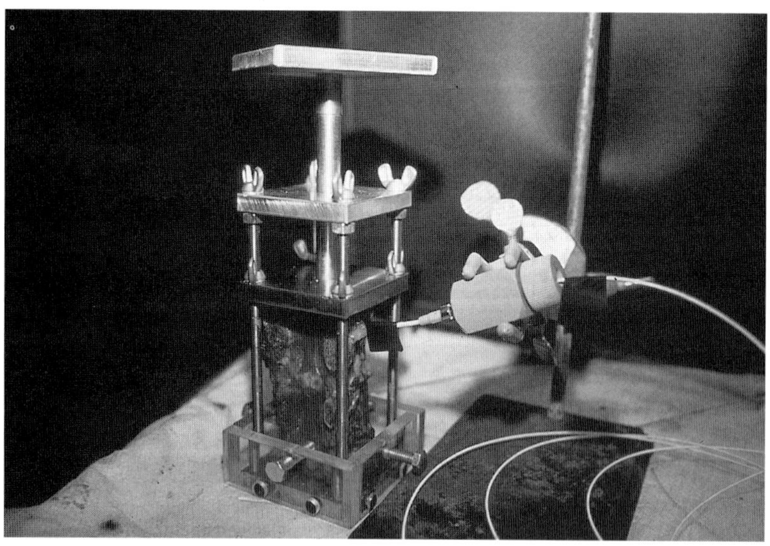

Figure 1.4. Metal frame designed to stabilize a portion of the lumbar spine in a vertical orientation. The loading platform accommodates a lead brick load. Four wing nuts provide a constant loading pressure on the discs when the lead weight is removed.

gauge needle at 90 degrees from the first needle. A 400 μm optical fiber was inserted into the 18-gauge needle and connected to the MBB Medilas Nd:YAG laser with an SMA connector. The laser was calibrated to deliver 20 watts at 1.0-second bursts with 5-second pauses to allow for heat dissipation; two 20-pound bricks were loaded onto the platform, and intradiscal pressures were recorded. When equilibration occurred, the four wing nuts were turned clockwise until no pressure change resulted when the lead bricks were removed. Static load was thus achieved. The laser was turned on until 1000 joules was delivered. Eighteen experiments were performed. The mean preload pressures were 1100 mmHg, the mean after-loading pressures were 2350 mmHg. The mean after-lasing pressures were 1120 mmHg, and final pressures 23 minutes after cessation of lasing were 1000 mmHg. The continued decline of pressure after cessation of lasing is probably due to continued denaturation of disc (Fig. 1.5). In a parallel series of 17 experiments, the laser was not turned on as a control. There was a negligible drop of pressure[5] (Fig. 1.6).

The elliptical laser tracts formed by 1000 joules of Nd:YAG energy measured 2 cm $\times$ 5 to 6 mm at the equator and were cal-

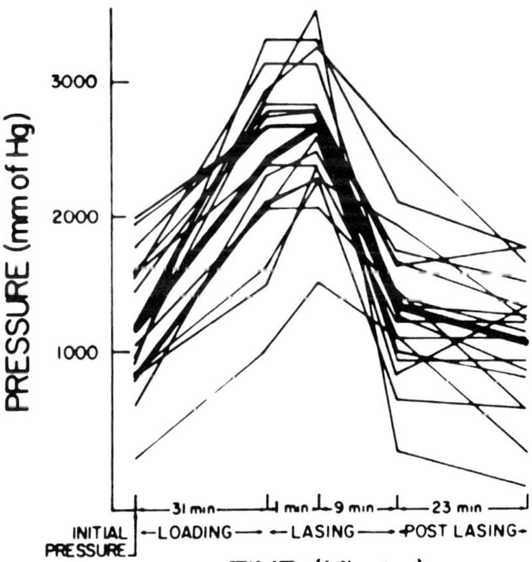

Figure 1.5. Plot of a loading phase with a preload pressure of 2419 mmHg, a stabilized after-loading pressure, against the fall of pressure in the first 9 minutes of lasing, and the continued fall in pressure during 23 minutes after lasing with stabilization at the end. The total fall of intradiscal pressure with laser ablation = 1344 $\pm$ 601 mmHg or 55.6% ($p < 0.0001$). (Reprinted with permission from Case RB, Choy DSJ, Altman P. Change of intradiscal pressure versus volume change. *J Clin Laser Med Surg* 1995;13:125–126.)

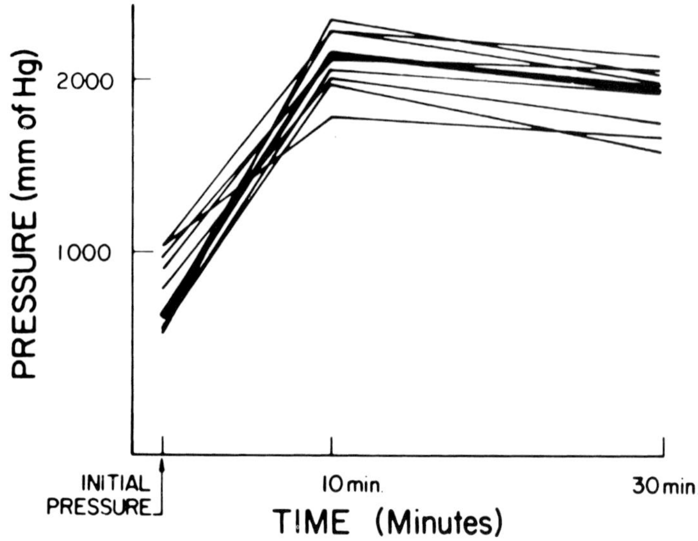

Figure 1.6. Control discs ($n = 9$) were subjected to the same conditions as those in Fig. 1.5 except that the laser was not turned on. The mean fall of intradiscal pressure was 143 mmHg in a 20-minute period. (Reprinted with permission from Case RB, Choy DSJ, Altman P. Change of intradiscal pressure versus volume change. *J Clin Laser Med Surg* 1995;13:125–126.)

culated to be 200 to 250 mm^3 (Fig. 1.7, see color plate). Microscopic sections revealed a *hole* surrounded by a thin zone of carbonization, then a collar of protein coagulation with small vacuoles containing steam from water vaporization[6] (Fig. 1.8, see color plate).

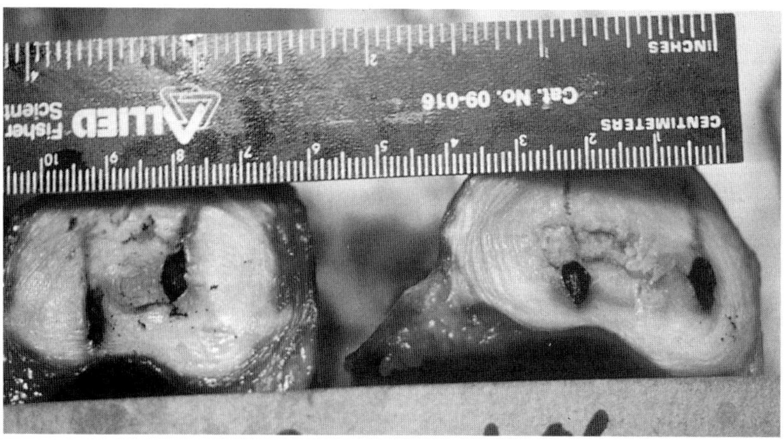

Figure 1.7. Laser tracts formed in nucleus pulposus by 1000 joules of laser energy at a 1.32 μm on the left and a 1.06 μm Neodymium (Nd:YAG) laser on the right. (See color insert)

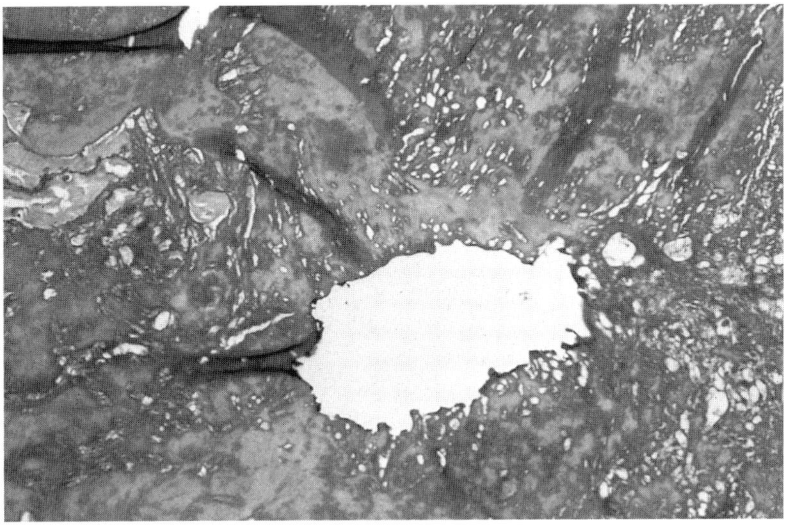

Figure 1.8. Histologic appearance of a laser tract in the nucleus pulposus. There is a central hole surrounded by a zone of protein denaturation and then vacuoles, which are probably steam pockets. (Hematoxylin and eosin stain.) (See color insert)

The in vitro intradiscal pressure decrease was subsequently verified on eight occasions when in vivo pre- and postlaser measurements were made in patients undergoing percutaneous laser disc decompression (PLDD). The average decrease of intradiscal pressure was from a baseline of 300 to 154 mmHg (Fig. 1.9).

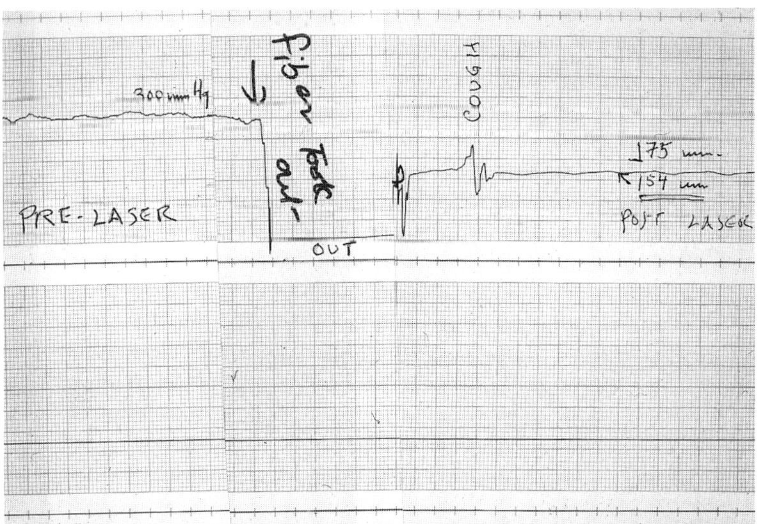

Figure 1.9. Pre- and post-PLDD (percutaneous laser disc decompression) intradiscal pressures, with handwritten notes. There is a fall from 300 mmHg to 154 mmHg. The "glitch," caused by a cough, demonstrates open manometrics.

These experiments benefited from Dr. Case's extensive experience in pressure measurements in his long and productive history of investigations in experimental cardiology.

With the large number of lasers of different wavelengths, it was next essential to ascertain which wavelengths would be best suited for decompressing intervertebral discs. Peter Altman, Dr. Stephen Trokel, and I studied the erbium:YAG (2940 nm) CO_2 (10,600 nm), Nd:YAG (1318 and 1064 nm), argon (488, 516 nm), holmium:YAG (2150 nm), and the excimer (193 nm) lasers. The results are indicated in Figure 1.10 in graphs showing mass of disc ablated by the different lasers.[7] The most efficient lasers in terms of energy absorption by water were the CO_2 and erbium:YAG lasers. To be fair to the holmium:YAG and excimer lasers, these early models did not have the power capacities of their present-day cousins. It is now known that the Ho:YAG laser is superior to the Nd:YAG laser where water absorption of power is concerned. However, it will be seen from later discussion that what works well in the laboratory is not necessarily the optimal

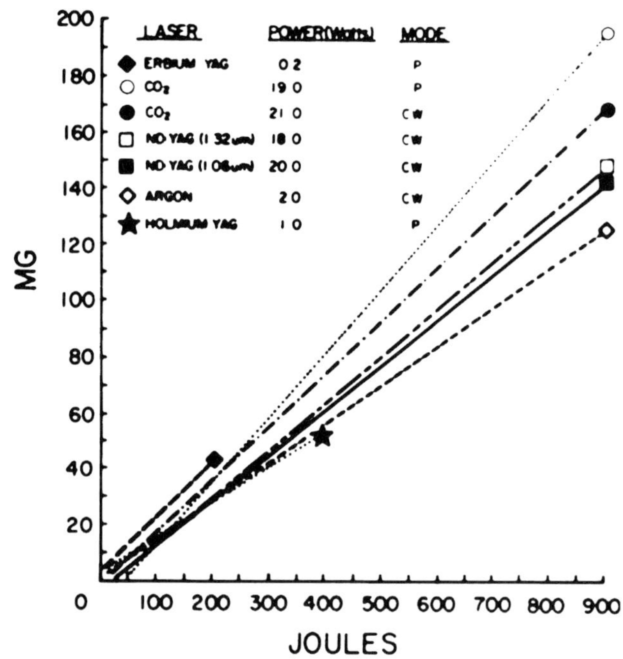

Figure 1.10. Composite graph of various wavelengths versus mass of disc ablated. The CO_2 in the pulsed (P) mode is the most efficient, and the least efficient is the argon in a continuous wave (CW) mode. The potassium triphosphide (KTP) wavelength is close to that of the argon laser.

laser in the operating room. On the basis of our studies, we chose the Nd:YAG laser emitting at 1064 nm for use in PLDD.

Thermal experiments used bovine spine segments immersed in 37°C saline baths with thermocouples placed at 1.0 cm from the laser fiber tip directly in the line of fire, laterally to the laser at the neural foraminae, and at the anterior surface of the spinal canal. The optical fiber/needle was inserted from a posterolateral direction with the needle tip just past the annulus. Application of laser energy (20 J) resulted in temperature rises not exceeding 2°C, well within the safety range.

In vivo animal studies using 13 mongrel dogs weighing 22 to 30 kg were next undertaken. Institutional review board (IRB) approval was obtained, and all humane animal treatment guidelines were meticulously followed. Under general anesthesia, and with C-arm radiographic guidance, 18-gauge, 9-inch-long needles were inserted under aseptic conditions through the shaved skin into a single lumbar disc of each animal. Canine discs are very difficult to enter because the vertebral anatomy differs significantly from that of the human. The spinous processes are angled cephalad, and the discs are one quarter as thick. If one is able to enter a canine disc percutaneously, the human disc presents no problem at all. One thousand joules were delivered to each disc at 20 watts in 1.0-second bursts with 5-second pauses for heat dissipation. Only one dog developed a limp. At 2 weeks all animals were humanely killed and autopsied. There were no instances of extradiscal injury.

I believe that ours is the only group in the world that worked so assiduously in the laboratory for 2 years to provide a solid scientific basis for the subsequent clinical work that started in mid-February 1986.

First Steps

How did I meet Peter Ascher? In 1980, President Jimmy Carter initiated a transfer of laser technology to China that involved sending one third of the best laser physicists in the United States together with nine medical doctors who were involved with lasers. The physicists were from MIT, the University of Chicago, the Bell Research Laboratories, the Lawrence Livermore Laboratory, the U.S. Naval Weapons Research Laboratory, and the Atomic Energy Laboratory in Los Alamos. I was privileged to be one of the medical/surgical group, having just invented laser angioplasty. I had yet to perform the first angioplasty on a human patient. At the meetings in China were Professor Carlo Sacchi of the Politecnico di Milano and Professor Peter Ascher of the Neurosurgical Institute, University of Graz, Graz, Austria. Ascher was already established as a leader in lasers in neurosurgery. With his alpine hat and feather, his lederhosen outfit, and his curved Austrian pipe, Ascher was a sight never before seen by the Chinese populace, and everywhere he went, the neurosurgeon was surrounded as though he were a Martian. The showman in Ascher loved the attention.

I was still a neophyte, but the concept of using an argon laser inside a coronary artery apparently stimulated the imagination of both the laser physicists and the laser surgeons, and I received an undeserved amount of attention. Not knowing much about lasers at the time, I attached myself to the 33 physicists for the entire month. It was like a crash course in postgraduate laser physics. Indeed, I was not invited to the welcoming party in Shanghai for the physicians because I was mistaken for a physicist. The next day, to her great mortification, the hostess discovered I was a medical doctor, so she set up a special private party at her parents' home at which I discovered that her father had been an employee of my father's in Shanghai.

Since it was a high-level mission, we were feted by the mayors of Shanghai and Hangzhou. Deng Xiaopeng himself gave us a banquet at the Great Hall of the People, and the chef of Madame Sun Yat Sen came out of retirement to cook. Afterward, Deng held a receiving line, and all the American professors lined up to shake the great man's hand and have their wives take pictures of the great moment. However, Deng's bodyguards, dressed as waiters, kept getting in the way to protect the chairman. Guess what? These important professors and chairmen of physics departments got back in line three or four times on the theory that to a Chinese all Americans look alike, until their wives succeeded in taking their pictures.

In November 1985, after my eight successful angioplasties in Toulouse, Peter Ascher and I were awaiting our turn to speak at a major laser symposium in Milan organized by Professor Sacchi. Before our talks, the simultaneous interpreter came over and told us that it took three words in Italian to express one word in English, and therefore, would we speak at one-third speed? Needless the say, the usual 10-minute presentations by our Italian colleagues were taking up to 30 to 45 minutes (because lecturer-time discipline seems to be lacking in Italy). It was then about 8 P.M., and both Ascher and I were dozing off. Out of boredom, Peter suddenly asked, "What's new, Choy?"

"I've been using Nd:YAG laser on cadaver and bovine discs and on canine discs in vivo."

He immediately woke up. "Ach du lieber! When can you come to Graz to do the first case with me?"

"When is the best skiing in Austria?"

"January and February."

"How about mid-February?"

"O.K."

In mid-February 1986 I arrived at his hospital in Graz. Peter was downcast.

"We have no cases," he announced.

"Then let's have lunch," I suggested.

During lunch a nurse burst into the room and announced with great excitement, "The ambulance just brought in a man who is thrashing about on the gurney with pain in his back and leg."

"Let's go see him," Peter said.

"No, no, order the MRI. Let's finish lunch, then we'll go see him," I replied. So that is what we did. The MRI showed a herniation of the L5-S1 disc.

Standing over the patient, an immigrant Turkish worker whose face was twisted in pain, Peter said, "You have a herniated lumbar disc."

"Can you help me?" he asked.

"This is Professor Choy from New York, and he has a new treatment with a laser through a needle put into your back with local anesthesia."

"What is the alternative?"

"The alternative is that I cut you open."

"I'll take the laser."

This could never have happened in the United States. The entire concept of PLDD would have had to be submitted to an IRB, endlessly argued and debated, and perhaps permission would have been granted in 1 or 2 years. In Austria, the doctor was still king. There was no IRB. There was no informed consent. The doctor just goes ahead and does his thing. I don't know if that is all good. Ascher, being a master of practical psychology, instinctively used the right words with the patient. No one likes to be "cut open."

Presently, all was ready. The Nd:YAG laser, the needle, the fiber, the patient, the sterilization, the draping, the gloves, the gowning. Under local anesthesia and with fluoroscopic guidance, a 14-gauge needle was inserted into the L5-S1 disc, then the optical fiber. We planned to deliver 1000 joules. At 600 joules, the patient suddenly exclaimed "Die Schmerzen sind vorbei!" (the pain is gone).

I took off my gloves and mask, went around to the front, and took a picture of the smiling patient (Fig. 1.11, see color plate), the first person to be treated with PLDD. This picture is shown because of its historical significance.

This pattern of immediate pain cessation was to become almost a norm in the following 17 years. It is really not so surprising, since as vaporization of water occurs, the fall of intradiscal pres-

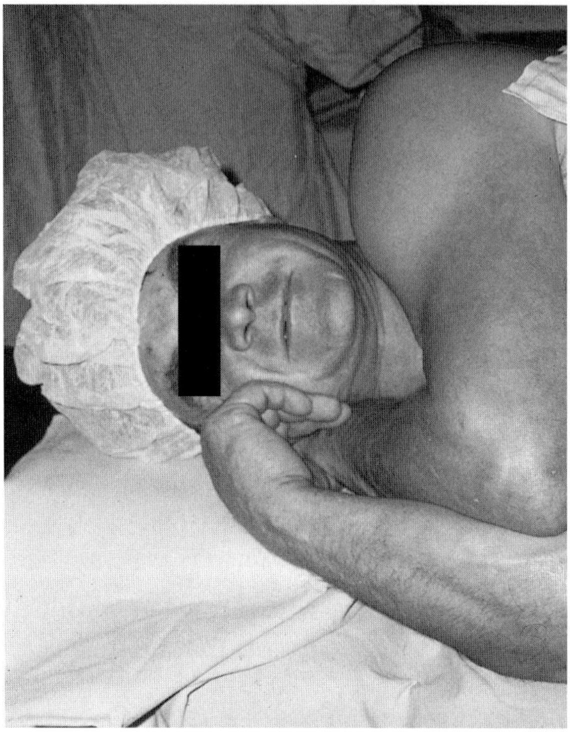

Figure 1.11. The first percutaneous laser disc compression (PLDD) patient after receiving 600 joules in Graz, Austria, February 1986. The patient is free of pain. (See color insert)

sure is simultaneous, so disc shrinkage also occurs. It is not amazing, it is simply physical laws at work.

Ascher and I held a small celebration at a weinstube after this first case (Fig. 1.12, see color plate).

On my return to New York, because of bureaucratic obstacles and endless paper work associated with obtaining an IRB approval at St. Luke's Hospital, PLDD did not start until September 1988. Meanwhile Peter Ascher was treating cases left and right. Peter flew by Concorde to New York to perform the first PLDD case at St. Luke's–Roosevelt. Our first peer-reviewed paper was a letter to the *New England Journal of Medicine*[8] with the title "Percutaneous Laser Disc Nucleolysis of Lumbar Disks." Soon I was asked by Professor Augustus White III, orthopedic-surgeon-in-chief at Harvard, to contribute a section to the forthcoming textbook *Clinical Biomechanics of the Spine*.[9] He suggested a change from "nucleolysis" to "decompression," a more accurate and descriptive term. Hence one quarter of the established name for the procedure was contributed by Augustus White III of Harvard: percutaneous laser disc decompression, *decompres-*

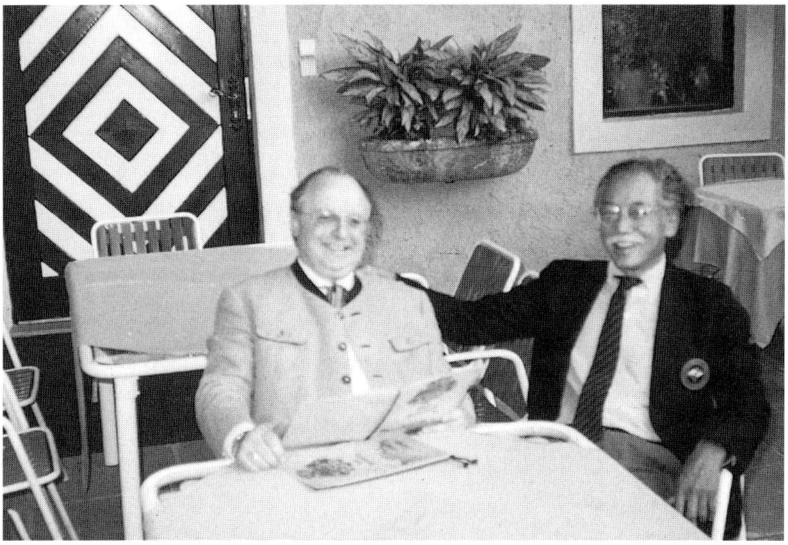

Figure 1.12. Drs. Ascher and Choy celebrating in a weinstube after the first successful procedure. (See color insert)

sion for the mechanism of action, hence PLDD. Subsequent publications have appeared in *Spine*,[10] *Clinical Orthopedics & Related Research*,[7] a State-of-the-Art review issue of *Spine*,[11d] and a number of updates in the *Journal of Clinical Laser Medicine and Surgery*.[12–15] A special issue of this journal[16] was devoted to PLDD in 1995. Some 146 presentations and workshops have been conducted worldwide by the author. Book chapters have appeared in seven texts.

Percutaneous laser disc decompression (PLDD) is being performed in almost every nation in western Europe, in the United Kingdom, in South and Central America, Cuba, Japan, China, India, Korea, and the United States. As of this writing (May 2002), some 35,000 cases have been treated worldwide; some 10,000 in the United States. Reported success rates according to the MacNab criteria (Table 1.2) from laser spine surgeons around the world average 75 to 85%, with a complication rate of 1%. My own figures from a database of some 2000 cases are 89% and 0.4%, respectively. PLDD received Food and Drug Administration (FDA) approval in 1991 and was awarded a Current Procedural Terminology (CPT) code by the American Medical Association in January 2000. It is being reimbursed by third-party payers in the United States.

The International Musculoskeletal Laser Society (IMLAS) was organized by Siebert, Gerber, Knight, and others in 1993 and has held annual meetings in Paris, Neuchatel, Kassel, Lake Tahoe, Seville, Bogotá, and Sydney.

Table 1.2 MacNab Criteria

Response	Criteria
Good	Resumed preoperative function Occasional backache or leg pain No dependency-inducing medications Activity appropriate No objective signs of nerve root involvement
Fair	May be nonproductive if unchanged from preoperative status Intermittent episodes of mild lumbar and/or low back pain No dependency-inducing medications Activity appropriate No objective signs of nerve root involvement
Poor	Subjective No productivity Continued pain behavior Medication abuse Inactive Compensation and/or litigation focus Objective signs of continuing radiculopathy

Subsequent chapters deal with anatomy and pathology of the intervertebral disc, laser physics, radiologic considerations, patient selection, the neurologic examination, the PLDD procedure, *keyhole surgery* (foraminotomy), magnetic resonance imaging (MRI) with the spine under compression, spinal stenosis, extruded discs, erectile dysfunction, complications of PLDD and

Table 1.3 The Critic and the New Idea

1. Idea stage: "It won't work." "It's been tried before."
2. Success in the laboratory: "Very lucky." "Beginner's luck."
3. After first abstract: "Too bad, a tragedy really, because now they'll continue."
4. After five successful cases: "Highly experimental." "Too risky, unethical, and immoral."
5. After 15 successful cases: "May occasionally succeed in carefully selected cases, but is generally not important or useful."
6. After many successes: "So-and-So has not been able to duplicate their results in Shangrila."
7. Final stage: "This is a very fine contribution. I predicted this; in fact, I had the same idea in 1929."

their treatment, postprocedure instructions, follow-up care including rehabilitation, the familial incidence of herniated disc disease with underlying genetic factors, and why PLDD should be the mainstream treatment of choice for herniated disc disease in the twenty-first century.

Every new idea is met with resistance. Table 1.3 describes how a critic typically greets a new idea.

References

1. Choy DSJ. Positive and negative gravitational forces and herniated disk sciatic pain. *N Engl J Med* 1997;337:19.
2. Choy DSJ, Stertzer SH, Rottedam HZ, Bruno MS. Laser coronary angioplasty: experience with 9 cadaver hearts. *Am J Cardiol* 1982;50: 1209–1211.
3. Choy DSJ, Stertzer SH, Myler RK, Marco J, Fournial G. Human coronary laser recanalization. *Clin Cardiol* 1984;7:377–381.
4. Choy DSJ, Case RB. Intervertebral disc pressure as a function of fluid volume infused. *Spine* 1993;7(1)(state-of-the-art review: laser discectomy):11–15.
5. Choy DSJ, Altman P. Fall of intradiscal pressure with laser ablation. *Spine* 1993;7(1)(state-of-the-art review: laser discectomy):23–29.
6. Choy DSJ. Percutaneous laser disc decompression using the 1.06 and 1.32 μm Nd:YAG lasers. *Spine* 1993;7(1)(state-of-the-art review: laser discectomy):41–47.
7. Choy DSJ, Altman PA, Case RB, Trokel SL. Laser radiation at various wavelengths for decompression of intervertebral disc. *Clin Orthop* 1991;267:245–250.
8. Choy DSJ, Case RB, Fielding WSD, Hughes J, Liebler W, Ascher P. Percutaneous laser nucleolysis of lumbar disks. *N Engl J Med* 1987;317:771–772.
9. White AA III, Panjabi MM. *Clinical Biomechanics of the Spine.* 2nd ed. Philadelphia: Lippincott; 1990:446.
10. Choy DSJ, Ascher PW, Saddekni S, Alkaitis D, Liebler W, Hughes J, Diwan S, Altman P. Percutaneous laser lumbar disc decompression—a new therapeutic modality. *Spine* 1992;178:949–956.
11. Scherk H. *Spine* 1993;7(1)(state-of-the-art reviews: laser discectomy).
12. Choy DSJ, Michelsen J, Getradjman G, Diwan S. Percutaneous laser disc decompression—an update. *J Clin Lasers Med Surg* 1992;4:177–184.
13. Choy DSJ. Percutaneous laser disc decompression update: focus on device and procedure advances. *J Clin Laser Med Surg* 1993;11(4):181–183.
14. Choy DSJ. Percutaneous laser disc decompression: 352 cases with an 8½ year follow-up. *J Clin Laser Med Surg* 1995(13);1:17–21.

15. Choy DSJ. Percutaneous laser disc decompression: twelve years' experience with 752 procedures in 518 patients. *J Clin Laser Med Surg* 1998(16);6:325–331.
16. Choy DSJ. Percutaneous laser disc decompression Special Issue. *J Clin Laser Med Surg* June 1995;13:100–202.

2

Principles of Lasers

Daniel S.J. Choy

Lasers are now ubiquitous. Before 1960, no working laser existed. First came Townes and Schawlow's concept of the **m**icrowave **a**mplification through **s**timulation of **e**mitted **r**adiation (MASER), followed by the slight change of "microwave" to "light." Then came Maiman's development of the first workable LASER, with a ruby crystal as the lasing medium in 1960.

Today, lasers are used in reading of bar codes at supermarket checkout counters, as pointers in the lecture hall, to guide smart bombs, to sculpt corneas, to open arteries, to transmit information bits through optical fibers, to identify **d**eoxyribo**n**ucleic **a**cid (DNA) in laser flow cytometry, to perform cellular microsurgery, to flip cells around using *laser tweezers,* to compress deuterium pellets in fusion experiments, to create light shows, and to assassinate intestinal worms.

In a fusion experiment at the Institute of Optics in Rochester, New York, 24 UV laser beams are aimed and fired at the same instant at a deuterium pellet suspended by a fiber from a spider web (Fig. 2.1). The instantaneous compression of the deuterium releases fusion energy; but so far, the amount of energy generated does not surpass the total input energy of the laser beams.

In another experiment illustrating the power and coherence of a laser beam, scientists on mountain tops in Arizona and California aimed two 3-watt argon lasers through telescopes at a dark portion of the moon in the earth's shadow, and the two spots were photographed by a circling spacecraft (Fig. 2.2). Imagine that an ordinary lightbulb is rated at 100 watts, and these two devices were rated only at *3* watts each. Three percent of energy

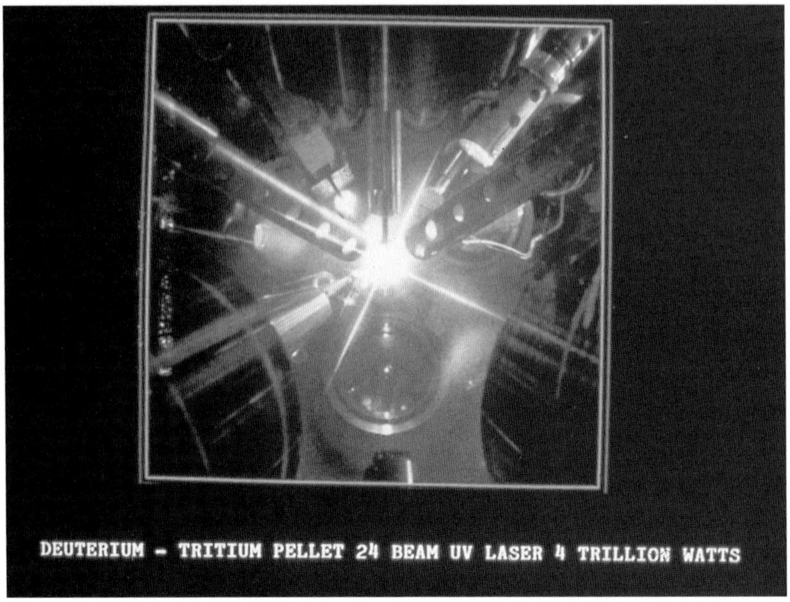

Figure 2.1. Array of 24 UV lasers aimed at a suspended deuterium pellet for a fusion experiment. (Courtesy of Institute of Optics, University of Rochester, Rochester, NY.)

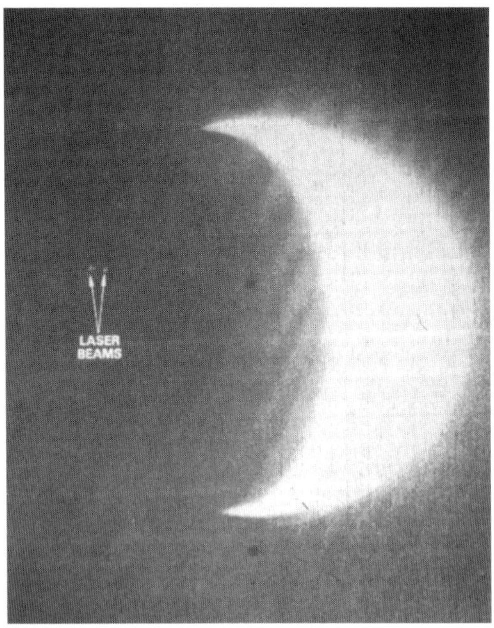

Figure 2.2. Two 3-watt argon laser spots projected on the moon, a distance of 230,000 miles from earth, photographed by *Surveyor VII*.

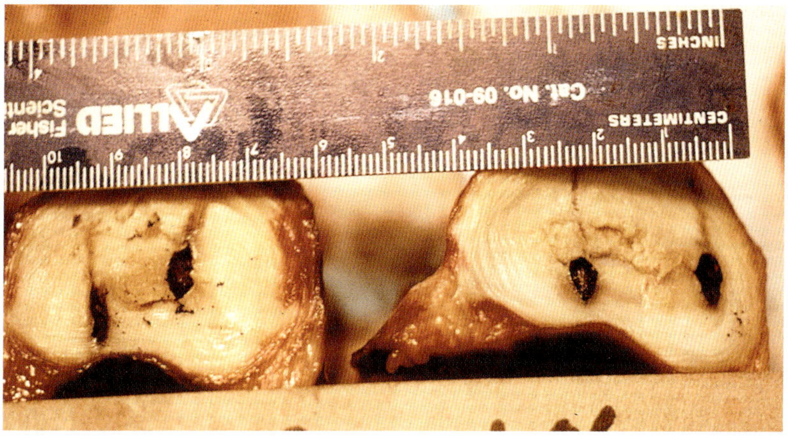

Figure 1.7. Laser tracts formed in nucleus pulposus by 1000 joules of laser energy at a 1.32 μm on the left and a 1.06 μm Nd:YAG laser on the right.

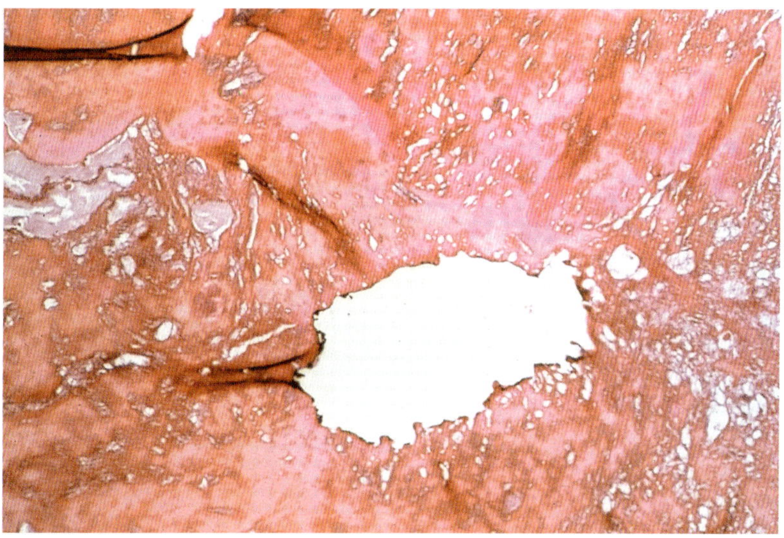

Figure 1.8. Histologic appearance of a laser tract in the nucleus pulposus. There is a central hole surrounded by a zone of protein denaturation and then vacuoles, which are probably steam pockets. (Hematoxylin and eosin stain.)

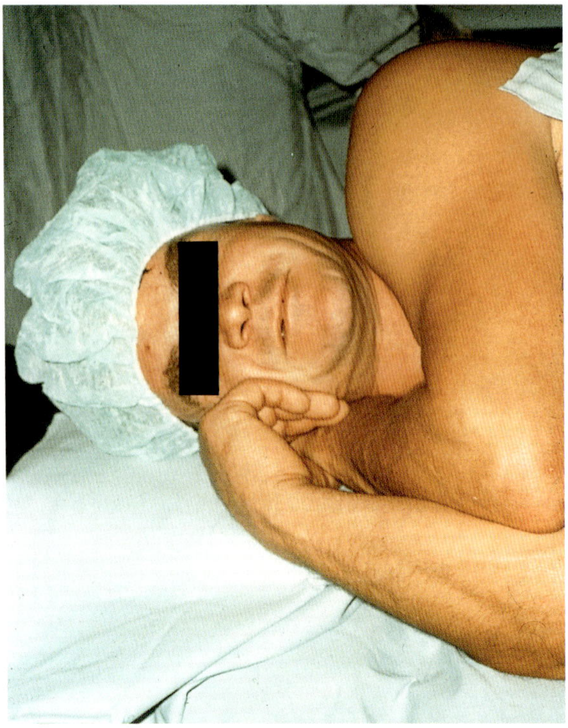

Figure 1.11. The first PLDD patient after receiving 600 joules. Graz, Austria, February 1986. The patient is free of pain.

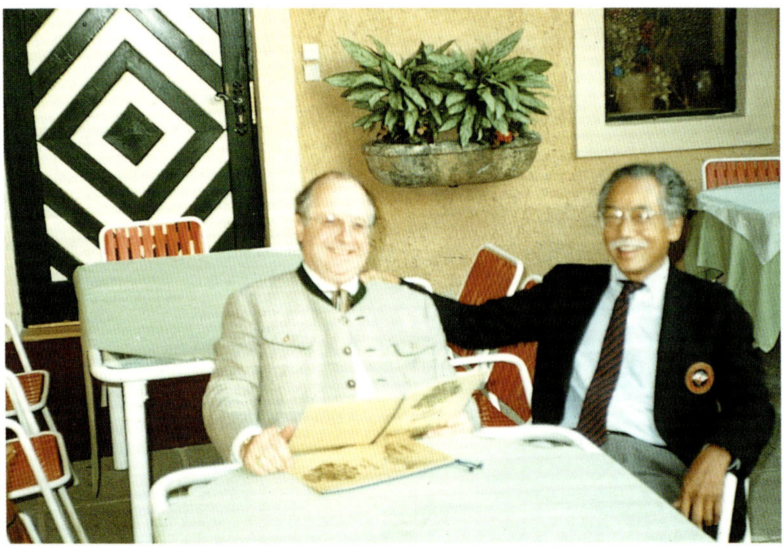

Figure 1.12. Drs. Ascher and Choy celebrating in a weinstube after the first successful procedure.

Color Plate III

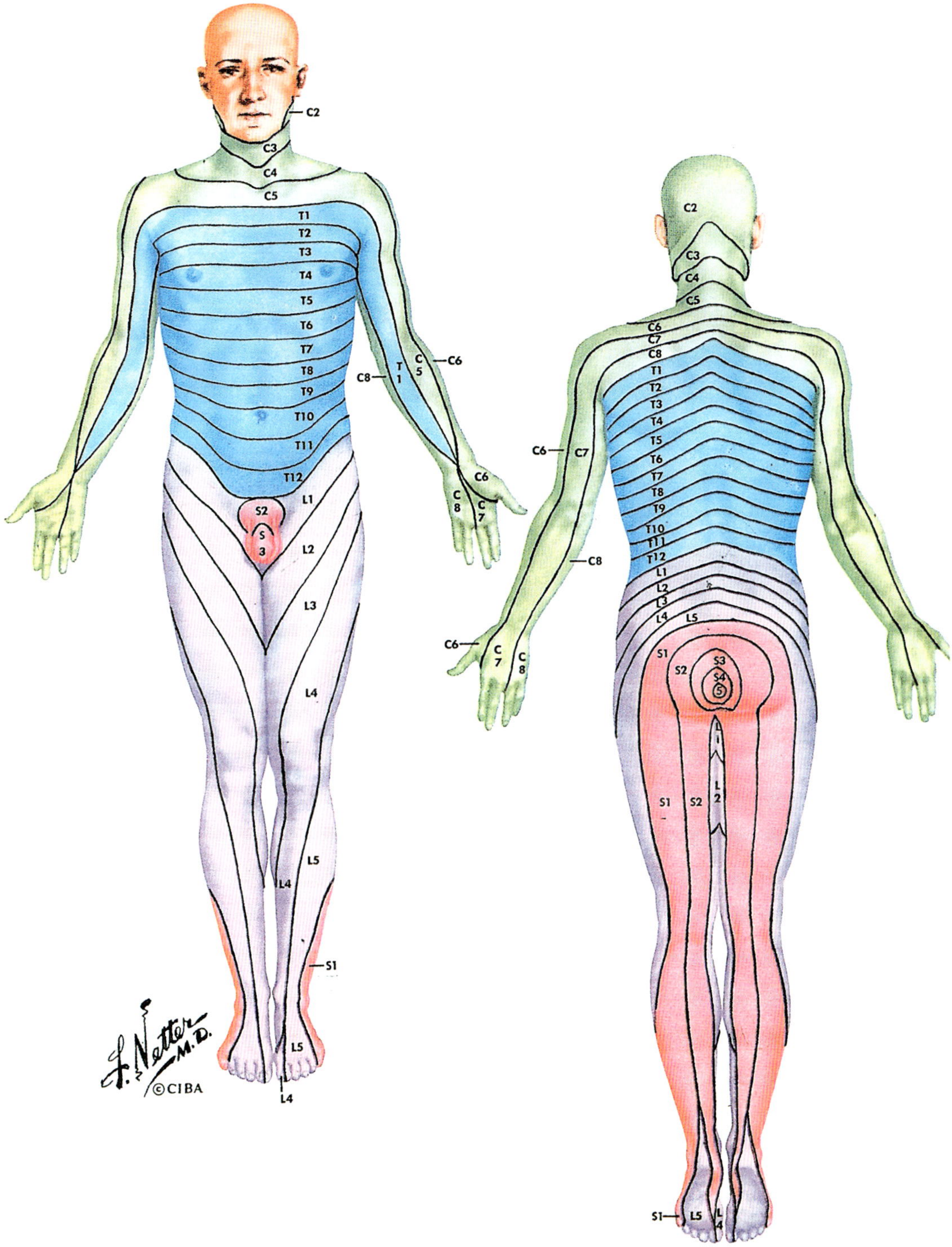

Figure 6.2. Dermatomal map. (From *The Netter Collection of Medical Illustrations, Vol I Nervous Sysem*. Copyright 1983. Icon Learning Systems, LLC, a subsidiary of MediMedia USA Inc. Reprinted with permission from Icon Learning Systems, LLC. Illustrated by Frank H. Netter, MD. All rights reserved.)

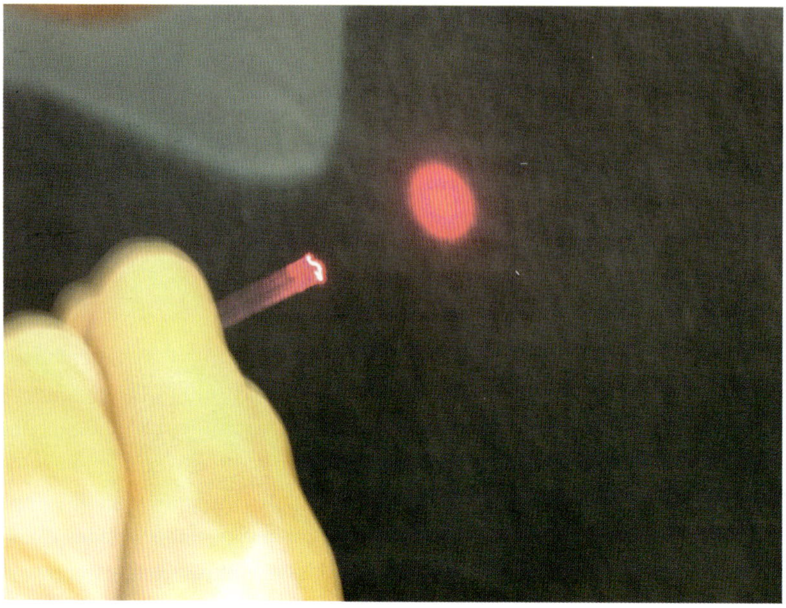

Figure 10.24. A sharp, round laser spot indicating good focus.

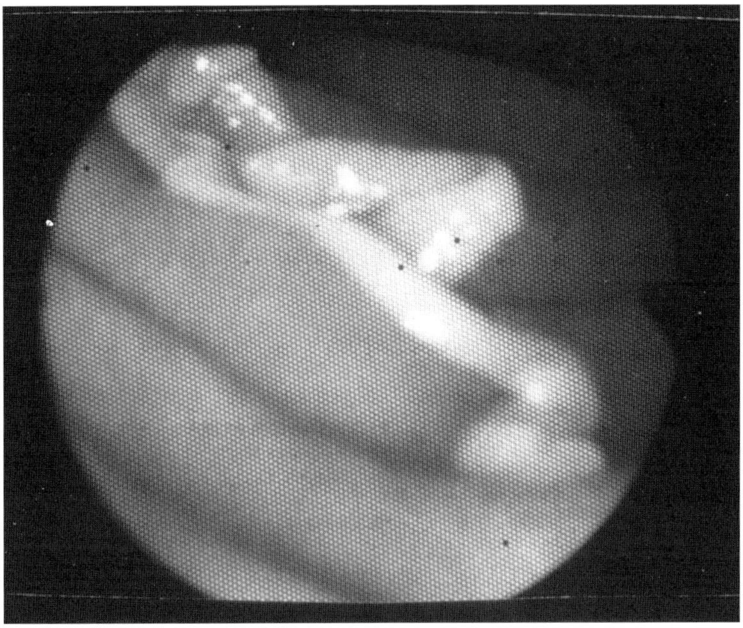

Figure 2.3. Endoscopic view of the body of *Taenia saginata* in the intestine of a French patient. (Courtesy of Phillipe Raimbert, MD.)

used by an ordinary lightbulb was enough to power a laser beam able to produce a spot on the moon—230,000 miles away—that could be photographed. Such is the power of a *coherent* light beam.

In a clinical experiment conducted, appropriately enough, in the City of Light, Paris, a gastroenterologist, Dr. Phillipe Raimbert, treated a patient infested with the common tapeworm *Taenia saginata* that had resisted all drug attempts at purging. A Neodymium:YAG (Nd:YAG) laser beam was aimed at the worm's body (Fig. 2.3) and fired at 5 joules. The worm did not like it and raised its head, whereupon the laser was aimed between the "eyes" and 20 joules promptly dispatched the worm (Fig. 2.4), prompting the following headline in a journal, "*Safari au Taenia*" (Fig. 2.5).

How does such a versatile tool work?

Essentially, a lasing medium, which may be a gas, liquid, or crystal, is contained in a cylindrical tube, or resonator, with a fully reflecting mirror on one end and a partially translucent mirror on the other (Fig. 2.6). External energy, usually in the form of electricity, or sometimes in the form of another laser, is applied to the medium. The electrons are excited and jump to a higher orbit. During decay, as each excited electron falls back to its home orbit, a photon is emitted. This photon is joined by other released

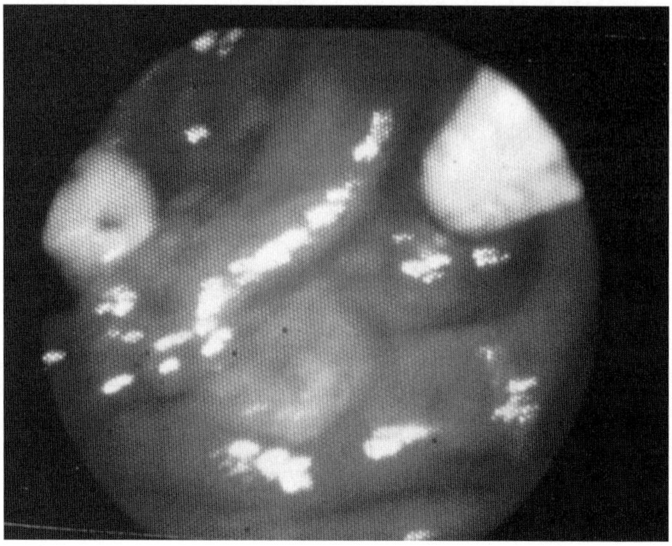

Figure 2.4. Right after a laser burst to the body, the worm has raised its head. The laser was then aimed between the *eyes,* effectively terminating the parasite. (Courtesy of Phillipe Raimbert, MD.)

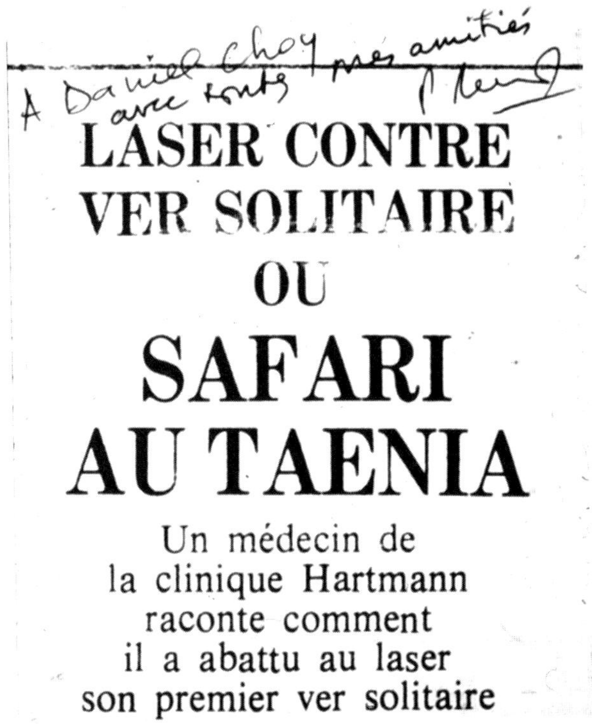

A Daniel Choy avec toutes mes amitiés

LASER CONTRE VER SOLITAIRE OU

SAFARI AU TAENIA

Un médecin de la clinique Hartmann raconte comment il a abattu au laser son premier ver solitaire

Figure 2.5. The headline in a French medical journal announcing the first successful in vivo assassination of a worm by laser. (Courtesy of Phillipe Raimbert, MD.)

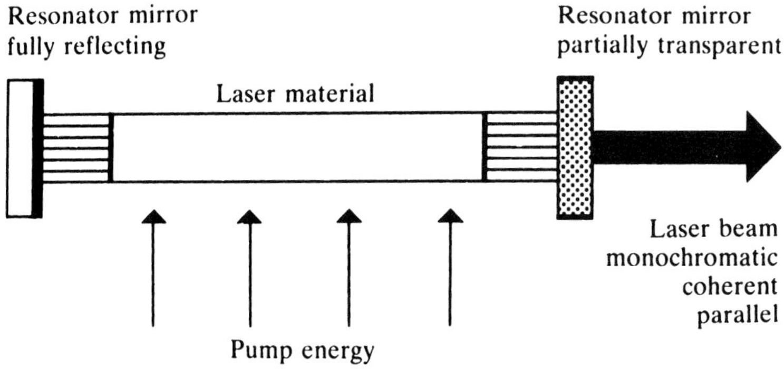

Figure 2.6. Diagram of a laser. The resonator tube has a fully reflective mirror on the left and a partially translucent one on the right. The laser beam emits through the right end of the tube as a coherent beam.

photons, and they bounce in all directions. The cylindrical tube favors those that travel along its long axis, and the stream of photons is reflected back and forth between the two mirrors until sufficient strength is achieved to break out through the translucent mirrored end as a coherent stream of photons vibrating in phase, at the same frequency. It is the phase-locked, monofrequency characteristic that gives the laser beam its power and coherence (Fig. 2.7).

Different lasing media produce different wavelengths. Thus the CO_2 laser generates a laser beam with a wavelength of 10,600 nm, the erbium:YAG 2940 nm, the argon 488–514 nm, the Holmium:YAG (Ho:YAG) 2150 nm, the excimer 193 nm, the Nd:YAG 1064 and 1318 nm, the KTP—532 nm, and the diode laser in the range of 800 to 900 nm.

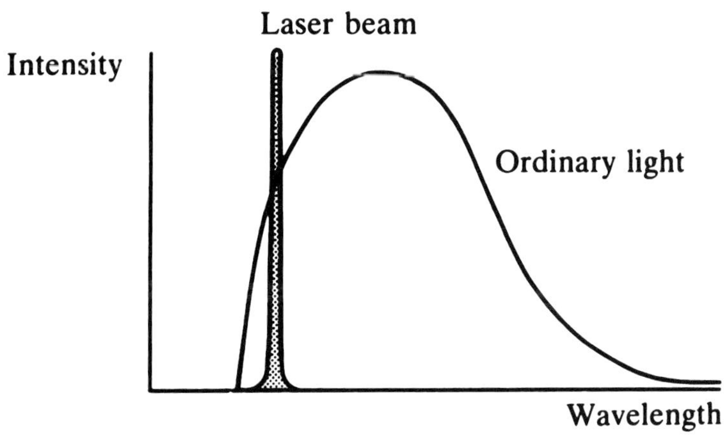

Figure 2.7. A laser beam is coherent (in phase) and has monofrequency.

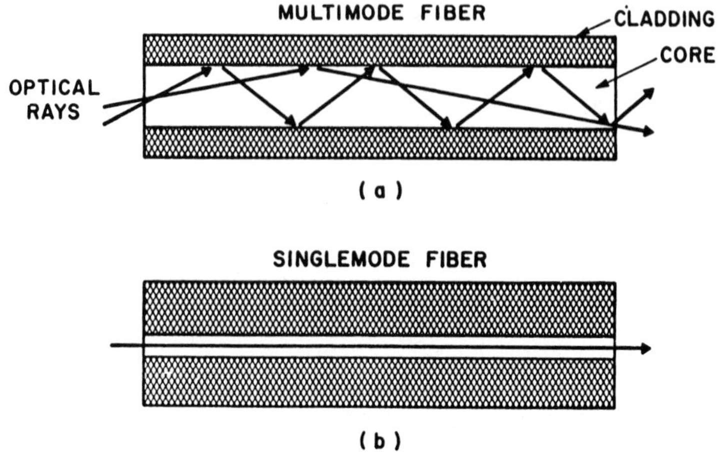

Figure 2.8. An optical fiber or waveguide, with a central transparent core and a reflective cladding. The laser beam is internally reflected whether the fiber is straight or curved.

Until the advent of waveguides, or optical fibers, lasers could be transmitted only through a vacuum or through air. In a liquid medium the beam would be rapidly dispersed. To date, there is still no practical waveguide for the CO_2 laser. Hence, the initial application of laser energy in medicine and surgery was not surprisingly in the field of ophthalmology. Argon lasers have been used to coagulate retinal vessels and to create drainage holes in the iris for the treatment of glaucoma. Corneal sculpting with the CO_2 and excimer lasers has made great strides and is Food and Drug Administration (FDA) approved.

In the early 1980s, single-mode and multimode optical fibers (Fig. 2.8) were developed. There is a transparent core, usually of quartz, and a reflective cladding, either of plastic or, to provide a higher melting point, quartz. Will a laser beam traveling down a fiber be continually reflected internally by the reflective cladding until it emerges from the terminal end as a laser beam, or as a noncoherent beam? When I began my first experiments with an argon laser fired through a "laser catheter" for coronary artery angioplasty in 1980, the answer to this question was not definitively known. Several physicists whom I consulted were not sure if the beam, entering the optical fiber as a laser, would emerge as a laser. In an early experiment I was able to show that a stream of water falling in an arc from a catheter would "bend" the laser (Fig. 2.9). Later when I could ignite a paper target with a 3-watt argon laser transmitted through a curved 120-degree quartz fiber, I was convinced that laser input = laser output. Simple as it may seem at this late date, the *transmissibility* of a laser beam through a waveguide *essentially unaltered* was the bedrock

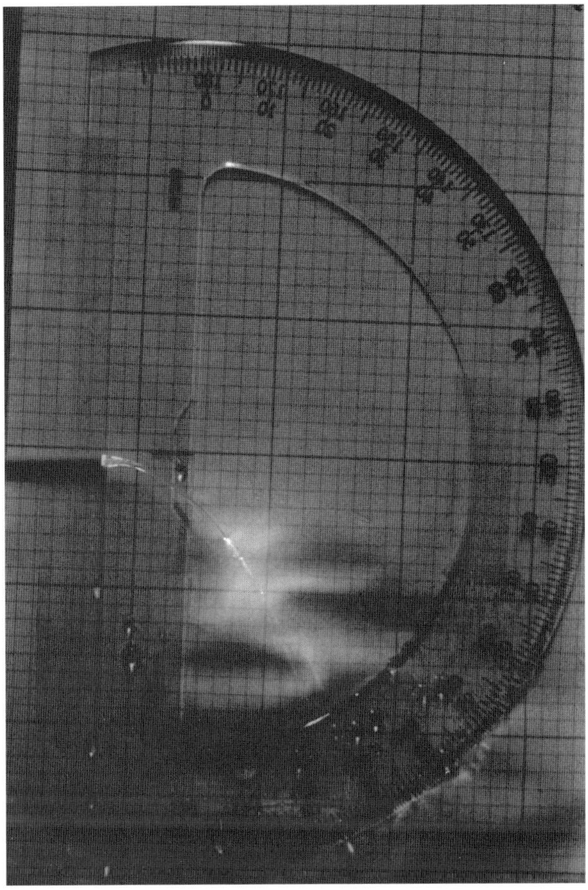

Figure 2.9. An early experiment illustrating how a laser beam emerging from a catheter is bent (through internal reflection by the water–air interface) as the water spout falls in a curve from the catheter tip. The critical angle for this continuous wave argon laser, at 3 watts, was 30 degrees. Beyond 30 degrees the laser "broke away" from the stream.

and foundation of present applications of laser in medicine and surgery. Not much has been written about this all-important phenomenon before, but I assure you, it is vital.

It was fine for physics to have developed the laser. But now, how to apply this new tool to medicine and surgery? Of concern to the laser surgeon (new specialty, hence a new name) is how each laser reacts with tissue. First, if a laser beam is absorbed by the tissue there will be heat generation. Thus, the argon laser (green-blue) is well absorbed by hemoglobin (red) and hence found its first application in the eye. When a tissue is transparent or nearly so, most of the laser beam will be transmitted and will therefore exert little effect on this tissue. The CO_2 laser can generate short pulses of great power and is primarily absorbed

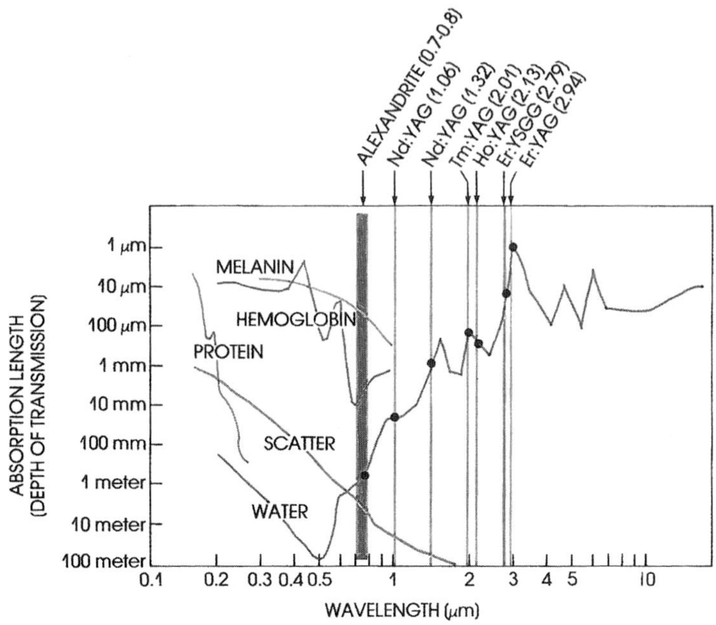

Figure 2.10. Laser–tissue interactions at different wavelengths.

by water. It therefore excels at surface cutting, with little penetration power. The Nd:YAG laser has greater penetration and is better suited for coagulation (Fig. 2.10). The excimer laser works through disruption of molecular bonds and excels at making fine cuts with little or no heat generation. It is also known as the "cold laser." Not all lasers are very efficient; for instance, the argon laser produces only approximately 0.1% of the electrical power needed to activate it.

The remainder of this chapter is devoted to highlighting the essential points made by the late Nobel laureate Arthur Schawlow in his chapter for the 1995 special issue of the *Journal of Clinical Medicine & Surgery* devoted to percutaneous laser disc decompression.

1. Only the free electron laser is adaptable to a wide range of wavelengths and power levels, but its large size and cost will keep it only in large research institutions for the foreseeable future.
2. Shock waves can arise from nonthermal processes such as laser spark breakdown from the high electric fields of a pulsed light beam focused inside a transparent medium.
3. The absorption of red light by the hematoporphyrin dye can activate singlet oxygen molecules that disrupt the cellular nuclei and lead to apoptosis. This is the basis for the photody-

namic therapy of cancer pioneered by Dr. Tom Dougherty, Roswell Park, New York.

4. The monochromaticity of the laser makes possible highly sensitive spectroscopy, in some instances the detection of as little as a single atom of an element.
5. The interference patterns of laser light make possible precise measurements by interferometry and also the emerging field of holography.
6. The helium–neon laser, invented by Ali Javan, is widely used as a handheld pointer in the lecture hall and as an aiming beam in surgical lasers, where the laser beam is invisible, as in the CO_2 and Nd:YAG lasers.

This, then, is the instrument, a product of man's inexhaustible ingenuity, that has revolutionized warfare, marketing, spectrometry, imaging, classroom teaching, holography, cancer therapy, ophthalmology, dermatology, and now spinal surgery.

3

Anatomy and Pathophysiology of Intervertebral Discs*

Sohail K. Mirza

The intervertebral disc is a unique and complex structure. It is the largest avascular structure in the body.[1] It imparts mobility to the spinal column while providing efficient load transfer across the vertebrae. The intervertebral disc has the most complex embryologic development of any joint.[2] Biomechanically, it exhibits complex dynamic properties of interchanging fluid and solid phases.[3] Disc degeneration is universal in the human spine.[4] The annual cost to society of disc-related conditions is estimated at $20 to $50 billion.[5] At the fundamental level, however, relatively little is known about the intervertebral disc which is the focus of intense research efforts worldwide. This chapter reviews the current understanding of the intervertebral disc at the basic science level.

Anatomy

Embryologic Development

The human intervertebral disc has a more complex developmental history than any other joint in the body.[3] It is derived from the notochord and somatocoele mesenchymal cells.[6] The noto-

*Adapted from Mirza, SK, and White, AA: Anatomy of intervertebral disc and pathophysiology of herniated disc disease. Journal of Clinical Laser Medicine and Surgery 1995;13:131–142.

chord plays a prominent part in the differentiation of disc.[3] Cotten et al. have clearly described the differentiation of the intervertebral disc, and the following description is derived from their work.[2]

The primitive disc is composed of two elements: the notochord and the fibrocartilaginous perinotochordal tissue. The notochord is continuous and uniform initially and occupies the central axis of the developing vertebral column. The mesenchymal tissue of the somites undergoes cellular proliferation and migration to the notochord, forming a continuous mesenchymal vertebral column. The notochord develops sinuous expansions dorsally in the intervertebral regions. The mesenchymal tissue, in turn, forms individual alternating areas of dense-celled zones and loose-celled zones. The dense-celled zones form the intervertebral disc and the loose-celled zones form the vertebral bodies.

The tissue immediately adjacent to the notochord forms cartilage with a matrix. The outer zone of the mesenchymal tissue forms fibroblasts that begin to assume a laminated pattern. The notochord cells in the region of the intervertebral discs proliferate and form an expansion. Notochord cells disappear from the regions of the vertebral body. This stage of differentiation is complete by 10 weeks.

In weeks 11 to 20, the dorsal expansion of the notochordal cellular mass forms the nucleus pulposus. The annulus region forms increased collagen fibers in inner zone (13th week) and assumes a cruciate arrangement in the outer zone with fibers crossing at 110 to 140 degrees. Little further modification goes on after 20 weeks. Notochord cells form a syncytium with a mucoid matrix and show progressive degeneration and decrease in number. Some networks of notochordal cells persist at birth. Numerous collagen fibers form in the annulus with cartilaginous matrix production in the inner zone.[3]

Thompson et al. observed that mature disc cells in tissue culture have been noted to possess the capacity to respond to growth factors and that disc repair can be modulated by growth factors.[7] These authors theorized that modulation of tissue repair by growth factors may become a therapeutic alternative to fusion or prosthetic replacement for intervertebral disc pathology.[7]

Morphologic Structure

Annulus

Marchand and Ahmed conducted a thorough, quantitative study of the structure of the annulus fibrosus.[8] The annulus consists of 15 to 25 layers of fiber bundles arranged in a crisscross pattern (Fig. 3.1). The layers are 0.14 to 0.52 mm thick. The layers are relatively thicker in the lateral portion of the annulus and in its in-

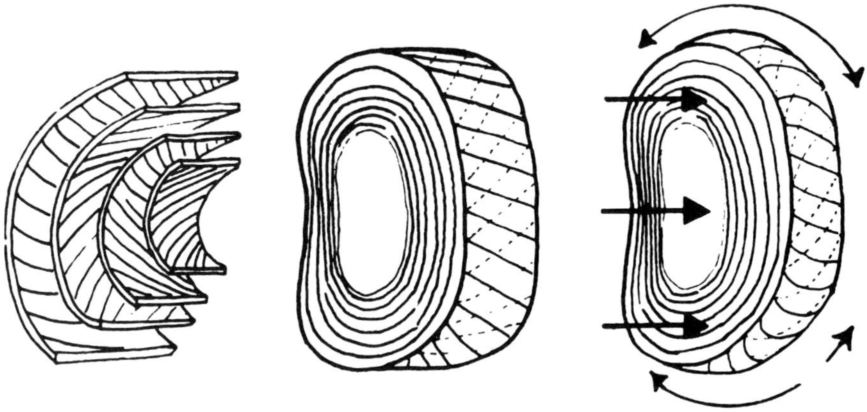

Figure 3.1. The intervertebral disc is an enclosed hydraulic structure composed of cephalad and caudal endplates, with multiple collagen fiber layers of the annulus fibrosus in a circular ring surrounding the nucleus pulposus. Composed of proteoglycans and water, the nucleus pulposus is poorly vascularized and devoid of neural fibers. The annular fibers are arranged at approximately 80 degrees from one layer to the next. This *basket* arrangement of fibers allows expansion and contraction to accommodate expansion and contraction of the nucleus, a bioengineering masterpiece.

ner layers. The total disc height comprises 20 to 62 fiber bundles. The fiber bundles are perpendicular in successive layers. They extend over the edge of the vertebral body. The inclination of the fiber bundles changes as the bundles extend over the vertebral edge. The average interbundle space is 0.22 mm wide and is filled with a gelatinous material. No layer-to-layer connections were identified. The total number of layers per annulus increases in lower lumbar levels.

Marchand and Ahmed noted that contrary to earlier assumptions, the structure of the annulus is highly irregular.[8] Irregularities in the laminar structure are present in both circumferential and radial directions. Forty percent of the layers are incomplete in any 20 degree circumferential sector of the disc. The inclination of the fiber bundles varies from 0 to 90 degrees near locations of these laminar irregularities. These structural irregularities are most frequent in the posterolateral regions of the annulus. Tsuji et al. also noted irregular laminate structure in the posterior parts of the annulus, with a greater proportion of incomplete laminar layers, increased fiber interlacing angle, and loose interlaminar connections.[9]

Nucleus

The nucleus pulposus moves within the disc with changes in posture.[10] It moves anteriorly in the normal disc with lumbar extension. The nucleus frequently communicates with the epidural space and surrounding neural structures. In their study involving methylene blue injection of the nucleus, McMillam et al.

noted that 14% of 105 discs showed leaks.[11] Ninety-three percent of the leaks were located in the posterolateral region, lateral to the posterior longitudinal ligament. The injected dye showed contact with the adjacent nerve root in 27% of the leaks.

Endplate

The endplate consists of a thin flat layer of hyaline cartilage, thinner in the center. Nutritional substances reach the disc through the endplate by diffusion.[12] Cells of the intervertebral disc and the cartilage endplate sit in fibrous capsules, forming chondrons.[13]

Nerve Root

Nerve roots differ from peripheral nerves. Nerve roots are bathed in cerebrospinal fluid (CSF) and do not contain endoneurium or perineurium.[14] The nerve root is located cephalad in the foramen.[15] With straight leg raising, the lumbar nerve roots move 0.5 to 5 mm and sustain 2 to 4% strain.[16] A more transverse course of the nerve root in the spinal canal may be associated with increased risk of sciatica.[17] Conjoined nerve roots are noted in 2 to 4% of the patients undergoing imaging studies[18] and 14% of those participating in anatomic studies.[19–21] Conjoined nerve roots may be associated with lumbosacral developmental anomalies and increased risk of disc herniation[18] or cases of failed back surgery.[19]

Posterior Longitudinal Ligament

The posterior longitudinal ligament (PLL) in the cervical area is double layered, with a venous plexus between the layers laterally.[22] The PLL in the lumbar region is loosely connected centrally in the upper lumbar levels and is smaller in diameter at the lower levels.[23]

Intervertebral Foramen

The normal intervertebral foramen is oval.[24] With disc degeneration, the foramen assumes an auricular shape.[24]

Facet Joints

The facet joints provide torsional rigidity and structural support in axial loading.[25] Posterior elements restrict the disc to 80% of its full range of flexion.[26] At the limit of flexion, the tensile stress in the posterior annulus is 44% of the value required to cause failure.[26]

Blood Supply

The normal intervertebral disc is avascular.[1,27] Segmental blood supply of the lumbar spine has been described by Parke and Watanabe.[28] The segmental vessels contribute to a capillary bed surrounding the annulus.[29] Blood vessels penetrate the subchondral bone of the vertebral body and the calcified region of the hyaline cartilage endplate.

Blood vessels are not observed in the discs of people under 30 years of age.[30] Invasion of blood vessels from the exterior is observed to begin in the fifth decade of life. Invasion of the interior of the intervertebral disc can be considered to be a sign of the aging of the intervertebral disc.[30]

Nerve Supply

The anterior annulus is innervated by nerves derived from the ventral rami and gray ramus communicans.[31] The posterior annulus is innervated by sinuvertebral nerve, a branch of the spinal nerve at the intervertebral foramen level.[32] No nerve fibers or neuropeptides have been identified in the normal nucleus pulposus.[32–34] Yoshizawa et al. identified nerve endings only in the outer half of the annulus in normal and degenerated discs.[33] Ashton et al. noted that nerve fibers ran between and across lamellae and extended at least 3 mm into the annulus.[34] No fibers were observed in the nucleus. Fibers were present in association with and distant from blood vessels surrounding the disc. Four neuropeptides were found to be associated with these fibers: calcitonin gene-related peptide (CGRP), substance P, vasoactive intestinal peptide (VIP), and C-flanking peptide of neuropeptide Y.

Coppes et al. reported that nerve endings in abnormal discs penetrated the annulus to reach the nucleus pulposus.[35] No relationship was identified between the presence of nerve endings and outgrowth or ingrowth of blood vessels. The same authors identified encapsulated nerve endings in the annulus as well as nerve endings containing substance P. Human cervical discs are supplied with both nerve fibers and mechanoreceptors in the annular regions, but no nerves are located in the nucleus pulposus.[36]

Yamashita et al. identified physiologically functioning mechanosensitive units in the anterolateral portion of the lumbar intervertebral discs of rabbits.[31] They reported a greater density of these receptors in the psoas muscle and facet joints. They concluded the disc may be less sensitive than the paravertebral muscle and facet joint.[31]

The anterior longitudinal ligament (ALL) and the PLL are richly supplied by the ventral neural plexus and reinforced by perivascular nerves of the segmental arteries.[37]

Biochemistry

Biochemical Structure

The nucleus pulposus contains 65% proteoglycan and 20% collagen.[12] The annulus contains 20% proteoglycan and 60% collagen. Elastic fibers are present throughout the disc.[12] Collagen con-

Table 3.1 Zones of Cartilage in the Matrix of the Intervertebral Disc

Zone	Type of Collagen
Pericellular	IV, sometimes III
Territorial	III
Interterritorial	I or II

tent is highest in cervical discs and lowest in lumbar discs.[38] Polyanion concentration is highest in lumbar discs.[38]

Eighty percent of the collagen in the intervertebral disc is type I and II.[13] Type I is localized to the annulus and type II to the nucleus. The annulus also contains small amounts of collagen types II, V, VI, IX, and XI. The nucleus contains small amounts of type IV, IX, and XI collagen. Types III and VI are concentrated in the pericellular spaces of the disc and the end plate. Types III and VI are highly organized into fibrous pericellular capsules (chondrons). Type IV is also present in blood vessels from vascularization in degenerative discs. Type IX collagen has been localized in human cartilage to regions of endochondral ossification. Roberts et al. also identified zones of distribution of collagen subtypes in the matrix of the intervertebral disc (Table 3.1).[13]

Tissue adaptation occurs in the annulus fibrosus and the nucleus pulposus with mechanical loading.[13,39] In addition, the distribution of collagen types I and II changes. Type I increases principally in the outer fibers of the posterior quadrant and on the concave side of scoliotic curves (areas of compression), and type II increases towards the central annulus. An overall increase in type I collagen is also noted.[38] Nucleus proteoglycan levels correlate with increasing compressive loads.[38,39]

Hydration, Pressure, and Permeability

The intervertebral disc shows diurnal variations in fluid content.[40] The normal disc shows an average 1.2 ± 0.7 mm daily variation and a degenerated disc 2.1 ± 1.1 mm.[41] A total diurnal height variation of 13 to 21 mm was recorded in healthy 22-year-old subjects.[42] Sixty-five percent of height loss occurs in the first 6 minutes after a 10 kg weight has been lifted in upright posture.[42]

Prolonged bed rest (5 to 17 weeks) has been associated with 22% expansion of the disc.[43] This expansion was reversed to baseline within a few days after termination of 5 weeks of bed rest. The disc height remained above baseline for 6 weeks following 17 weeks of bed rest. This study also reported rapidly reversible changes in disc height after an 8-day space flight. Considering the marginal nutritional status of the normal disc, increased disc height may increase diffusion distances to a level sufficient to alter disc metabolism and lead to disc degeneration.[44] The authors speculated that intervertebral disc expansion may account for back pain experienced by astronauts during space flight.[44] Loss of height has been noted in association with certain sports.[45,46]

Intradiscal pressure is lowest in the supine position and rises markedly in the sitting, leaning-forward position.[47] Axial traction applied to the pelvis decreases intradiscal pressure.[48]

Antibiotics can penetrate the intervertebral disc.[49] Some medications (e.g., cisplatin, levodopa, and methyldopa) have been incidentally noted to accumulate in disc tissue.[50,51]

Metabolism

The intervertebral disc is the largest avascular structure in the body.[52] Metabolism of the disc is mainly anaerobic.[53] Nutrients pass by flow and diffusion through the endplates and the periannular route.[54] The diffusion distance can be as large as 8mm in the human disc.[55] Although the nutrient supply of the annulus is adequate, the supply to the nucleus is precarious. Endplate sclerosis in disc degeneration may result in a compromised nutrient supply to the intervertebral disc. Nutrient consumption rate, exchange area, and disc thickness are the parameters that most influence nutrient concentrations.[29] Maximum cell density in the disc is determined by nutrient supply. Oxygen and glucose concentrations in the center of the disc can fall to very low values.[29] Concentration of oxygen at the center of the disc is 1/20 to 1/50 that at periphery.[29] Lactate concentration at the center of the disc is 8 to 10 times the plasma concentration.

The metabolism of the disc is also dependent on the loads across the disc.[54] In their study of bovine discs, Oshima et al. noted that metabolism was highest with loads of 5 to 10 kg and in the inner layers of the annulus fibrosus.[56]

Biomechanics

Laboratory Models of Disc Pathology

Animal Models

Kaapa et al. studied injury to the porcine annulus.[57–59] After making an annular incision through a retroperitoneal approach, they noted that the nucleus became small and fibrotic, and developed yellowish discoloration. The annulus showed replacement of lamellae with granulation tissue. The lamellar structure was not restored in the area of injury 3 to 5 months following disc injury.

The vertebral body developed ventral osteophytes. Biochemically, collagen synthesis and total collagen increased, collagen cross-links decreased, and water content decreased.[58] Fibrosis of the nucleus pulposus involved the appearance of type I and type III collagens and fibroblast-like cells. Healing of the wounds in the annulus also show increased synthesis of type I and type III collagen.[59] Kaapa et al. concluded that trauma to the annulus fibrosus can initiate a progressive degenerative process in the disc tissue.[58]

The desert sand rat has been used to study disc degeneration.[60] The earliest changes in intervertebral disc disease in this animal model are related to the subchondral bone. Subchondral bony sclerosis was the only change noted by 18 months. No difference in biomechanical testing and histology was observed at up to 18 months. The authors concluded that increased compliance due to subchondral sclerosis may be a predegenerative response.[60]

Osti, Vernon-Roberts, and Fraser studied injury to the annulus in a sheep model.[61] An incision 5 mm deep was made in the left anterolateral annulus adjacent to the inferior endplate in an effort to reproduce a rim lesion. Progressive failure of the inner annulus was seen in all animals at 4 to 12 months. The outermost annulus showed some ability to heal. The inner annulus failed to heal. Deformation and bulging of collagen bundles was noted following the incision, with subsequent inner extension of the tear and complete failure of the disc. The authors concluded that a tear of the outer annulus leads to formation of concentric clefts and acceleration of radial clefts.[61]

Computer Models

There is no simple relationship between structure and function in disc tissues: the same portion of the annulus may behave as a fluid or as a tensile structure.[3,62] Finite-element analyses have been useful in understanding disc mechanics.[63–65]

Nataranjan et al. modeled motion segment without posterior elements.[63] They concluded that annular injuries are unlikely with pure compressive loads and that failure always starts at the endplates. They also noted that discrete peripheral tears can form concentric annular tears and accelerate degeneration.[63]

Kim et al. used a finite-element model to study the effect of degeneration at one level on the adjacent level. Degeneration at the L4-5 level disc predicted decreased loads on the facet joints, increased intradiscal pressure (by 10%), and disc bulge at the L3-4 level disc.[64]

Mechanisms of Disc Injury

Most of the information on the mechanical behavior of the intervertebral disc is based on cadaver studies. Keller et al. have cautioned that the biomechanical response of the vertebral unit is altered by animal death.[66] Respiration plays an important role in the mechanical and nutritional behavior of the disc. In the absence of normal physiologic conditions, one may not be able to reliably predict the mechanical response of the lumbar spine.[66]

The laminate structure of the posterior parts of the annulus is considered to predispose the disc to injury in this region.[8,9] These localized structural irregularities are thought to decrease strength of the annulus and increase local stresses and strains, predisposing the annulus to rupture.[67] Ito et al. have noted increased frequency of radial ruptures in the annulus in older specimens.[68]

Gordon et al. presented a laboratory model to reliably produce disc rupture under physiologically reasonable stresses.[69] They loaded cadaveric lumbar spine specimens (1.5 Hz for 6.9 hours) under 1,334 N compression in 7 degrees of flexion and less than 3 degrees of rotation. Annular protrusions were produced in 10 of 14 specimens; nuclear extrusion through the annular tear occurred in 4 specimens. The authors concluded that intervertebral disc prolapse is peripheral in origin, with the annulus being the site of primary pathologic change (Fig. 3.2).[69] Bending in addition to axial compression is important in predisposing a disc to

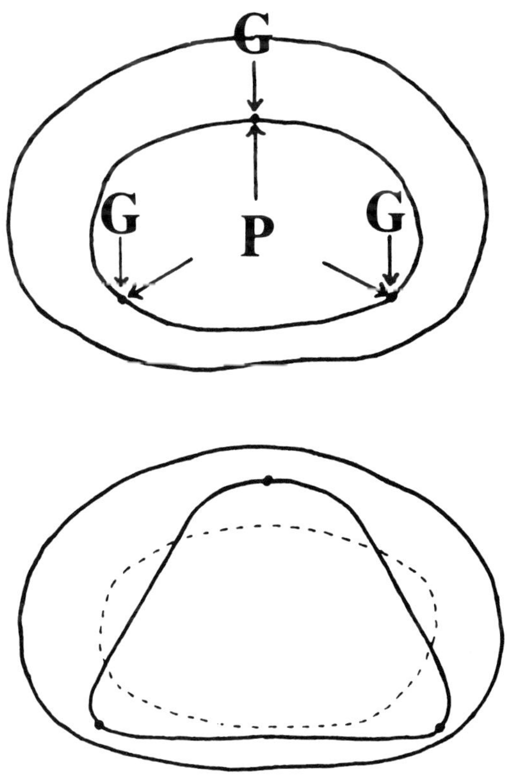

Figure 3.2. Increase of intradiscal pressure deforms the annulus in three chief directions: dorsally, ventrally, and dorsolaterally. Most herniations thus occur in the dorsolateral direction.

prolapse.[70] Disc failure in bending occurs through overstretching of the posterior annulus in the vertical direction.[26] The normal disc is protected by the posterior elements from overstretching.[26] The posterior elements would sustain damage before the disc in traumatic loading. The posterior elements may not, however, protect the posterior annulus from fatigue failure.[26] Fatigue loading has also been shown to produce radial fissures and extrusion of nuclear material.

Brinckmann and Porter explored the role in disc prolapse of loose fragments in the disc.[71] They made a ventral incision in human cadaveric specimens and created a 10 mm × 10 mm posterolateral radial fissure extending to 1 mm of the periphery. Fragments of nuclear material from other discs were inserted into the nucleus, and the annular incision was repaired. The discs were compressed to failure. The authors concluded that the key to the pathology of disc protrusion and prolapse is the loose fragment. They stated that prolapse appears to be a late event during the course of a long-term degenerative process.[71] This has been criticized for its methodology and conclusions.[70] Adams has cautioned that it should not be presumed that degeneration precedes prolapse.[70]

Posterior longitudinal ligament (PLL) morphology has also been correlated with the type of disc herniation: central herniation with intact PLL in the upper lumbar levels and posterolateral extrusion with ruptured PLL in the lower levels.[23]

Asymmetry of facet joints has been associated with disc degeneration and disc herniation at the thoracolumbar junction.[72] This association has not been validated in subsequent studies.[73–75]

Pathophysiology

Age-Related Changes

Disc

The most marked change in disc degeneration is loss of proteoglycan.[53] Altered loading of the spine exerts significant alterations in the disc proteoglycan levels.[76] Proteoglycan synthesis also results in decreases in pH. Proteoglycan synthesis appears to be more affected by low pH than by protein synthesis. The pH in healthy discs is 6.9 to 7.1 and in degenerative discs below 6.5.[76] Smoking increases intradiscal lactate level and decreases pH.[53,77] A low pH has been noted in the perineural tissues at the site of disc herniations.[78] Proteoglycan synthesis is also inhibited by nonsteroidal anti-inflammatory drugs (NSAIDs).[79]

Scott et al. have studied age-related changes in the proteoglycans.[38] They noted that many of the changes had occurred before maturity. Collagen in the nucleus increases in thoracic and lumbar regions and remains high in cervical discs. Collagen in the annulus increases with age. Water content of the disc decreases with aging. Chondroitin sulfate (CS) and polyanion concentration also decrease. Hyaluronic acid (HA) and keratin sulfate (KS) increase. Oversulfated KS, absent in fetal discs, reaches mature levels by age 10 years. Scott et al. noted that the occurrence, location, and concentration of KS, and its ratio to CS, correlate well with the ambient oxygen concentration in the cornea, the cartilage, and the intervertebral disc. They concluded that since KS requires less oxygen during biosynthesis, it is a functional substitute for CS when oxygen is lacking.[38]

An increase in the ratio of elastin to proteoglycan is noted in the first four decades.[80] The elastin-to-collagen ratio in nuclei decreases with aging.[80]

Degenerated discs differ from controls in the amount and distribution of collagen types and the organization of the pericellular capsule.[13] Staining for type IV collagen is changed: pericellular staining is less intense, and the fibrous pattern is more widespread. Multiple pericellular rings and formation of chondrocyte clusters are seen. Similar changes are observed in the cervical and lumbar spine.[81]

Annulus

Age-related changes lead to a loss of integrity of the disc.[82] Annuli in specimens from persons less than 40 years old show obliquely oriented fibers in laminae in pennate arrangements. Annuli in persons older than 40 years show breakdown of laminae: fraying, splitting, loss of collagen fibers, spaces filled with material showing an intense positive periodic acid–Schiff stain (proteoglycan), and deposition of chondroid material in the annulus. Circumferential and radial ruptures are noted in the annulus in older specimens.[68]

The thickness of the laminar layers of the annulus is increased in older specimens.[8] Amyloids of immunoglobulin origin are produced in the intervertebral discs because of abnormalities in the enzyme system.[83] Progressive amyloid deposition is noted in the annuli of persons over the age of 15 years. Deposition first occurs in outer layers of annulus and at attachment sites to vertebral bodies in the inner layers. Amyloid is not found in the nucleus.

Peripheral tears of the annulus alter the biomechanics of the entire disc tissue.[84] Osti, Vernon-Roberts, and Fraser noted that peripheral tears of the annulus may play an important role in the degeneration of the intervertebral joint complex.[61]

Nucleus

Age-related changes in the nucleus include loss of water, decrease in CS and HA, increase in KS/CS ratio, increase in lower molecular weight sugar fractions of glycoproteins, fibrosis, chondroid changes, and the appearance of areas of calcification.[82,85]

Fujita et al., who identified leukocyte elastase in degenerated intervertebral discs, concluded that in pathologic conditions, proteinases, normally present in the vertebral body, flow into and degrade the matrix of the intervertebral disc.[12]

Lipofuscin (age pigment) is produced from oxidation of lipids.[83] It is deposited in increasing amounts with age in various organs. Lipofuscin has been identified in the nucleus pulposus and in the middle and inner layers of annulus fibrosus.[83] Lipofuscin deposition corresponds to regions of strong histologic degeneration. Lipofuscin is also found in surgical specimens of herniated discs from younger patients more often than expected from autopsy studies. This finding may indicate that herniated discs are in a state of more advanced degeneration.[83] The nucleus pulposus does not move within the disc with changes in posture of the lumbar spine in degenerative discs as in normal discs.[10] Range of motion of the moving segment decreases with disc degeneration.[86]

Endplate

Endplates become calcified with age and subsequently are replaced by bone.[82] The endplate is separated from the subchondral bone in 51.1% of persons aged 77 years.[87] The endplate can, therefore, herniate with the annulus in elderly patients.

Irregularities of the endplate are common in degenerative discs. Fujita et al. found that bone marrow tissues often penetrate the endplate into the nucleus.[12] They proposed that this bone marrow invasion leads to a flow of proteinases from the vertebral body into the disc. Cytokines such as interleukin I may then activate these enzymes and initiate matrix degradation.

Facet Joint

Loss of fluid from the nucleus increases contact forces across the facet joints.[65] Butler et al., who reviewed the records of 68 patients who had undergone both computed tomography (CT) scans and magnetic resonance imaging (MRI) of the lumbar spine, noted that both disc degeneration and facet osteoarthritis increase with age.[88] No difference was noted between men and women. Disc degeneration was present in 144 of 330 discs; no facet osteoarthritis was noted in 108 of these levels. Facet osteoarthritis was present at 41 of 330 levels; except for one patient with Paget's disease, all these levels also had disc degeneration. Butler et al. concluded that disc degeneration occurs before facet osteoarthritis. Facet osteoarthritis may be secondary to mechanical changes in facet loading with disc degeneration.[88]

Radiographic studies using x-rays suggested a possible association of facet tropism with disc herniation. Studies using MRI and CT films have shown no association. The risk of disc degeneration, however, is increased in the presence of facet joint tropism.[89]

Biologic Basis of Risk Factors

Genetic

Lumbar disc herniation in patients aged 18 years or younger shows familial predisposition and clustering with an odds ratio of 5.61.[90] Matsui et al. reported on disc herniation in two monozygotic twins and suggested that genetic factors are involved in the development of lumbar disc herniation in young patients.[91]

Researchers do not know why some individuals develop disc degeneration earlier than others. Proposed theories include factors related to injury, physical environmental exposure, and genetic predisposition.[92,93] Recent studies suggest that genetic polymorphisms may be a risk factor for symptomatic lumbar disc disease.[94–96] The strongest association identified to date is a single amino acid substitution in collagen type IX, a structural protein in the intervertebral disc.[97,98]

The intervertebral disc contains many different forms of collagen.[99,100] Each collagen molecule is composed of three coiled polypeptide chains, each chain containing highly repetitive sequences of three amino acids: glycine, proline, and hydroxyproline.[101] The individual chains within a collagen molecule and chains of adjoining collagen molecules are linked together by strong bonds, such as hydrogen bonds or disulfide bonds.[102] Collagen type IX is important in cross-linking between collagen molecules in the intervertebral disc.[103–105] A mutation in the genes coding for collagen type IX may diminish collagen cross-linking in disc tissue, making it more susceptible to mechanical damage or degeneration.[106]

Two specific variations in genes that code for collagen type IX, *Col9A2* and *Col9A3*, each involving substitution of a single amino acid (tryptophan), have been identified as putative disease-causing sequence variations for intervertebral disc disease.[97,98] Annunen et al. reported that a variation that converted a codon for glutamine to one for tryptophan was present in the gene *Col9A2* in 6 out of 157 individuals with disc disease and none of 174 control subjects.[98] They further noted that the tryptophan allele cosegregated with the disease phenotype in four families studied. In a subsequent study, Paassilta et al. reported that another polymorphism in collagen type IX, this one involving a tryptophan substitution for arginine in *Col9A3*, was present in

12.2% of 171 individuals with lumbar disc disease and only in 4.7% of 341 controls.[97] They estimated that the presence of one *Trp3* allele increases the risk of lumbar disc disease approximately threefold. Researchers, however, do not know whether these tryptophan-encoding allelic polymorphisms in collagen type IX genes (*Col9A2* and *Col9A3*) are expressed at the protein level in the fabric of disc tissue. Also, if these changes are expressed at the protein level, it is not known whether they have any functional consequences in terms of extracellular matrix assembly.

Atherosclerosis

Atherosclerosis of the abdominal aorta may play a part in disc degeneration.[107] A correlation has been noted between the grade of disc degeneration and stenosis of the ostia of arteries supplying the disc. Compression of epidural veins with dilatation of noncompressed veins also correlates with the degree of disc degeneration and prolapse.[108]

Smoking

Exposure to cigarette smoke increases intradiscal lactate level,[109] lowers intradiscal pH,[77] and degrades hyaluronic acid.[110] All these changes may accelerate disc degeneration.

In a study of twin pairs with high smoking discordance, smoking was associated with increased scores for intervertebral disc degeneration as documented by MRI.[111] The effect was present across the entire lumbar spine, implicating a systemic mechanism. Smokers had 18% greater mean disc degeneration scores in the lumbar spine than nonsmokers.

Vibration

The resonant frequency of the human spinal system is 5 Hz. The vibration generated by common construction vehicles is 3.5 to 9 Hz.[112] The rate of proteoglycan synthesis in the nucleus decreases upon exposure to vibrations having a frequency of 10 to 35 Hz.[112] Vibration alone, however, does not induce matrix degradation.[113] The presence of structural abnormalities, such as narrowing of neural foramina, accelerates the degradation by vibration of proteoglycan and collagen in the annulus.

Sports

A high frequency of radiologic changes in spine and disc degeneration has been noted in athletes who specialize in wrestling, gymnastics, and water-ski jumping.[114,115]

Pathology of Disc Herniation

In a review of 508 cases, Boutin and Hogshead noted that the pathologist's report had no discernible influence on patient man-

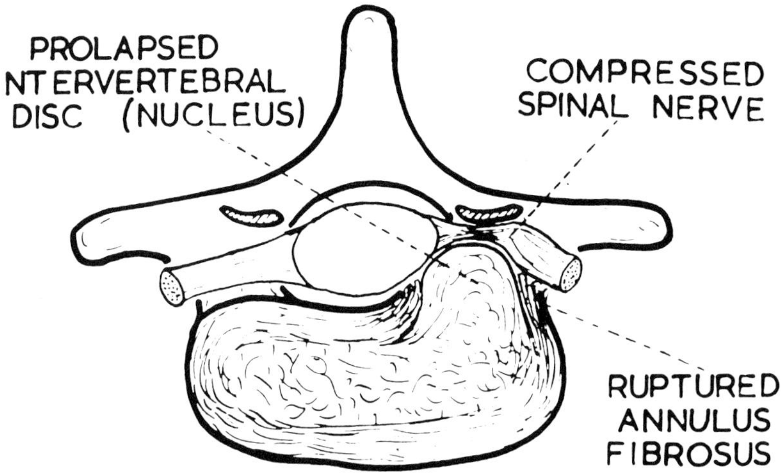

Figure 3.3. Cross-sectional view of a disc herniation: the disc protrusion has extended dorsally to compress a nerve root.

agement.[116] Only nuclear material is found in 85% of extruded discs; the remaining 15% contain both nuclear and annular material.[117] Protruded discs contain both nucleus and annulus (Fig. 3.3). No differences have been observed between extruded and protruded discs at the histochemical level.[117] Most recurrent disc herniations and herniations with multiple extruded fragments contain portions of the end plate.[118] Lipson has proposed that herniation of the disc may entail metaplasia of the herniated material.[119]

Discs surgically removed have a lower fluid content in the nucleus and a higher fluid content in the annulus compared with discs taken at autopsy.[120]

Chitkara reported on neovascularization observed in the edges of extruded herniated disc fragments.[121] A direct relationship was noted between presence of neovascularization and the duration of symptoms: neovascularization was observed in 12.5% of herniated discs of patients with symptoms for less than 1 month and in 82% of patients with symptoms that had lasted longer than 6 months. Neovascularization was also more frequent in lumbar (61.2%) than in cervical disc herniations (3.8%). Blood vessels have also been observed in surgical specimens of protrusion type of disc herniation.[30] The authors concluded that blood vessels in surgical specimens of the protrusion type of herniation are a sign of degeneration of the intervertebral disc.[30] The origin of these blood vessels, however, is unclear. Two case reports describe the vessels as originating in the extradural fat and scar tissue and penetrating the extruded fragment.[122,123]

Mechanisms of Pain Generation

Disc

Neuropeptides involved in transmission of pain have been identified in the intervertebral disc.[124] Calcitonin gene-related peptide (CGRP), VIP, and substance P have been mapped in the outer annulus in dogs.[124] Concentrations of these substances in the dorsal root ganglion (DRG) changed with manipulation of the intervertebral disc. Substance P and VIP increased with discography, and substance P but not VIP decreased with injection of local anesthetic.[124] Weinstein et al. hypothesized that the intervertebral disc may be sensitized by chemical alterations following injury. Chemical events in the disc following injury may also sensitize the DRG and generate pain.[124]

Nerve Root

Contact pressure on a nerve root with disc protrusion is estimated to be approximately 400 mmHg.[125] Acute compression of the nerve root causes numbness, paresthesia, and weakness, but not pain.[14,126] Nerve root compression causes impairment of nutritive blood flow (at 5–10 mmHg compression), increased permeability of blood vessels, edema, increased tissue pressure, altered local ion balance, and altered impulse conduction (at 50–75 mmHg compression).[127,128] Inflamed nerve roots cause pain when compressed.[14] Radicular pain without image-documented evidence of nerve root compression has also been described, implicating a nonmechanical mechanism of nerve root dysfunction.[129,130]

Disc degeneration has been implicated as a source of nerve root inflammation and chemical radiculitis.[126] The mechanism of nerve root inflammation is not known. Proposed irritants include low pH, breakdown products from nucleus,[131] proteoglycans from discs,[132] and autoimmune reaction to exposed disc tissue.[14,133,134]

Saal et al. reported that phospholipase A_2 activity is 20- to 100,000-fold more than any other phospholipase activity that has been described. Extruded discs had higher levels than contained herniations. Phospholipase A_2 is involved in prostaglandin and leukotriene synthesis. Phospholipase A_2 extracted from human lumbar disc has a powerful inflammatory effect in vivo.[135] Saal et al. concluded that these data established biochemical evidence of inflammation at the site of lumbar disc herniations.[136] They postulated that loss of integrity of the outer annulus leads to the escape into epidural space of inflammatogenic material, including phospholipase A_2, producing a local inflammatory response.

Willburger and Wittenberg also reported increased phospholipase A_2 activity in disc tissue.[137] They reported phospholipase A_2 activity 50 times higher in disc tissue than in synovial tissue. However, prostaglandin release from disc tissue was 1/30 that released from synovial tissue. The authors stated that because prostaglandin release from a sequestered disc is rather low, the inflammatory effect observed might be more heavily attributable to immunologic reactions.[137]

Biologic Basis for Diagnostic Studies

Laboratory Studies

No laboratory studies exist for diagnosis of disc related conditions. Skouen et al. reported elevated CSF protein levels in patients with sciatica whose myelographic exam results indicated nerve root compression.[138] They stated that plasma albumin and IgG leaked from the nerve root into the CSF and speculated on the possibility of a diagnostic test for radiculopathy based on this finding. None has been developed thus far. Communication between the CSF and the peripheral nerve interstitial fluid has been observed.[139] Compounds injected into the central nervous system can be traced to the epineural–perineural sheaths and the endoneurium of the peripheral nerves.

CT Studies

Bulging greater than 2.5 mm may represent a pathologic annular tear.[140] Conjoined nerve roots may be mistaken as asymmetrical disc protrusion.[141] CT-myelogram evidence is more helpful than MRI in patients who have had prior surgery.[142]

MRI Studies

Longitudinal (T1) and transverse (T2) relaxation time MRI signals have characteristic relationships with water content in the normal intervertebral disc.[143] A T1 signal shows a positive linear relationship with water content of the nucleus. A T2 signal shows no linear relationship but exhibits a transition point at 75% total water content. Intradiscal pressure measurements do not correlate with MRI signal changes.[144]

Tertti et al. compared MRI findings to biochemical and histologic changes found in cadaveric spine specimens.[145] Low T2 signal was associated with dehydration, decreased total protein, and a decreased C/K ratio in the nucleus. No histologic differences were noted for MRI findings. The authors concluded that a low T2 signal probably reflects true biochemical disc degeneration, but its relation to structural change is uncertain.

Early degenerative disc disease may exist before the loss of disc height or signal intensity is noticed.[146] Magnetic resonance imaging (MRI) is less specific than discography in detecting disc pathology.[147]

Discography

The mechanism that produces pain during disc injection is not known.[148] Discography produces a mechanical stimulus. Disc injection has been noted to decrease disc bulge and to deflect the endplate. Impingement on the endplate by the discography needle can cause exquisite back pain. The endplate itself, or events within the bone, are possible sources of pain during clinical discography.[148]

Indications for discography are listed as follows: pain lasting more than 4 months, and pain unresponsive to conservative treatment; a prior CT, MRI, or myelogram is necessary to exclude other sources of pain, and in postoperative patients, there must be localization of symptomatic level and determination of levels for fusion.[149] For discography, the rate of false positives has been reported as 0.0.

Not all peripheral annular lesions are detected by discography.[147] Specificity of discography may be 31% and sensitivity 81 to 100%; validity is unknown. Radiation exposure, if involved, may be significant.[150] It should be recognized that when a study with less than 100% specificity is used to decide on operative management, the result will be unnecessary surgery and its associated morbidity and cost.

Classification of Disc Pathology

The terminology used to describe disc-related conditions and disc pathology is confusing.[151–153] Spine surgeons employ a wide variety of terms to describe relatively few conditions and pathologic states.[154] In their survey of 51 respondents, Fardon et al. noted that 50 terms were offered to describe the four most common diagnoses for back problems and 53 terms listed to classify eight specific categories of surgical findings describing herniated discs.[154]

In imaging studies, the size of disc herniation in relation to the size of the spinal canal has been reported to provide the best positive correlation to the clinical findings.[155,156] The sagittal plane ratio of disc herniation to canal size has also correlated with the degree of sciatic pain in this study. Imaging studies, however, have been shown to have high rates of false positive findings in asymptomatic individuals.

Adams et al. have developed a reliable and reproducible five-stage classification of disc morphology.[157] This classification, however, can accurately be applied only to spines that can be sectioned in the midsagittal plane; it is not clinically useful. A variation of this scale has been employed in classification of disc pathology with discography.[157]

Consequences of Disc Surgery

Disc Injury

Brinckman and Grootenboer have observed that loss of disc tissue results in a decrease of disc height, an increase of the radial disc bulge, and a decrease of the intradiscal pressure.[158] Removal of 1 g of tissue decreased disc height by 0.8 mm and increased radial bulge by 0.2 mm. Removal of 3 g of tissue decreased the intradiscal pressure to 40% of the initial value. Motion segments had a slack appearance after discectomy. The authors cautioned that discectomy may have disadvantageous side effects.[158]

Smith and Walmsley reported that an incision in the outer part of the injured annulus heals in 3 to 4 weeks.[159] Keller et al. showed that any injury to the annulus leads to disc degeneration.[66] A small defect in the annulus (3.6 mm coring tool to 15 mm depth) was just as deleterious as removing a large section of annular material. Ahlgren et al., however, noted that severe early disc degeneration was associated with excision of a full-thickness annular window but not with annular penetration with a 2.5 mm trochar.[160]

Adhesions

Adhesions between the posterior annulus and the nerve root are common following discectomy.[161] Also, patients with postoperative scar tissue have been reported to have more severe complications.[162] Scar formation may be due to presence of foreign material.[162–164] Placement of a fat graft does not prevent adhesions anterior to the nerve root.[161] Gelfoam increases fibrosis. Instillation of sodium hyaluronate, an inert, biodegradable, viscous solution, decreases the area of fibrosis and the tenacity of adhesions.[161]

Conclusions

The intervertebral disc is considered to be the primary focus of pathology for the majority of patients with low back pain. The structure of the disc has been well described in the literature. The metabolism and nutrition of the intervertebral disc remain unclear. Physicochemical changes in disc tissue with mechanical loading and aging have been identified to a limited extent. Innervation of the normal and abnormal disc and neurochemical changes within the disc in pathologic conditions are the focus of current investigations. The mechanism of pain generation and the pathway of pain conduction in low back pain and sciatica, however, are not known.

References

1. Coventry MB, Ghormley RK, Kernohan JW. The intervertebral disc: its microscopic anatomy and pathology, II: changes in the intervertebral disc concomitant with aging. *J Bone Joint Surg Am* 1945; 27:233–247.
2. Cotten A, Sakka M, Drizenko A, Clarisse J, Francke JP. Antenatal differentiation of the human intervertebral disc. *Surg Radiol Anat* 1994;16(1):53–56.
3. McNally DS, Adams MA. Internal intervertebral disc mechanics as revealed by stress profilometry. *Spine* 1992;17(1):66–73.
4. Kraemer, J. Presidential address: natural course and prognosis of intervertebral disc diseases. *Spine* 1995;20(6):635–639.
5. Nachemson A. Newest knowledge of low back pain. A critical look. *Clin Orthop* 1992;271:8–20.
6. Huang R, Zhi Q, Wilting J, Christ B. The fate of somitocoele cells in avian embryos. *Anat Embryol Berl* 1994;190(3):243–250.
7. Thompson JP, Oegema TR Jr, Bradford DS. Stimulation of mature canine intervertebral disc by growth factors. *Spine* 1991;16(3):253–260.
8. Marchand F, Ahmed AM. Investigation of the laminate structure of lumbar disc anulus fibrosus. *Spine* 1990;15(5):402–410.
9. Tsuji H, Hirano N, Ohshima H, Ishihara H, Terahata N, Motoe T. Structural variation of the anterior and posterior anulus fibrosus in the development of human lumbar intervertebral disc. A risk factor for intervertebral disc rupture. *Spine* 1993;18(2):204–210.
10. Beattie PF, Brooks WM, Rothstein JM, Sibbitt WL Jr, Robergs RA, MacLean T, Hart BL. Effect of lordosis on the position of the nucleus pulposus in supine subjects. A study using magnetic resonance imaging. *Spine* 1994;19(18):2096–2102.
11. MacMillan J, Schaffer JL, Kambin P. Routes and incidence of communication of lumbar discs with surrounding neural structures. *Spine* 1991;16(2):167–171.
12. Fujita K, Nakagawa T, Hirabayashi K, Nagai Y. Neutral proteinases in human intervertebral disc. Role in degeneration and probable origin. *Spine* 1993;18(13):1766–1773.
13. Roberts S, Menage J, Duance V, Wotton S, Ayad S. 1991 Volvo Award in basic sciences. Collagen types around the cells of the intervertebral disc and cartilage end plate: an immunolocalization study. *Spine* 1991;16(9):1030–1038.
14. Rydevik B, Brown MD, Lundborg G. Pathoanatomy and pathophysiology of nerve root compression. *Spine* 1984;9:7–15.
15. Rauschning W. Normal and pathologic anatomy of the lumbar root canals. *Spine* 1987;12(10):1008–1019.
16. Smith SA, Massie JB, Chesnut R, Garfin SR. Straight leg raising. Anatomical effects on the spinal nerve root without and with fusion. *Spine* 1993;18(8):992–999.
17. Sato K, Kikuchi S. An anatomic study of foraminal nerve root lesions in the lumbar spine. *Spine* 1993;18(15):2246–2251.
18. Okuwaki T, Kunogi J, Hasue M. Conjoined nerve roots associated with lumbosacral spine anomalies. A case report. *Spine* 1991;16(11): 1347–1349.

19. Gomez JG, Dickey JW, Bachow TB. Conjoined lumbosacral nerve roots. *Acta Neurochir Wien* 1993;120(3–4):155–158.
20. Piatt JH Jr. The frequency of intradural conjoined lumbosacral dorsal nerve roots found during selective dorsal rhizotomy [letter; comment]. *Neurosurgery* 1994;34(2):380.
21. Phillips LH 2d, Park TS. The frequency of intradural conjoined lumbosacral dorsal nerve roots found during selective dorsal rhizotomy. *Neurosurgery* 1993;33(1):88–90; discussion 90–91.
22. Kubo Y, Waga S, Kojima T, Matsubara T, Kuga Y, Nakagawa Y. Microsurgical anatomy of the lower cervical spine and cord. *Neurosurgery* 1994;34(5):895–890; discussion 901–902.
23. Ohshima H, Hirano N, Osada R, Matsui H, Tsuji H. Morphologic variation of lumbar posterior longitudinal ligament and the modality of disc herniation. *Spine* 1993;18(16):2408–2011.
24. Stephens MM, Evans JH, O'Brien JP. Lumbar intervertebral foramens. An in vitro study of their shape in relation to intervertebral disc pathology. *Spine* 1991;16(5):525–529.
25. Zimmerman MC, Vuono-Hawkins M, Parsons JR, Carter FM, Gutteling E, Lee CK, Langrana NA. The mechanical properties of the canine lumbar disc and motion segment. *Spine* 1992;17(2):213–220.
26. Adams MA, Green TP, Dolan P. The strength in anterior bending of lumbar intervertebral discs. *Spine* 1994;19(19):2197–2203.
27. Taylor TK, Akeson WH. Intervertebral disc prolapse: a review of morphologic and biochemical knowledge concerning the nature of prolapse. *Clin Orthop* 1971;76:54–79.
28. Parke WW, Watanabe R. The intrinsic vasculature of the lumbosacral spinal nerve roots. *Spine* 1985;10:508–515.
29. Stairmand JW, Holm S, Urban JP. Factors influencing oxygen concentration gradients in the intervertebral disc. A theoretical analysis. *Spine* 1991;16(4):444–449.
30. Yasuma T, Arai K, Yamauchi Y. The histology of lumbar intervertebral disc herniation. The significance of small blood vessels in the extruded tissue. *Spine* 1993;18(13):1761–1765.
31. Yamashita T, Minaki Y, Oota I, Yokogushi K, Ishii S. Mechanosensitive afferent units in the lumbar intervertebral disc and adjacent muscle. *Spine* 1993;18(15):2252–2256.
32. McCarthy PW, Carruthers B, Martin D, Petts P. Immunohistochemical demonstration of sensory nerve fibers and endings in lumbar intervertebral discs of the rat. *Spine* 1991;16(6):636–653.
33. Yoshizawa H, O'Brien JH, Smith WT, Trumper M. The neuropathology of intervertebral discs removed for low back pain. *J Pathol* 1980;132:95.
34. Ashton IK, Roberts S, Jaffray DC, Polak JM, Eisenstein SM. Neuropeptides in the human intervertebral disc. *J Orthop Res* 1994;12(2):186–192.
35. Coppes MH, Marani E, Thomeer RT, Oudega M. Innervation of annulus fibrosis in low back pain. *Lancet* 1990;336:189–190.
36. Mendel T, Wink CS, Zimny ML. Neural elements in human cervical intervertebral discs. *Spine* 1992;17(2):132–135.
37. Groen GJ, Baljet B, Drukker J. Nerves and nerve plexuses of the human vertebral column. *Am J Anat* 1990;188:282–296.

38. Scott JE, Bosworth TR, Cribb AM, Taylor JR. The chemical morphology of age-related changes in human intervertebral disc glycosaminoglycans from cervical, thoracic and lumbar nucleus pulposus and annulus fibrosus. *J Anat* 1994;184(pt 1):73–82.
39. Brickley-Parsons D, Glimcher MJ. Is the chemistry of collagen in intervertebral discs an expression of Wolff's law? A study of the human lumbar spine. *Spine* 1984;9:148–163.
40. Neufeld JH. Induced narrowing and back adaptation of lumbar intervertebral discs in biomechanically stressed rats. *Spine* 1992;17(7): 811–816.
41. Botsford DJ, Esses SI, Ogilvie-Harris DJ. In vivo diurnal variation in intervertebral disc volume and morphology. *Spine* 1994;19(8): 935–940.
42. Paajanen H, Lehto I, Alanen A, Erkintalo M, Komu M. Diurnal fluid changes of lumbar discs measured indirectly by magnetic resonance imaging. *J Orthop Res* 1994;12(4):509–514.
43. Krag MH, Cohen MC, Haugh LD, Pope MH. Body height change during upright and recumbent posture. *Spine* 1990;15(3):202–207.
44. LeBlanc AD, Evans HJ, Schneider VS, Wendt RE 3rd, Hedrick TD. Changes in intervertebral disc cross-sectional area with bed rest and space flight. *Spine* 1994;19(7):812–817.
45. Glover MG, Hargens AR, Mahmood MM, Gott S, Brown MD, Garfin SR. A new technique for the in vitro measurement of nucleus pulposus swelling pressure. *J Orthop Res* 1991;9(1):61–67.
46. Fowler NE, Lees A, Reilly T. Spinal shrinkage in unloaded and loaded drop-jumping. *Ergonomics* 1994;37(1):133–139.
47. Reilly T, Chana D. Spinal shrinkage in fast bowling. *Ergonomics* 1994;37(1):127–132.
48. Nachemson A. Lumbar intradiscal pressure. *Acta Orthop Scand* 1960;40:1077–1092.
49. Ramos G, Martin W. Effects of vertebral axial decompression on intradiscal pressure. *J Neurosurg* 1994;81(3):350–353.
50. Boscardin JB, Ringus JC, Feingold DJ, Ruda SC. Human intradiscal levels with cefazolin. *Spine* 1992;17(6 suppl):S145–S148.
51. Minami T, Hashii K, Tateyama I, Kadota E, Tohno Y, Tohno S, Utsumi M, Yamada MO, Ichii M, Namikawa K, et al. Accumulation of platinum in the intervertebral discs and vertebrae of ovarian tumor–bearing patients treated with cisplatin. *Biol Trace Elem Res* 1994;42(3):253–257.
52. Rausing A, Rosen U. Black cartilage after therapy with levodopa and methyldopa. *Arch Pathol Lab Med* 1994;118(5):531–535.
53. Ohshima H, Urban JP. The effect of lactate and pH on proteoglycan and protein synthesis rates in the intervertebral disc. *Spine* 1992;17(9):1079–1082.
54. Holm S, Maroudas A, Urban JPG, Selstam G, Nachemson A. Nutrition of the intervertebral disc: solute transport and metabolism. *Connect Tissue Res* 1981;8:101–119.
55. Urban JPG, Holm S, Maroudas A, Nachemson A. Nutrition of the intervertebral disc: effect of fluid flow on solute transport. *Clin Orthop* 1982;170:296–302.

56. Ohshima H, Urban JP, Bergel DH. Effect of static load on matrix synthesis rates in the intervertebral disc measured in vitro by a new perfusion technique. *J Orthop Res* 1995;13(1):22–29.
57. Kaapa E, Holm S, Han X, Takala T, Kovanen V, Vanharanta H. Collagens in the injured porcine intervertebral disc. *J Orthop Res* 1994;12(1):93–102.
58. Kaapa E, Han S, Holm S, Peltonen J, Takala T, Vanharanta H. Collagen synthesis and types I, III, IV, VI collagens in an animal model of disc degeneration. *Spine* 1995;20(1):59–65.
59. Kaapa E, Zhang LQ, Muona P, Holm S, Vanharanta H, Peltonen J. Expression of type I, III, and VI collagen mRNAs in experimentally injured porcine intervertebral disc. *Connect Tissue Res* 1994; 30(3):203–214.
60. Ziran BH, Pineda S, Pokharna H, Esteki A, Mansour JM, Moskowitz RW. Biomechanical, radiologic, and histopathologic correlations in the pathogenesis of experimental intervertebral disc disease. *Spine* 1994;19(19):2159–2163.
61. Osti OL, Vernon-Roberts B, Fraser RD. 1990 Volvo Award in experimental studies. Annulus tears and intervertebral disc degeneration. An experimental study using an animal model. *Spine* 1990;15:762–767.
62. Laible JP, Pflaster DS, Krag MH, Simon BR, Haugh LD. A poroelastic-swelling finite element model with application to the intervertebral disc. *Spine* 1993;18(5):659–670.
63. Natarajan RN, Ke JH, Andersson GB. A model to study the disc degeneration process. *Spine* 1994;19(3):259–265.
64. Kim YE, Goel VK, Weinstein JN, Lim TH. Effect of disc degeneration at one level on the adjacent level in axial mode. *Spine* 1991; 16(3):331–335.
65. Shirazi-Adl A. Finite-element simulation of changes in the fluid content of human lumbar discs. Mechanical and clinical implications. *Spine* 1992;17(2):206–212.
66. Keller TS, Holm SH, Hansson TH, Spengler DM. 1990 Volvo Award in experimental studies. The dependence of intervertebral disc mechanical properties on physiologic conditions. *Spine* 1990;15(8): 751–761.
67. McNally DS, Adams MA, Goodship AE. Can intervertebral disc prolapse be predicted by disc mechanics? *Spine* 1993;18(11):1525–1530.
68. Ito S, Yamada Y, Tsuboi S, Yamada Y, Muro T. An observation of ruptured annulus fibrosus in lumbar discs. *J Spinal Disord* 1991;4(4): 462–466.
69. Gordon SJ, Yang KH, Mayer PJ, Mace AH Jr, Kish VL, Radin EL. Mechanism of disc rupture. A preliminary report. *Spine* 1991;16(4): 450–456.
70. Adams M. Laboratory model of lumbar disc protrusion: fissure and fragment. *Spine* 1994;19(17):2015–2017.
71. Brinckmann P, Porter RW. A laboratory model of lumbar disc protrusion. Fissure and fragment. *Spine* 1994;19(2):228–235.
72. Farfan HF, Cosette JW, Robertson GH, Wells RV, Kraus H. The effects of torsion on the lumbar intervertebral joints: the role of tor-

sion in the production of disc degeneration. *J Bone Joint Surg Am* 1970;52:468–497.
73. Hagg O, Wallner A. Facet joint asymmetry and protrusion of the intervertebral disc. *Spine* 1990;15(5):356–359.
74. Cassidy JD, Loback D, Yong-Hing K, Tchang S. Lumbar facet joint asymmetry. Intervertebral disc herniation. *Spine* 1992;17(5):570–574.
75. Duncan NA, Ahmed AM. The role of axial rotation in the etiology of unilateral disc prolapse. An experimental and finite-element analysis. *Spine* 1991;16(9):1089–1098.
76. Puustjarvi K, Lammi M, Helminen H, Inkinen R, Tammi M. Proteoglycans in the intervertebral disc of young dogs following strenuous running exercise. *Connect Tissue Res* 1994;30(3):225–240.
77. Hambly MF, Mooney V. Effect of smoking and pulsed electromagnetic fields on intradiscal pH in rabbits. *Spine* 1992;17(6 suppl): S83–S85.
78. Nachemson A. Intradiscal measurements of pH in patients with lumbar rhizopathies. *Acta Orthop Scand* 1969;40:23–42.
79. Yoo JU, Papay RS, Malemud CJ. Suppression of proteoglycan synthesis in chondrocyte cultures derived from canine intervertebral disc. *Spine* 1992;17(2):221–224.
80. Olczyk K. Age-related changes of elastin content in human intervertebral discs. *Folia Histochem Cytobiol* 1994;32(1):41–44.
81. Oda J, Tanaka H, Tsuzuki N. Intervertebral disc changes with aging of human cervical vertebrae, from the neonate to the eighties. *Spine* 1988;13:1205–1211.
82. Bernick S, Walker JM, Paule WJ. Age changes to the anulus fibrosus in human intervertebral discs. *Spine* 1991;16(5):520–524.
83. Yasuma T, Arai K, Suzuki F. Age-related phenomena in the lumbar intervertebral discs. Lipofuscin and amyloid deposition. *Spine* 1992;17(10):1194–1198.
84. Osti OL, Vernon-Roberts B, Fraser RD. Annular tears and disc degeneration in the lumbar spine. *J Bone Joint Surg Br* 1992;74:678–682.
85. Vasan NS, Gutteling EW, Lee CK, Cibischino M, Parsons JR. A preliminary study of mechanically stress-induced changes in the extracellular matrix of the canine intervertebral disc. *Spine* 1991;16(3): 317–320.
86. Mimura M, Panjabi MM, Oxland TR, Crisco JJ, Yamamoto I, Vasavada A. Disc degeneration affects the multidirectional flexibility of the lumbar spine. *Spine* 1994;19(12):1371–1380.
87. Tanaka M, Nakahara S, Inoue H. A pathologic study of discs in the elderly. Separation between the cartilaginous endplate and the vertebral body. *Spine* 1993;18(11):1456–1462.
88. Butler D, Trafimow JH, Andersson GB, McNeill TW, Huckman MS. Discs degenerate before facets. *Spine* 1990;15(2):111–113.
89. Noren R, Trafimow J, Andersson GB, Huckman MS. The role of facet joint tropism and facet angle in disc degeneration. *Spine* 1991;16(5):530–532.
90. Matsui H, Terahata N, Tsuji H, Hirano N, Naruse Y. Familial predisposition and clustering for juvenile lumbar disc herniation. *Spine* 1992;17(11):1323–1328.

91. Matsui H, Tsuji H, Terahata N. Juvenile lumbar herniated nucleus pulposus in monozygotic twins. *Spine* 1990;15(11):1228–1130.
92. Heliovaara M. Risk factors for low back pain and sciatica. *Ann Med* 1989;21(4):257–264.
93. Lotz JC, Colliou OK, Chin JR, Duncan NA, Liebenberg E. Compression-induced degeneration of the intervertebral disc: an in vivo mouse model and finite-element study. *Spine* 1998;23(23):2493–2506.
94. Kawaguchi Y, Osada R, Kanamori M, Ishihara H, Ohmori K, Matsui H, Kimura T. Association between an aggrecan gene polymorphism and lumbar disc degeneration. *Spine* 1999;24(23):2456–2460.
95. Heikkila JK, Koskenvuo M, Heliovaara M, Kurppa K, Riihimaki H, Heikkila K, Rita H, Videman T. Genetic and environmental factors in sciatica. Evidence from a nationwide panel of 9365 adult twin pairs. *Ann Med* 1989;21(5):393–398.
96. Videman T, Leppavuori J, Kaprio J, Battie MC, Gibbons LE, Peltonen L, Koskenvuo M. Intragenic polymorphisms of the vitamin D receptor gene associated with intervertebral disc degeneration. *Spine* 1998;23(23):2477–2485.
97. Paassilta P, Lohiniva J, Goring HH, Perala M, Raina SS, Karppinen J, Hakala M, Palm T, Kroger H, Kaitila I, Vanharanta H, Ott J, Ala-Kokko I. Identification of a novel common genetic risk factor for lumbar disk disease. *JAMA* 2001;285(14):1843–1849.
98. Annunen S, Paassilta P, Lohiniva J, Perala M, Pihlajamaa T, Karppinen J, Tervonen O, Kroger H, Lahde S, Vanharanta H, Ryhanen L, Goring HH, Ott J, Prockop DJ, Ala-Kokko L. An allele of COL9A2 associated with intervertebral disc disease. *Science* 1999;285(5426):409–412.
99. van der Rest M, Garrone R. Collagen family of proteins. *Faseb J* 1991;5(13):2814–2823.
100. van der Rest M, Aubert-Foucher E, Dublet B, Eichenberger D, Font B, Goldschmidt D. Structure and function of the fibril-associated collagens. *Biochem Soc Trans* 1991;19(4):820–824.
101. Diab M. The role of type IX collagen in osteoarthritis and rheumatoid arthritis. *Orthop Rev* 1993;22(2):165–170.
102. Eyre D. Collagen cross-linking amino acids. *Methods Enzymol* 1987;144:115–139.
103. Eyre DR, Apon S, Wu JJ, Ericsson LH, Walsh KA. Collagen type IX: evidence for covalent linkages to type II collagen in cartilage. *FEBS Lett* 1987;220(2):337–341.
104. Diab M, Wu JJ, Eyre DR. Collagen type IX from human cartilage: a structural profile of intermolecular cross-linking sites. *Biochem J* 1996;314(Pt 1):327–332.
105. Pihlajamaa T, Perala M, Vuoristo MM, Nokelainen M, Bodo M, Schulthess T, Vuorio E, Timpl R, Engel J, Ala-Kokko L. Characterization of recombinant human type IX collagen. Association of alpha chains into homotrimeric and heterotrimeric molecules. *J Biol Chem* 1999;274(32):22464–22468.
106. Bonnemann CG, Cox GF, Shapiro F, Wu JJ, Feener CA, Thompson TG, Anthony DC, Eyre DR, Darras BT, Kunkel LM. A mutation in the alpha 3 chain of type IX collagen causes autosomal dominant

multiple epiphyseal dysplasia with mild myopathy. *Proc Natl Acad Sci USA* 2000;97(3):1212–1217.
107. Kauppila LI, Penttila A, Karhunen PJ, Lalu K, Hannikainen P. Lumbar disc degeneration and atherosclerosis of the abdominal aorta. *Spine* 1994;19(8):923–929.
108. Hoyland JA, Freemont AJ, Jayson MIV. Intervertebral foramen venous obstruction. A cause of periradicular fibrosis? *Spine* 1989;14:558.
109. Holm S, Nachemson A. Nutrition of the intervertebral disc. Acute effects of smoking. *Uppsala J Med Sci* 1988;93:91–99.
110. McDevitt CA, Beck GJ, Ciunga MJ, O'Brien J. Cigarette smoking degrades hyaluronic acid. *Lung* 1985;167:237–245.
111. Battie MC, Videman T, Gill K, Moneta GB, Nyman R, Kaprio J, Koskenvuo M. 1991 Volvo Award in clinical sciences. Smoking and lumbar intervertebral disc degeneration: an MRI study of identical twins. *Spine* 1991;16(9):1015–1021.
112. Ishihara H, Tsuji H, Hirano N, Ohshima H, Terahata N. Effects of continuous quantitative vibration on rheologic and biological behaviors of the intervertebral disc. *Spine* 1992;17(3 suppl):S7–S12.
113. Pedrini-Mille A, Weinstein JN, Found EM, Chung CB, Goel VK. Stimulation of dorsal root ganglia and degradation of rabbit annulus fibrosus. *Spine* 1990;15(12):1252–1256.
114. Sward L, Hellstrom M, Jacobsson B, Nyman R, Peterson L. Acute injury of the vertebral ring apophysis and intervertebral disc in adolescent gymnasts. *Spine* 1990;15(2):144–148.
115. Sward L, Hellstrom M, Jacobsson B, Nyman R, Peterson L. Disc degeneration and associated abnormalities of the spine in elite gymnasts. A magnetic resonance imaging study. *Spine* 1991;16(4):437–443.
116. Boutin P, Hogshead H. Surgical pathology of the intervertebral disc. Is routine examination necessary? *Spine* 1992;17(10):1236–1238.
117. el-Hefnawy M, Yehia A, Farahat HM, el-Feky H, Mangoud AM, Aly MA, Essia MH, Abdel-Wahab RM. Extruded and protruded lumbar discs: combined clinical, histopathological, histochemical, immunopathological, histochemical, immunopathological and ultrastructural studies. *J Egypt Public Health Assoc* 1991;66(5–6):519–543.
118. Brock M, Patt S, Mayer HM. The form and structure of the extruded disc. *Spine* 1992;17(12):1457–1461.
119. Lipson SJ. Metaplastic proliferative fibrocartilage as an alternative concept to the herniated disc. *Spine* 1988;13:1055–1060.
120. Johnstone B, Urban JP, Roberts S, Menage J. The fluid content of the human intervertebral disc. Comparison between fluid content and swelling pressure profiles of discs removed at surgery and those taken postmortem. *Spine* 1992;17(4):412–416.
121. Chitkara YK. Clinicopathologic study of changes in prolapsed intervertebral disks. *Arch Pathol Lab Med* 1991;115(5):481–483.
122. Hirabayashi S, Kumano K, Tsuiki T, Eguchi M, Ikeda S. A dorsally displaced free fragment of lumbar disc herniation and its interesting histologic findings. A case report. *Spine* 1990;15(11):1231–1233.

123. Yamashita K, Hiroshima K, Kurata A. Gadolinium-DTPA–enhanced magnetic resonance imaging of a sequestered lumbar intervertebral disc and its correlation with pathologic findings. *Spine* 1994;19(4):479–482.
124. Weinstein JN, Claverie W, Gibson S. The pain of discography. *Spine* 1988;13:1344–1348.
125. Spencer DL, Mailler JA, Bertolini JE. The effect of intervertebral disc space narrowing on the contact force between the nerve root and a simulated disc protrusion. *Spine* 1984;9:422–426.
126. Garfin SR, Rydevik BL, Brown RA. Compressive neuropathy of spinal nerve roots. A mechanical or biological problem? *Spine* 1991;16(2):162–166.
127. Olmarker K, Rydevik B, Holm S, Bagge U. Effects of experimental graded compression on blood-flow in spinal nerve roots. *J Orthop Res* 1989;7:817–823.
128. Lind B, Massie JB, Lincoln T, Myers RR, Swenson MR, Garfin SR. The effects of induced hypertension and acute graded compression on impulse propagation in the spinal nerve roots of the pig. *Spine* 1993;18(11):1550–1555.
129. Naftulin S, Fast A, Thomas M. Diabetic lumbar radiculopathy: sciatica without disc herniation. *Spine* 1993;18(16):2419–2422.
130. Hasue M. Pain and the nerve root. An interdisciplinary approach. *Spine* 1993;18(14):2053–2058.
131. McCarron RF, Wimpee MW, Hudkins PG, Laros GS. The inflammatory effect of nucleus pulposus: a possible element in the pathogenesis of low back pain. *Spine* 1987;10:134–137.
132. Marshall LL, Treththewie ER, Curtain CC. Chemical radiculitis. *Clin Orthop* 1977;129:61–67.
133. Spiliopoulou I, Korovessis P, Konstantinou D, Dimitracopoulos G. IgG and IgM concentration in the prolapsed human intervertebral disc and sciatica etiology. *Spine* 1994;19(12):1320–1323.
134. Bobechko WP, Hirsch C. Autoimmune response to nucleus pulposus in the rabbit. *J Bone Joint Surg Br* 1965;47:574–580.
135. Franson RC, Saal JS, Saal JA. Human disc phospholipase A2 is inflammatory. *Spine* 1992;17(6 suppl):S129–S132.
136. Saal JS, Franson RC, Dobrow R, Saal JA, White AH, Goldthwaite N. High levels of inflammatory phospholipase A2 activity in lumbar disc herniations. *Spine* 1990;15(7):674–678.
137. Willburger RE, Wittenberg RH. Prostaglandin release from lumbar disc and facet joint tissue. *Spine* 1994;19(18):2068–2070.
138. Skouen JS, Larsen JL, Vollset SE. Cerebrospinal fluid proteins as indicators of nerve root compression in patients with sciatica caused by disc herniation. *Spine* 1993;18(1):72–79.
139. Pettersson CA. Drainage of molecules from subarachnoid space to spinal nerve roots and peripheral nerve of the rat. A study based on Evans blue–albumin and lanthanum as tracers. *Acta Neuropathol Berl* 1993;86(6):636–644.
140. Yu S, Haughton VM, Sether LA, Wagner M. Annulus fibrosus in bulging intervertebral discs. *Radiology* 1988;169:761–763.
141. Peyster RG, Teplick JG, Haskin ME. Computed tomography of lumbosacral conjoined nerve root anomalies. Potential cause of

false positive reading for herniated nucleus pulposus. *Spine* 1985;10:331–337.

142. Epstein NE, Epstein JA, Carras R, Hyman RA. Far lateral lumbar disc herniations and associated structural abnormalities. An evaluation in 60 patients of the comparative value of CT, MRI, and myelo-CT in diagnosis and management. *Spine* 1990;15(6):534–539.
143. Chatani K, Kusaka Y, Mifune T, Nishikawa H. Topographic differences of ^{1}H-NMR relaxation times T1, T2 in the normal intervertebral disc and its relationship to water content. *Spine* 1993;18(15):2271–2275.
144. Castagnera L, Grenier N, Lavignolle B, Greselle JF, Senegas J, Caille JM. Study of correlation between intradiscal pressure and magnetic resonance imaging data in evaluation of disc degeneration. Therapeutic issue with percutaneous nucleotomy. *Spine* 1991;16(3):348–352.
145. Tertti M, Paajanen H, Laato M, Aho H, Komu M, Kormanc M. Disc degeneration in magnetic resonance imaging. A comparative biochemical, histologic, and radiologic study in cadaver spines. *Spine* 1991;16(6):629–634.
146. Schiebler ML, Camerino VJ, Fallon MD, Zlatkin MB, Grenier N, Kressel HY. In vivo and ex vivo magnetic resonance imaging evaluation of early disc degeneration with histopathologic correlation. *Spine* 1991;16(6):635–640.
147. Gunzburg R, Parkinson R, Moore R, Cantraine F, Hutton W, Vernon-Roberts B, Fraser R. A cadaveric study comparing discography, magnetic resonance imaging, histology, and mechanical behavior of the human lumbar disc. *Spine* 1992;17(4):417–426.
148. Heggeness MH, Doherty BJ. Discography causes end plate deflection. *Spine* 1993;18(8):1050–1053.
149. Executive committee of the North American Spine Society. Position statement on discography. *Spine* 1988;13(12):1343.
150. Nachemson A. Lumbar discography—where are we today? *Spine* 1989;14(6):555–557.
151. Lord P. Definitions of disc disease [letter; comment]. *Br J Hosp Med* 1991;46(3):142.
152. Breton G. Is that a bulging disk, a small herniation or a moderate protrusion? [editorial; comment]. *Can Assoc Radiol J* 1991;42(5):318.
153. Milette PC. Radiculopathy, radicular pain, radiating pain, referred pain. What are we really talking about? [letter; comment]. *Radiology* 1994;192(1):280–282.
154. Fardon D, Pinkerton S, Balderston R, Garfin S, Nasca R, Salib R. Terms used for diagnosis by English-speaking spine surgeons. *Spine* 1993;18(2):274–277.
155. Thelander U, Fagerlund M, Friberg S, Larsson S. Describing the size of lumbar disc herniations using computed tomography. A comparison of different size index calculations and their relation to sciatica. *Spine* 1994;19(17):1979–1984.
156. Thompson JP, Pearce RH, Schechter MT, Adams ME, Tsang IK, Bishop PB. Preliminary evaluation of a scheme for grading the gross morphology of the human intervertebral disc. *Spine* 1990;15(5):411–415.

157. Adams MA, Dolan P, Hutton WC. The stages of disc degeneration as revealed by discograms. *J Bone Joint Surg Br* 1986;68:36–41.
158. Brinckmann P, Grootenboer H. Change of disc height, radial disc bulge, and intradiscal pressure from discectomy. An in vitro investigation on human lumbar discs. *Spine* 1991;16(6):641–646.
159. Smith JW, Walmsley R. Experimental incision of the intervertebral disc. *J Bone Joint Surg Br* 1951;33:12–25.
160. Ahlgren BD, Vasavada A, Brower RS, Lydon C, Herkowitz HN, Panjabi MM. Anular incision technique on the strength and multidirectional flexibility of the healing intervertebral disc. *Spine* 1994;19(8):948–954.
161. Songer MN, Ghosh L, Spencer DL. Effects of sodium hyaluronate on peridural fibrosis after lumbar laminotomy and discectomy. *Spine* 1990;15(6):550–554.
162. Jayson MIV. The role of vascular damage and fibrosis in the pathogenesis of nerve root damage. *Clin Orthop* 1992;279:40–48.
163. Hoyland JA, Freemont AJ, Denton J, Thomas AMC, McMillan JJ, Jayson MIV. Retained surgical swab debris in post-laminectomy arachnoiditis and peridural fibrosis. *J Bone Joint Surg Br* 1988;70:659.
164. Kawakami M, Weinstein JN, Spratt KF, Chatani K, Traub RJ, Meller ST, Gebhart GF. Experimental lumbar radiculopathy. Immunohistochemical and quantitative demonstrations of pain induced by lumbar nerve root irritation of the rat. *Spine* 1994;19(16):1780–1794.

4

Familial Incidence of Disc Herniation. Epidemiologic and Genetic Evidence: A Hypothesis Suggesting That Laminectomy and Discectomy Are Counterproductive

Daniel S.J. Choy

Herniations of any structure require a force pushing the herniating structure against a weakened restraining wall. Thus, an inguinal hernia requires an increase of intra-abdominal pressure pushing a viscus against a weak anterior abdominal wall; a myocardial herniation requires an event such as a transmyocardial infarction weakening the ventricular wall and allowing the systolic pressure in the ventricle to push out a pocket; the repeated shoulder dislocations of Marfan's syndrome occur because of a weak anterior capsule; a diaphragmatic hernia occurs in the context of a weak esophageal–gastric diaphragmatic ring; and the longitudinal aortic aneurysms and tears seen in the Ehlers–Danlos syndrome happen because of defective elastic tissue.

Intervertebral disc herniations are subject to the same physical laws. From the base of the skull to the top of the sacrum stretches a fibrous band—the posterior longitudinal ligament (PLL). The fibers in the midline, which attach horizontally to the midpoints of the disc margins, narrow and thin out at the L4-L5 and L5-S1 levels. The transverse breadth of the PLL varies from 21.4 ± 3.0 mm at the L1-2 to 11.5 ± 2.9 mm at the L5-S1 level, and the axial breadth ranges from 25.3 ± 4.7 mm at the L1-2 to 14.3 ± 3.5 mm at the L5-S1 level.[1] The considerably greater incidence of disc herniations at the L4-5 and L5-S1 levels compared with the L1-2 level may be partially related to this variation. The higher loading at the lower discs may also play a role. If the PLL and the annulus are weak, an increase in intradiscal pressure can push part of the nucleus pulposus through the thin points of these two structures. A Valsalva event caused by a cough, a sneeze, lifting a heavy load, a sudden compression of adjacent vertebral bodies in a motor vehicle accident, falling on the coccyx, an unanticipated step off a curb, or a rotational injury caused by teeing off on a golf course all can cause disc herniation, usually in a posterolateral direction. If the PLL is strong, a herniation may occur cephalad or caudad, through the end plate, which is composed of hyaline cartilage. Many authors describe "degeneration" of the annulus fibrosus and PLL as antecedent to herniation of the nucleus pulposus. Gordon et al. stated "intervertebral disc prolapse is peripheral in origin; the annulus fibrosus is the site of primary pathologic change."[2]

Incidence

When one considers that the incidence of disc herniation in the United States is 1.7%,[3] the remaining 98.3% must have strong PLLs, since certainly more than 1.7% of the population often experiences sudden and large increases of intradiscal pressure. It would then seem reasonable to postulate that the 1.7% who develop herniated nucleus pulposus (HNP) may have a congenital weakness of the PLL, and if this is so, there must be a familial incidence of disc protrusions. There would also be a significant incidence of disc herniations at multiple levels.

Table 4.1 A Review of the Author's 621 Patients*

Number of herniated discs	Number of patients	Percent
1	385	62.00
2	179	28.82
3	48	7.74
4	6	0.96
5	2	0.32
8	1	0.16

*Published in 2000.

These hypotheses were tested in a retrospective study of 200 patients with known HNP. These patients were contacted by telephone and mail. There were 174 respondents. Of these, 74 patients had first-order relatives with documented HNPs; 25 had more than one relative (second or third order). This was an incidence of 43%. The commonest occurrence was in fathers (42), then mothers (26), brothers (17), and sisters (14).

The review of multiple discs in 621 patients in Table 4.1 indicates that 62% had single discs, 29% had two, 7.7% had three, 1% had four, 0.3% had five, and 0.16% had eight.

Discussion

The 43% incidence of HNP in first-order relatives, compared with a national incidence of 1.7%, is highly significant, with $p < 0.0001$. The hypothesis just outlined appears to be accurate.

Others have found similar data. Simmons et al.[4] found in 65 patients a positive family history in 44.6%. Postacchini et al.[5] found 35% incidence of first-order relatives in a group of 284 patients with discogenic pain, and 37% in 114 patients who had open surgery for HNP. Four brothers whose parents both had had surgery for HNP were reported by Varughese et al.[6] to have the same condition. HNP in a pair of 16-year-old monozygotic twins was reported by Matsue et al.[7] Hurxthal[8] and Nelson et al.[9] reported multiple Schmorl's nodes in young twins.

With reference to the incidence of multiple discs, Gibson et al.[10] found that 75% of 20 patients had multiple disc involvement. The author's finding of 38% of patients with multiple discs was unexpected, but I suspect that most spine surgeons have the same experience. The frequency of these multiple herniations suggests that the PLL and the annulus are defective, and fail to hold the protrusions in place.

Finally, Annunen et al.[11] found an allele of *COL9A2* that was associated with herniated disc disease. Discs are composed of a matrix of collagen and proteoglycans. The annulus is predominantly collagen type I, and the nucleus pulposus is approximately 50% proteoglycan and 20% collagen II. Small amounts of collagen IX are found in both. In mice, mutations of collagen IX cause age-related disc degeneration and herniation.[12,13] Collagen IX is a heterotrimer of three alpha chains: α_1 (IX), α_2 (IX), and α_3 (IX), encoded by the genes *COL9A1*, *COL9A2*, and *COL9A3*, respectively. Collagen IX is a bridge between collagens and noncollagenous tissue. Collagen IX was studied in 157 unrelated Finnish patients with L4-5 and L5-S1 disc herniations. Sequencing by gel electrophoresis found heterozygous substitution of tryptophan (Trp) for either glycine (Gln) or arginine (arg) in the *COLA2* domain.[14]

This finding was surprising, since Trp is rarely found in collagenous domains of collagen IX in humans or mice. In 10 patients, there was heterozygous substitution for either Gln or Arg. Of the remaining 147 patients, 5 had Trp substitution. All 26 patients carrying the Trp substitution had intervertebral disease. The authors concluded that genetic risk factors contribute to the 5% prevalence of HNP in the Finnish population.[14] In addition, these factors consisted of Trp substitution disrupting the collagen triple helix, thus interfering with the interaction between collagen IX and II or preventing the action of lysyl oxidase, a catalyst of cross-link formation. These findings about collagen may well apply to the PLL and the annulus fibrosus. There is thus a strong molecular basis for suggesting that genetic or familial factors predispose people to HNP.

Microdiscectomy, chymopapain therapy, and percutaneous laser disc decompression (PLDD) are all directed toward reducing intradiscal pressure, and produce minimal, if any, weakening of the posterior wall of the spine. On the other hand, laminectomy and discectomy, by unroofing the lamina and creating a large hole in the annulus, further weakens an already compromised structure. In this procedure, one would expect to see a high incidence of recurrent disc herniation, and such is unfortunately the case.

One study[15] showed a 21% reherniation rate. Malter et al.[16] found a 15% reoperation rate in 6376 patients within 5 years. Eleven disc reherniations occurred in 30 patients who had anterior cervical decompressions in the series of Matsunaga et al.[17] Grane[18] found a reoperation rate of 3 to 19%. In 560 patients, Weir and Jacobs[19] reported that 18% required second operations.

Hirabayashi et al.[20] had 214 patients with a 7.5% reoperation rate. This is close to the results of Moore et al.,[21] namely 10%. Lindgren[22] reported 14% in 375 patients. The author's poll of nine neurosurgeons and orthopedic surgeons produced reoperation figures of 10 to 15%, respectively.

By contrast, in the author's 16-year experience, the reherniation rate has been 5%, usually caused by reinjury.

Occam's razor states that the simplest theory that explains a phenomenon is the best theory. In this case the simplest hypothesis is that intervertebral disc herniations are due to an increase in intradiscal pressure, together with a congenitally weakened annulus fibrosus and posterior longitudinal ligament.

Conclusion

Perhaps it is time to reassess an operation that has been in existence for 69 years, taught unchallenged from generation to generation of spine surgeons. Perhaps it is time to abandon a procedure that further weakens an already weakened posterior wall, resulting in relatively high rates of reherniation and failed back syndrome, and replace it with a minimally invasive procedure that is safe and effective. In 1991 Williams presciently stated: "As any structural engineer could have predicted, the once accepted standard lumbar surgical concepts and techniques of the past have finally proved to be destructive to the future competence of the lumbar anatomy."[23]

References

1. Oshima H, Hirano N, Osada R, Matsue H, Tsuje H. Morphologic variation of lumbar posterior longitudinal ligament and the modality of disc herniation. *Spine* 1993;18:2408–2411.
2. Gordon SJ, King HY, Mayer P, Mace AH, Kish VL, Radin EL. Mechanism of disc rupture. *Spine* 1991;6:450–456.
3. National Center for Health Statistics. National Interview Health Survey data tapes. 1985–1988, USA.
4. Simmons ED, Guntupalli M, Kowalski JM, Braun F, Seidel T. Familial predisposition for degenerative disc disease: a case-control study. *Spine* 1996;21:1527–1527.
5. Postacchini F, Lami R, Pugliese O. Familial predisposition to discogenic low back pain, an epidemiologic and immunogenetic study. *Spine* 1988;13:1403–1406.
6. Varughese G, Quartey G. Familial lumbar spinal stenosis with acute herniation. *J Neurosurg* 1979;51:234–236.
7. Matsui H, Tsuji H, Terahara N. Juvenile lumbar herniated nucleus pulposus in monozygotic twins. *Spine* 1990;5:1228–1230.
8. Hurxthal L. Schmorl's nodes in identical twins. *Lahey Clin Found Bull* 1966;15:89–92.
9. Nelson CL, Janecki CL, Gildenberg PL, Sava G. Disc protrusions in the young. *Clin Orthop* 1972;88:142–150.
10. Gibson MJ, Szypryt EP, Buckley JH, Worthington BS, Mulholland RC. Magnetic resonance imaging of adolescent disc herniation. *J Bone Joint Surg Am* 1987;69:699–703.
11. Annunen S, Paassilsta P, Lohiniva J et al. An allele of *COL9A2* associated with intervertebral disc disease. *Science* 1999;285:409–412.
12. Kimura T, Kakata T, Tsumaki N, et al. Progressive degeneration of articular cartilage and intervertebral discs. An experimental study in transgenic mice bearing a type IX collagen mutation. *Int Orthop* 1995;20:177–181.
13. Watanabe H, Nakata K, Kimata K, Nakanishe I, Yamada Y. Dwarfism and age-associated spinal degeneration of heterozygote and mice defective in aggrecan. *Proc Natl Acad Sci U S A* 1997;94:6943–6947.
14. Heliovaara M, Impiraara O, Slevers K. Lumbar disc syndrome in Finland. *Community Health J Epidemiol* 1987;41:251–258.
15. Delamarter RB, Bohlman HH. Failed microdiscectomies. American Association of Orthopedic Surgeons, 1990. Paper 515.
16. Malter AD, McNeney B, Loeser JD, Deyo RA. Five-year reoperation rates after different types of lumbar spine surgery. *Spine* 1998;23: 814–820.

17. Matsunaga S, Kabayama S, Yamamoro T, Yone K, Sakou T, Nakanishi K. Strain on intervertebral discs after anterior cervical decompression and fusion. *Spine* 1999;24:670–675.
18. Grane P. The postoperative spine: a radiological investigation of the lumbar spine after discectomy using MT imaging and CT. *Acta Radiol Suppl* 1998;414:1–23.
19. Weir BKA, Jacobs GA. Reoperation rate following lumbar discectomy. *Spine* 1980;5:366–370.
20. Hirabayashi S, Kumano K, Ogawa Y, Aoa Y, Machiro S. Microdiscectomy and second operation for lumbar disc herniation. *Spine* 1993;18:2206–2131.
21. Moore AJ, Chilton JD, Uttley D. Long-term results of microlumbar discectomy. *Br J Neurosurg* 1994;8:319–326.
22. Lindgren S. Some problems concerning the herniated intervertebral disc from a clinical point of view. *Acta Chir Scand* 1949;98:295–314.
23. Williams RW. Microdiscectomy—myth, mania, or milestone: an 18-year surgical adventure. *Mt Sinai J Med* 1991;58:139–145.

5

Patient Selection

Daniel S.J. Choy

The absolute requirement for performing percutaneous laser disc decompression (PLDD) is that the patient have a bulging, protruded, herniated intervertebral disc that is symptomatic. The remainder of the chapter is devoted to modifications of this statement.

Since PLDD is directed only at a symptomatic patient, a patient with an image-documented disc protrusion is not necessarily a candidate. Let us first consider the symptoms. These may consist of back pain in association with radiation down one or both extremities, or back pain alone. In the first few years of PLDD, the author excluded patients with back pain without radiation. Dr. William Black, of Scranton, Pennsylvania, began treating patients with Schmorl's nodes who had localized back pain with salutory results. In the past 10 years the author has treated a number of patients with the combination of image-documented disc protrusion and solitary, nonradiating back pain. The results are reported in Chapter 17.

The semantics of the words *bulge, protrusion,* and *herniation* require clarification. Some radiologists call the same lesion by one of the three terms. Since *herniation* carries overtones of anything from an associated annular bulge to an annular tear, I do not use the term any longer. *Bulge* sounds too innocuous and subclinical, and I tend to avoid that term also. I prefer *protrusion,* since it seems to denote a middle position that can be extended in either direction to encompass bulging or herniation.

Those who practice spine surgery or actively read MRIs and CT scans know that there is considerable overlap and much leeway in whether a radiologist will use one of the three terms.

Pain Reports and Magnetic Resonance Imaging Findings

Another point must be made forcefully. One does not treat a magnetic resonance image (MRI); one treats a patient. The MRI does not feel pain; the patient does. Hence, a patient presenting with a set of MRI films revealing multiple disc protrusions does not necessarily need PLDD to all the protruding discs. If the pain dermatome (see Chapter 6, Fig. 6.1 and 6.2) clearly demonstrates only, for instance, L5-S1 involvement, then only that disc needs to be treated. The reverse is also true. If a patient's MRI shows only a protrusion at L5-S1, but the history and examination clearly demonstrate an L4-5 component, then that disc should be treated as well. Such a decision requires judgment and courage on the part of the physician and is based on the bond of physician–patient trust that one hopes to have developed by the end of the consultation.

I stress this because all standard MRIs of the spine are unphysiologic. Most patients with protruded intervertebral disc disease are most comfortable lying down; they experience pain when sitting or standing. This is based on Nachemson and Morris's classic studies of intradisc pressure in the supine, standing, and sitting positions of 50, 100, and 200 kPa, respectively.[1] Consider this: all standard spine MRIs are performed in the supine position and are hence unphysiologic. Dr. Ferenc Jolecsz of Harvard clearly demonstrated this with three slides at the 1995 meeting in Salzburg of the Laser Association of Neurosurgery International (LANSI): a supine MRI showing a small bulge of the L5-S1 disc, the same patient 5 minutes later with a much larger protrusion of the same disc, and the second MRI being performed in a *sitting* position. At that time only two facilities for sitting MRIs existed, one in Zurich and the other at Harvard. The author's invention of MRI of the spine performed with spine compression is described in Chapter 8.

For these reasons I have come to rely less and less on the standard supine MRI and to place greater emphasis on history and physical findings. If the MRI does not agree with my clinical impression, it assumes a position of secondary importance, and I treat the patient based more on the clinical findings than on the MRI. This has been my policy over the past 5 years, and so far, the results seem to confirm the correctness of this approach.

In the patient with multiple-disc disease, where one or two seem to be *definite* culprits, and the others seem to be less likely but still possible candidates, I choose to perform PLDD on the *definite* discs and defer the others for 3 months. If, at the end of that time, the patient remains symptomatic, I then consider treating the remaining discs. This line of reasoning is fully explained to the patient, carefully recorded in the chart, and shown to the patient, so that he or she will remember 3 months down the line. Whenever possible, an accompanying relative or friend is told, as well, so that there is a witness, and also an additional memory at work.

Symptoms

During the first interview I perform a mental triage, rating the patient's pain on a scale of 1 to 10. I am inclined not to accept for PLDD a patient whose pain rating is below a 5.

I have had two patients, avid golfers (a redundancy), who were essentially pain free when not playing golf. Each wanted PLDD to be able to play without pain. I turned both down. Then there are a few patients with *litigation* backs, people who are in the midst of lawsuits seeking economic gain, who had minimal signs and symptoms both by radiographic imaging and examination. Such patients should also be rejected, not only because the situation is less than ethical, but because of the enormous amounts of time required on your part subsequent to the procedure in filling out legal reports, depositions, and the like.

Symptoms become less important if the patient has serious neurologic deficits such as weakness of the extensor hallucis longus muscle, the anterior tibialis, quadriceps, supraspinatus or infraspinatus, deltoids, interosseous muscles, digital extensors or separation flexors, with or without atrophy of muscle groups, foot drop, gait abnormalities, fixed trunk forward flexion, or genitourinary or anal sphincter problems. Such patients deserve early PLDD.

Patients with first-degree spondylolisthesis, mild scoliosis, and low-grade osteoarthritis are acceptable.

Previous back surgery is no longer a contraindication if enhanced imaging and examination determine recurrent *herniation* and absence of significant scar tissue nerve entrapment.

Previous fusion makes the disc inaccessible, as do cages.

Patients with spinal stenosis typically report increasing pain on walking a short distance. In spinal stenosis, discussed in Chapter 13, a protruding disc plays an etiologic role, and the condition can be successfully treated with PLDD.

Extruded discs, also discussed in Chapter 13, are acceptable if they maintain an anatomic connection to the parent disc.

Unstable angina, mild congestive heart failure, and mild pulmonary insufficiency are not contraindications.

Neither type I nor type II diabetes is a contraindication provided there is good control of glucose level.

Contraindications

The following conditions are contraindications for PLDD; cardiac and pulmonary disease are also addressed.

1. Patients with recent onset of symptoms, who have not had adequate conservative treatment for 3 months. It is well known that approximately 80 to 85% of patients with disc disease respond well to conservative therapy such as a short period of bed rest, muscle relaxants, anti-inflammatory drugs, and physiotherapy. Apropos of conservative management, I am not in favor of epidural blocks. A definitive paper on epidural blocks agreeing with my position appeared in the *New England Journal of Medicine* in 1997.[2] When epidural blocks work, they do so only temporarily. They are expensive, invasive, and can be painful; moreover, the steroids injected may weaken collagen.
2. Patients with severe spondylolisthesis.
3. Patients with severe scoliosis.
4. Patients with metastatic cancer.
5. Patients with vertebral compression fracture.
6. Bone spurs pressing on nerve roots.
7. Patients with a free fragment. It is known that 20% of free fragments are not detected by the best MRIs.[3–5] If there is no connection between the fragment and the parent disc, no matter how much pressure reduction is achieved in the parent disc by the laser, there will be no physical reason for the fragment to migrate toward the parent disc.
8. Moderate to severe vacuum phenomenon. This is a gas bubble in the disc, and therefore tends to negate the change in hydraulic forces on which PLDD is based.
9. Male patients over 80. My last five male patients over age 80 were all failures of PLDD. The apparent reason is that the water content of the nucleus pulposus at this age level, at least in men, is low. The proscription does not apply to female patients. I have had a good response in a 92-year-old woman.
10. Patients with a hemorrhagic diathesis that cannot be reversed.
11. Patients with a hemangioma adjacent to the disc.
12. Patients with multiple sclerosis.
13. Patients with other demylinating disease of the central nervous system.
14. Patients with systemic infections.

15. Patients with other diseases that project a life expectancy of less than 1 year.
16. Rarely, a severely disturbed patient, with "pains all over" presents herself (these patients are preponderantly women) in consultation. Often she confesses to a great fear of needles. Other phobias may also be expressed. It is best to disengage yourself. One such patient winced as I was marking her back with a felt-tipped pen. The slightest touch produced a spasm of withdrawal. Subsequently, she thrashed about on the table so that the procedure had to be aborted.

References

1. Nachemson A, Morris J. In vivo measurements of intradiscal pressure. Discometry, a method for the determination of pressure in the lower lumbar discs. *J Bone Joint Surg Am* 1964;46:1077–1092.
2. Carette S, Leclaire R, Sylvie M, et al. Epidural corticosteroid injections for sciatica due to herniated nucleus pulposus. *N Engl J Med* 1997;336:1634–1640.
3. Thornbury JR, Fryback DG, Turski PA, et al. Disk-caused nerve compression in patients with acute low back pain. Diagnosis with MR, CT, mylelography, and plain CT. *Radiology* 1993;186:731–738.
4. Greenspan A. CT discography vs MRI in intervertebral disk herniation. *Appl Radiol* March 1993:34–40.
5. Joubert JM, Laredo JD, Ziza JM, et al. Gadolinium-enhancing MR images in the preoperative evaluation of lumbar disc herniations. Presented at: 78th Scientific Assembly and Meeting of the Radiological Society of North America; November 29–December 4, 1992; Chicago. Abstract 304.

6

The Neurologic Examination

Daniel S.J. Choy

After the general thoughts expressed in the preceding chapter on patient selection, the single most important next step is the neurologic examination.

This should begin as soon as the patient enters your consultation room. Is he or she smiling? Frowning? Sad? Angry? Is the gait normal? Is the patient limping or striding forward with apparent comfort? Are the steps small and hesitant? Is a cane or crutch in use? Is the trunk bent forward? To one side? Does the patient decline your invitation to have a seat and prefer to remain standing (a position of greater comfort)?

Often the patient is accompanied by a family member. If a spouse, does he or she try to dominate the interview? Is the relationship a supportive one, or one of antagonism? These small signs can reveal a great deal and should not be ignored.

Pain Diagram

By then you will have seen the pain dermatome (Fig. 6.1). Some patients render this diagram in a sketchy manner, with a single line indicating the location of pain. An effort should be made to have such a patient describe, with one finger, in the standing position, on his or her own body, exactly where the pain is. You can then fill in the appropriate areas on the diagram. Areas of numbness and tingling should also be drawn in.

Figure 6.2 (see color plate) is the best dermatomal map I have seen and has been invaluable in my practice.

NAME_______________________________DATE__________CHART__________

Using the symbols given below, mark the areas on your body where you feel the described sensations.
Include all affected areas. Just to complete the picture, please draw your face

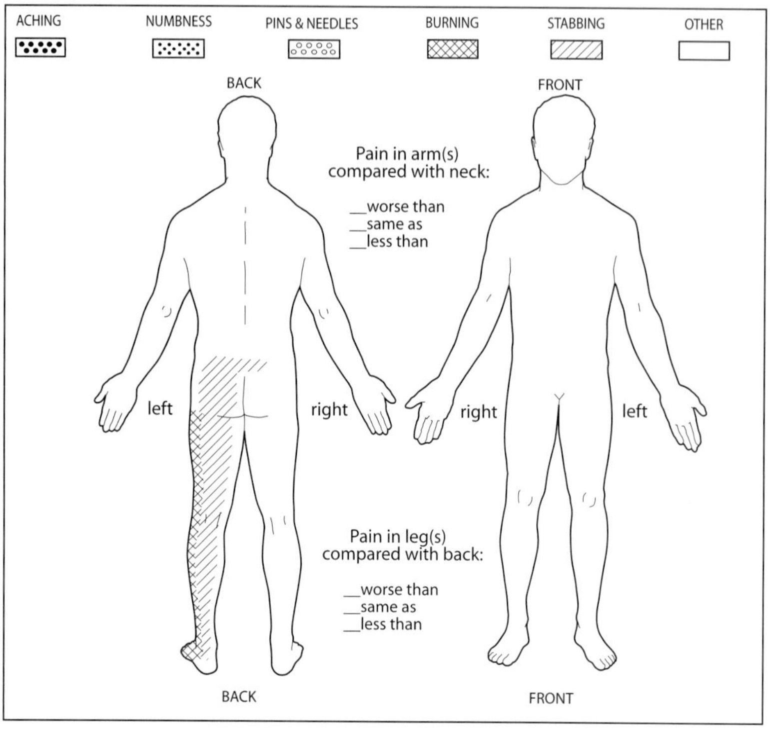

Does the following increase/decrease/no change in your symptoms?
Sitting__________Standing__________Lying Down__________

How long is your sitting tolerance?__________
Standing tolerance?__________
Walking tolerance?__________

Do you get calf pain/numbness that gets worse when you walk and that goes away
when you sit down?__________Lean forward?__________
How far do you walk before this happens?__________
How long does it take for the symptoms to resolve?__________

What is your position of comfort?__________

Figure 6.1. Posterior and anterior view of the human body, with the areas of pain for a particular patient appropriately marked. What is marked is characteristic of an L5-S1 lesion.

It is my practice to then tell the patient that part of the fun of practicing medicine is to try to make a diagnosis *without* looking at the magnetic resonance imaging (MRI) films. Most of the time one can be fairly accurate in predicting the offending disc(s). I then commit myself by writing on the pain diagram which disc(s) I think are responsible for the patient's pain, at the same time telling the patient and the family that I could be wrong. If it turns

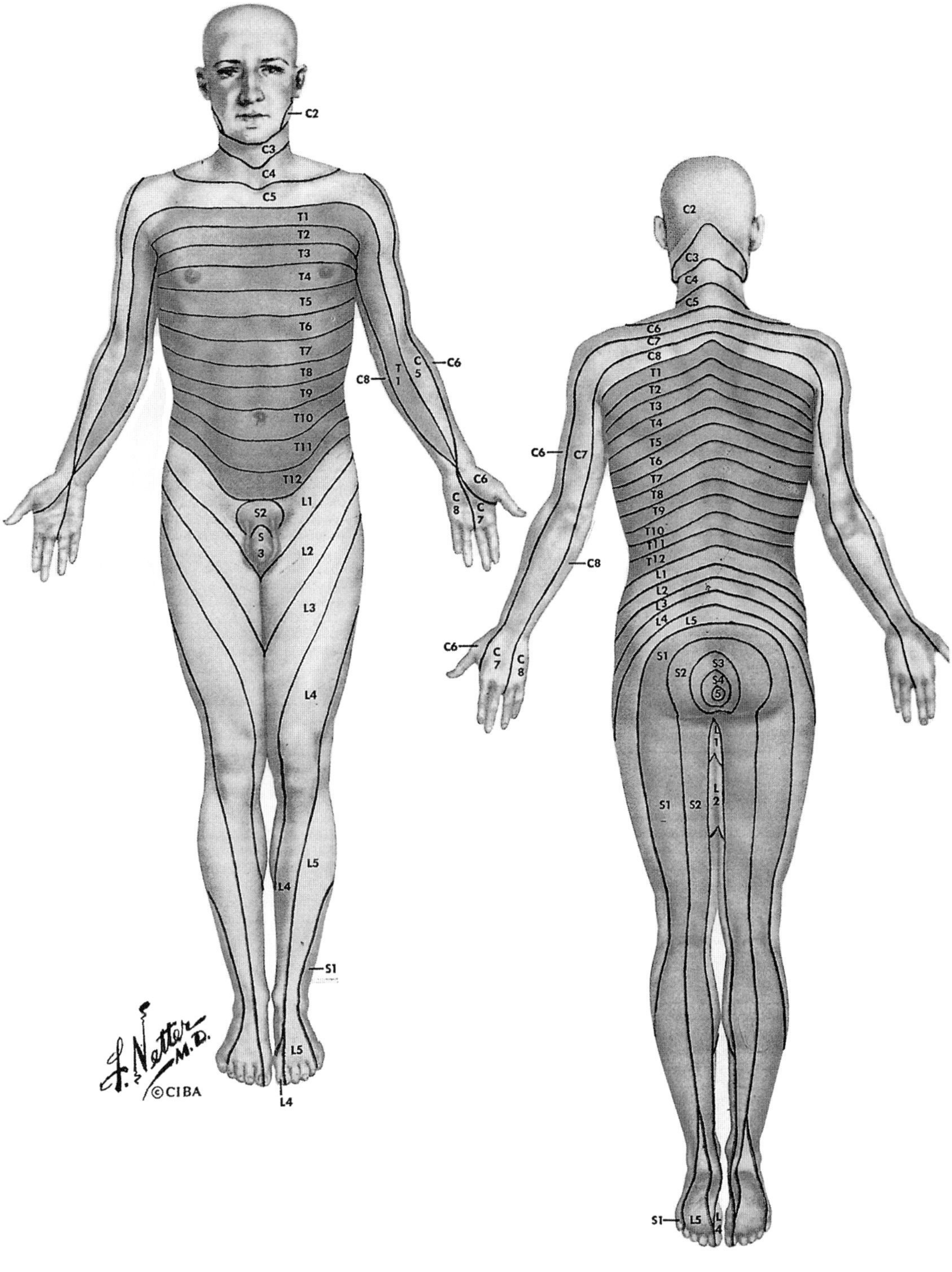

Figure 6.2. Dermatomal map. (From *The Netter Collection of Medical Illustrations, vol 1, Nervous System.* Copyright 1983. Icon Learning Systems, LLC, a subsidiary of MediMedia USA Inc. Reprinted with permission from Icon Learning Systems, LLC. Illustrated by Frank H. Netter, MD. All rights reserved.) (See color insert)

out that I am wrong, I have lost nothing; but if I am right then the patient and family are impressed with my clinical acumen. I do this only when there is a sciatic component to the pain. When there is only low back pain, one has no clue to the identity of the offending disc(s).

The History

The history is then taken. How long has the patient had the pain? What is the character of the pain? Burning? Sharp, knifelike? A dull ache? How did it start? Suddenly, gradually? Any precipitating incident, such as lifting some heavy object? Twisting the body? Golf? Tennis? Following severe coughing or sneezing? Reaching for an object high up? Running the marathon? After doing martial arts? Following a long car trip? Getting into or out of a car? A long airplane trip? Unloading luggage from a carousel? An auto accident? Stepping off a curb? Falling into the water during water skiing? A fall from downhill skiing? After yard work? Taking a jolting ride in an amusement park? I have had positive answers to each of these questions.

Is there concomitant onset of impotence? Are there genitourinary or anal sphincter problems?

What actions exacerbate and what maneuvers relieve the pain? Does walking exacerbate the pain and rest relieve it? Think of spinal stenosis. Which of the three positions is best: supine, sitting, or standing? If supine, is the lateral decubitus position best? Is the patient helped by flexing the thigh? A lateral decubitus po-

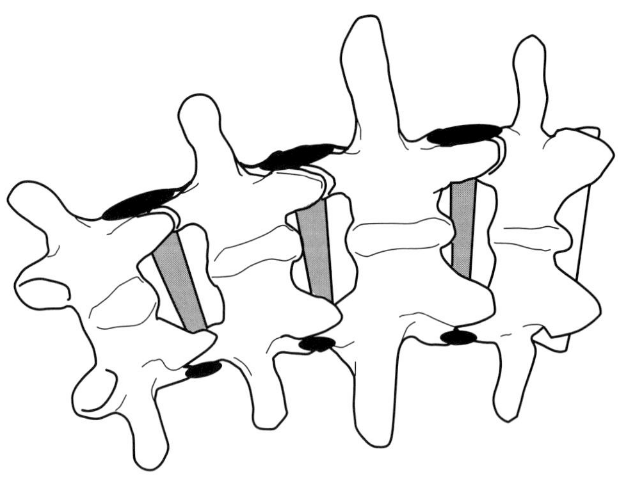

Figure 6.3. Diagram of how lateral flexion of the spine *opens up* the neural foramina on the convex side.

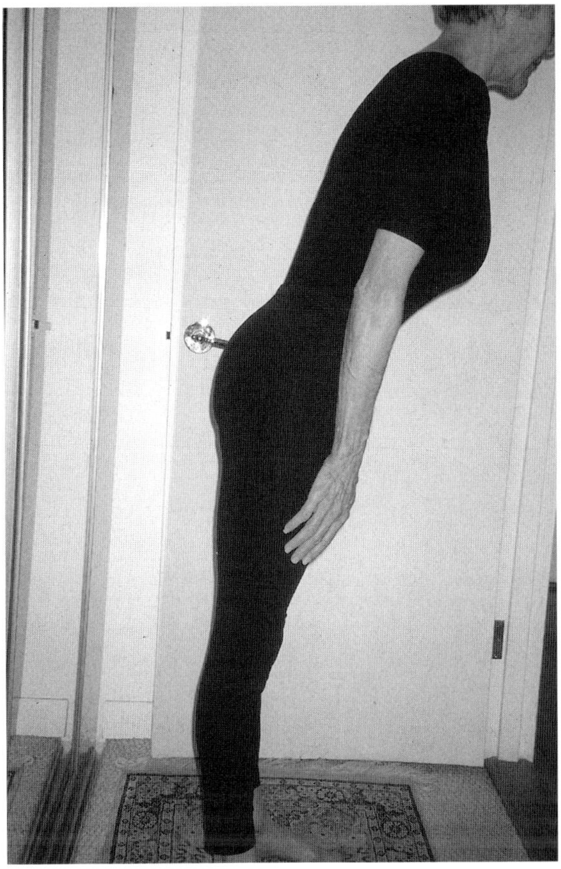

Figure 6.4. Patient's anteflexed posture, which relieves pressure on the nerve roots.

sition, with a pillow on the dependent side, with the upper leg flexed at the hip is indicative of a herniation on the superior side, since this maneuver opens up the facet joint and relieves pressure on the nerve root (Fig. 6.3). Similarly, if the trunk is bent forward (Fig. 6.4) during walking, the posterior disc space is opened up. Trunk flexion to one side (Fig. 6.5) caused by muscle spasm opens up the opposite side of the disc space, and is a protective mechanism. One can diagnose which side the sciatic pain is on by observing these postures. Similar protective mechanisms cause patients to walk with the affected leg partially flexed at the hip, with the foot in a plantar flexed position, thus shortening the sciatic nerve (Fig. 6.6).

Does coughing or sneezing bring on the pain? Does straining during bowel movements? These Valsalva maneuvers sharply elevate intradiscal pressure, and when present, are almost diagnostic of discogenic pain.

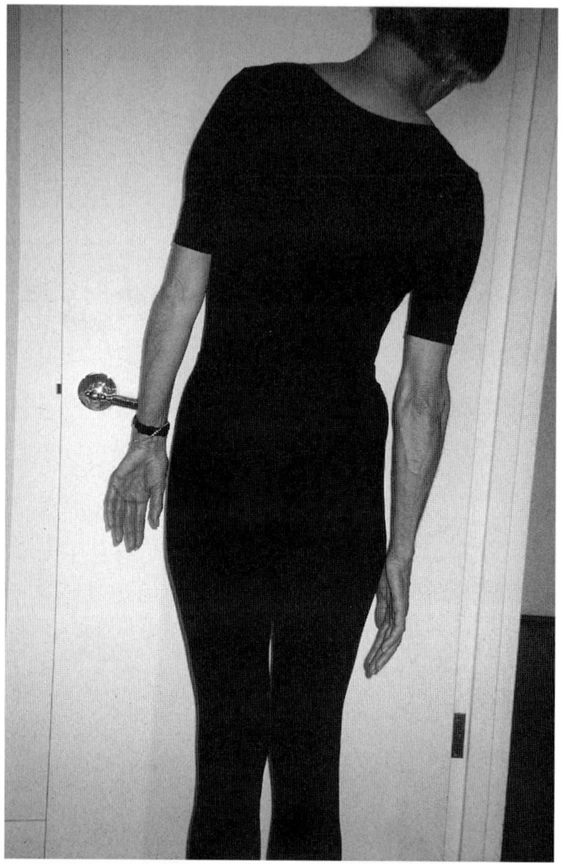

Figure 6.5. Patient's posture bent over to one side, opening up the neural foramina as in Figure 6.3.

The Examination

Weakness of the anterior tibialis and the extensor hallucis longus interferes with heel walking (L4-5) (Fig. 6.7); weakness of the gastrocnemius (L5-S1) interferes with toe walking (Fig. 6.8). In the case of foot drop, if the patient is wearing a favorite pair of old shoes, examination of the shoes reveals excessive wear of the toe of the sole on the affected side (Fig. 6.9).

Often the lumbar lordosis is lost; the patient will have a stiff back. Flexion to the affected side increases radicular pain, as does posterior trunk flexion.

In the cases of low back pain without a radicular component, I have found deep palpation on either side of the spinal column to be useful in eliciting tenderness over the affected disc. Radiation down a leg always makes one's diagnostic efforts easier; but if there is tenderness at a certain level with trunk flexion/extension

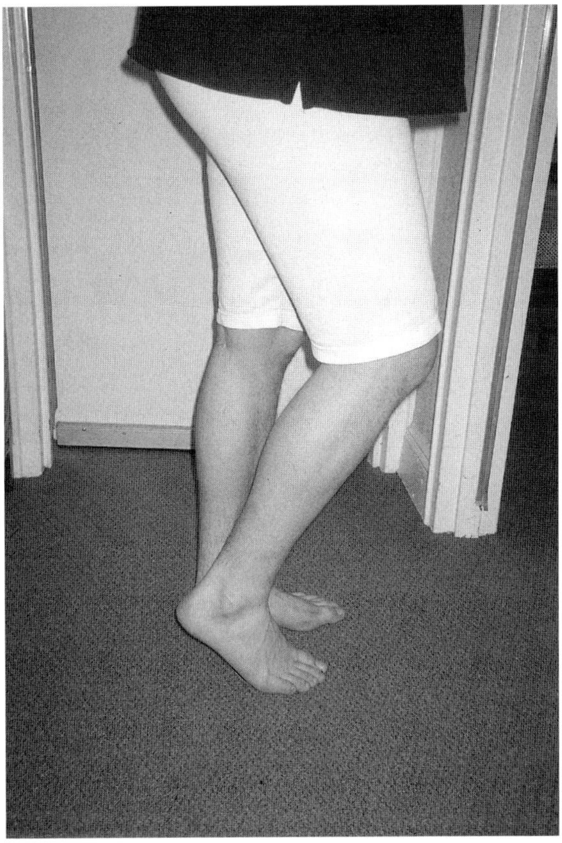

Figure 6.6. Patient's posture with affected leg flexed at the thigh and lower leg and with the foot plantar flexed, all of which tend to shorten the sciatic nerve.

and deep palpation, one can be fairly sure there is pathology at that level.

So much for observing the patient's stance, posture, and gait.

With the patient sitting, the examiner looks for signs of muscle atrophy. Quadriceps atrophy indicates an L4-5 lesion. The muscle groups are tested against resistance. Extensor hallucis longus weakness and/or foot drop are not uncommon in L4-5 lesions.

Asymmetry of deep tendon reflexes, or absence of patellar or Achilles reflexes are noted, the former being associated with L4-5 and the latter with L5-S1 lesions. Sometimes one can see both patellar and Achilles reflexes affected by L4-5 protruded discs, especially if it is large and central.

Straight leg raising (SLR) is performed with the patient supine. Often the patient keeps the affected leg flexed (Fig. 6.10) and resists efforts of the examiner to place the leg flat on the table. The patient is asked not to resist or to help the examiner, and to keep the knees straight. The heel is slowly lifted up until the patient

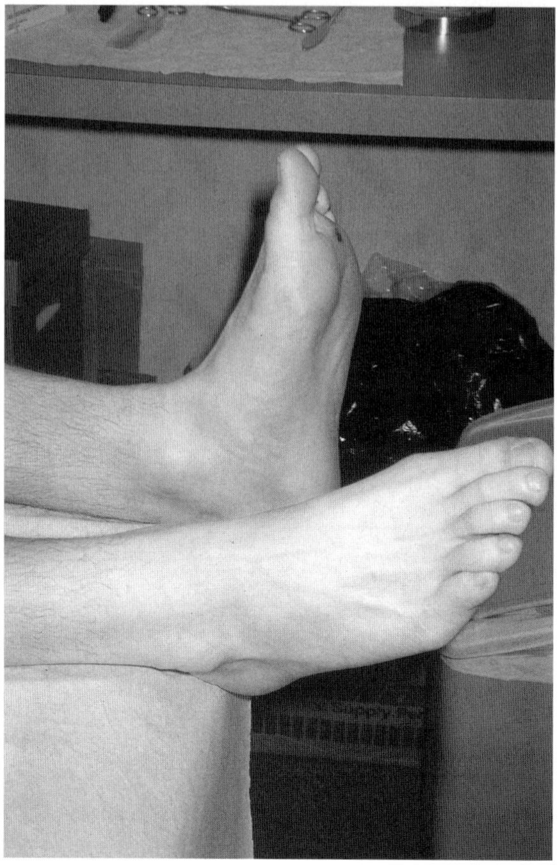

Figure 6.7. Foot drop. The right foot cannot be dorsiflexed for heel walking because of weakness of the tibialis anterior (L4-5).

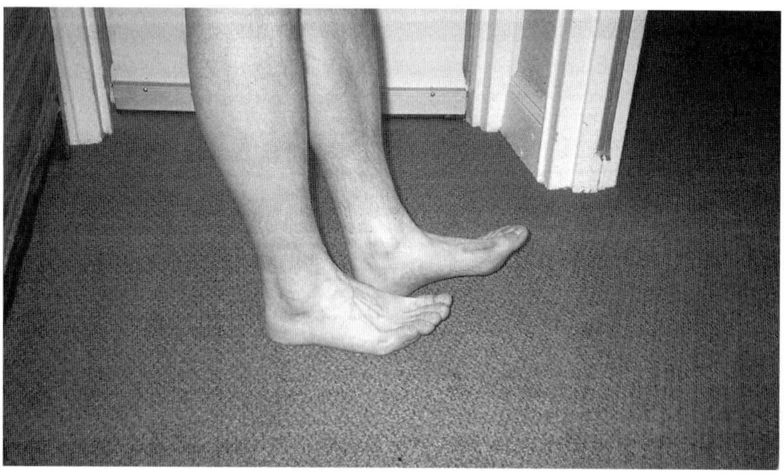

Figure 6.8. The right foot cannot be plantar flexed for toe walking because of weakness of the gastrocnemius muscle (L5-S1).

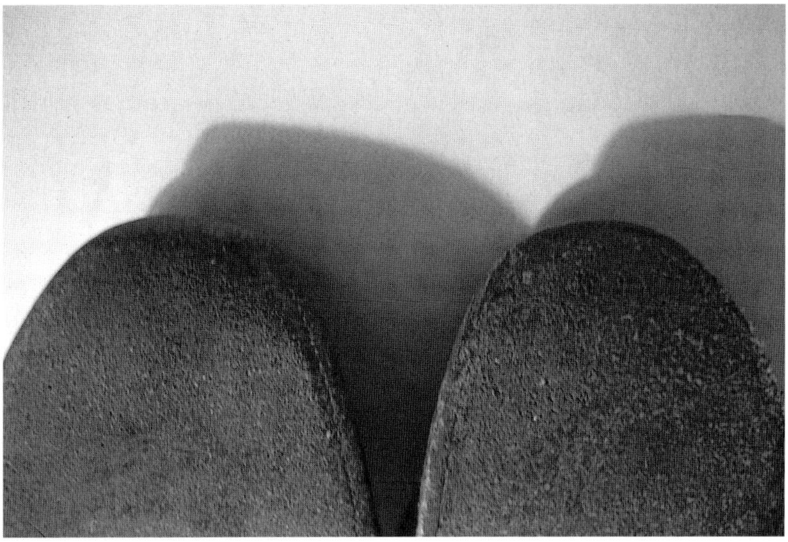

Figure 6.9. The toe of the left sole is worn more than that of the right because of foot drop. This sign is seen only if the patient has been wearing the same pair of shoes for some time.

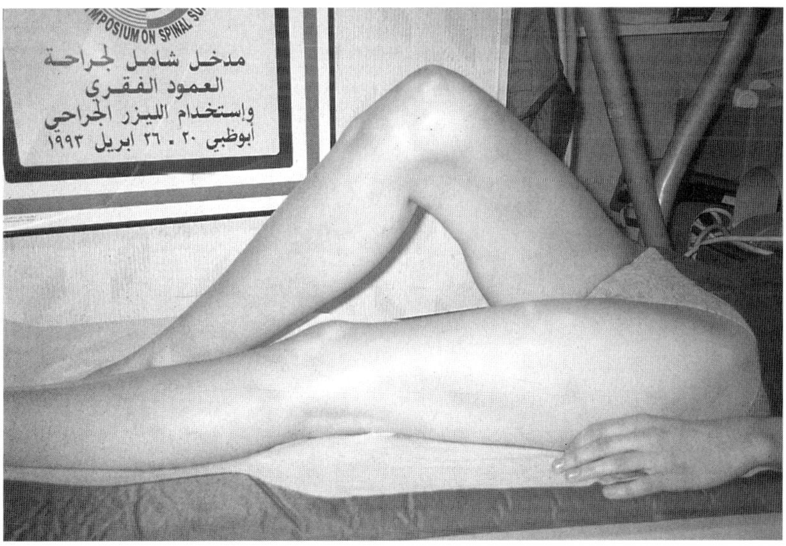

Figure 6.10. In the supine position, the patient automatically flexes the affected leg and resists efforts to straighten it. This is an attempt to shorten the sciatic nerve.

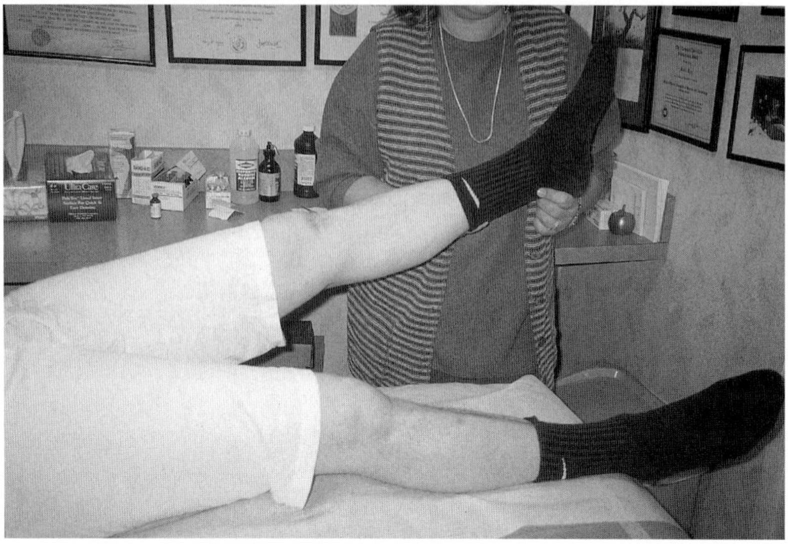

Figure 6.11. Here straight leg raising is limited to 20 degrees.

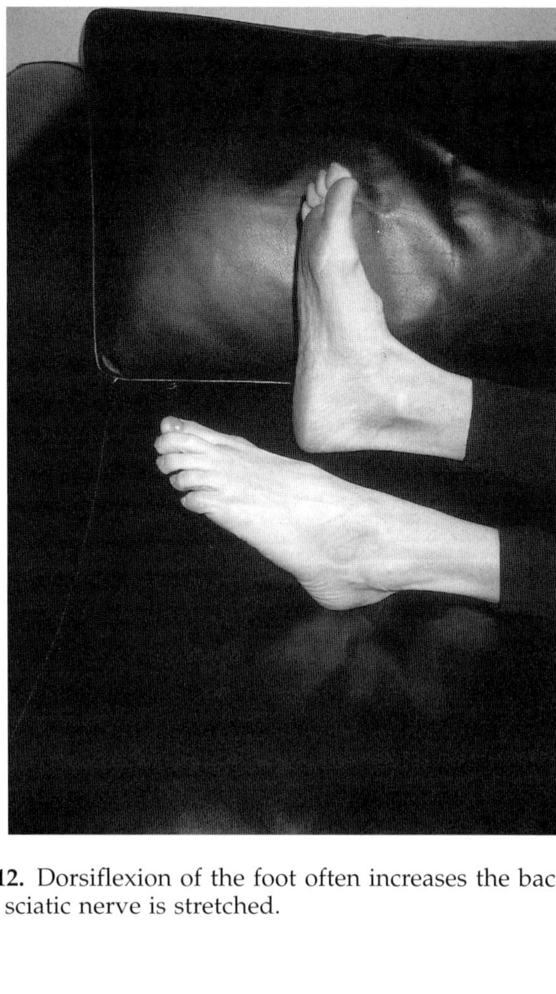

Figure 6.12. Dorsiflexion of the foot often increases the back pain, because the sciatic nerve is stretched.

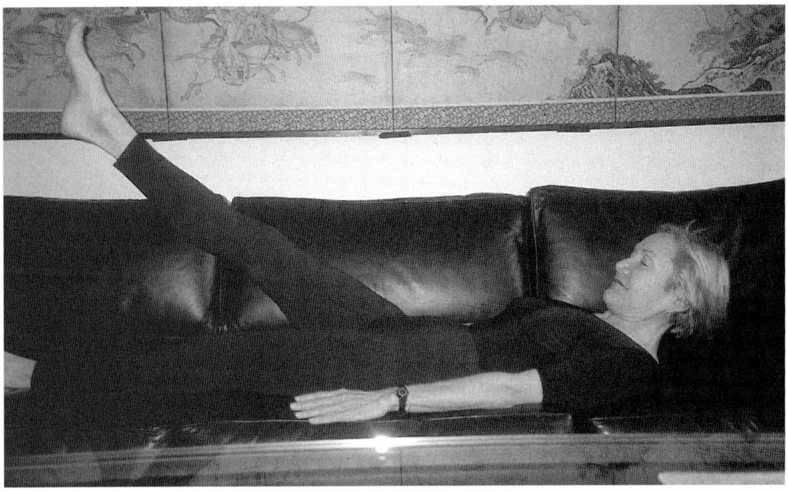

Figure 6.13. Raising the head also increases the back pain while the leg is kept in the raised position.

experiences pain in the low back, buttocks, or upper posterior thighs (Fig. 6.11). Pain in the popliteal fossa is not a positive SLR sign. Dorsiflexion of the foot (Fig. 6.12) and/or raising the head (Fig. 6.13) at this point will increase the pain. The angle of the leg with respect to the horizontal is noted. Bilateral positive SLR can be seen when the disc protrusion is large and central.

In the case of the L5-S1 disc, the bowstring sign can be positive. With the knee partially flexed, one hand palpates and "plucks" the popliteal nerve while the other hand slowly extends the knee (Fig. 6.14). It has been my experience that testicular pain is usually caused by the L5-S1 disc.

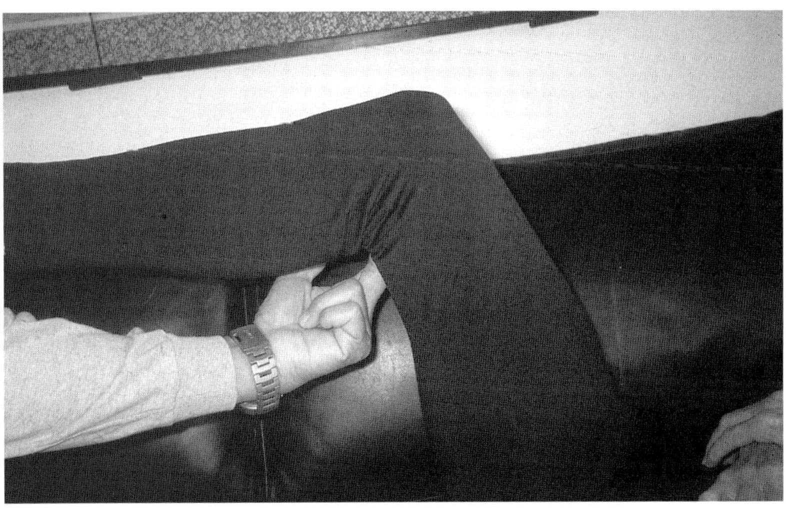

Figure 6.14 The *bowstring sign.*

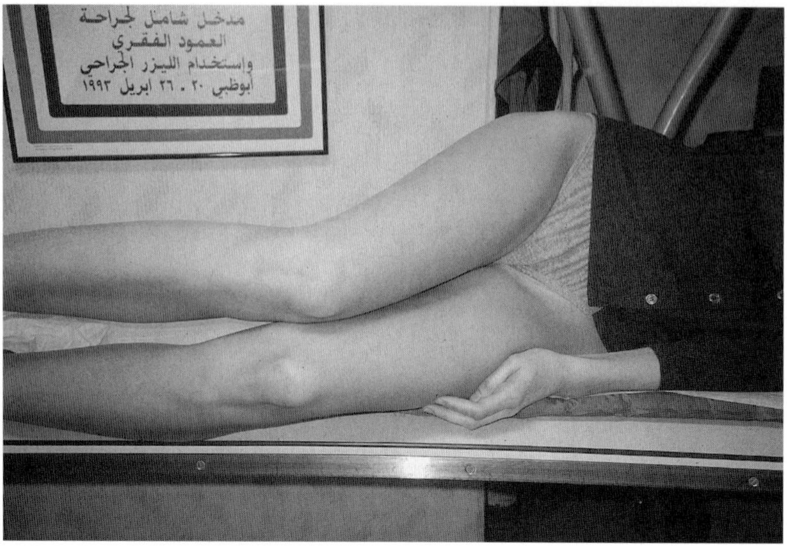

Figure 6.15. The so-called Choy sign: the patient, on being asked to sit up from a supine position, rolls over to the nonaffected side, bends the opposite leg, and pushes himself or herself up with the hands.

Patients with discogenic pain, on being asked to assume the erect position, often roll onto the side away from the protrusion, lift up the affected leg, and push up with both hands. This has been called the *Choy sign* (Fig. 6.15) by the neurologist Dr. Robert April. This is a learned maneuver and is not used by malingerers. Hence it is useful in detecting malingering.

I have not found sensory testing to be of much value in patients with disc disease because there is overlap, and the areas served are not as well delineated in dermatomes as is the case with pain fibers.

Similarly, I have not found electromyography (EMG) testing to be of much value because of the frequency of false negative results.

Differential Diagnosis

Conditions that may mimic disc disease are osteoarthritis of the hip, spinal cord tumors, pelvic pathology, and tumors of the cauda equina. Hip osteoarthritis is characterized by pain usually originating in the trochanteric area and radiating anteriorly only to the knee. Internal and external hip rotation (Figs. 6.16 and 6.17) exacerbate the pain. Tumors of the spinal cord are often accompanied by long tract signs, such as positive Babinski's sign (Fig. 6.18), and subjective symptoms tend to be bilateral. Vibration sense may be impaired. Pelvic pathology is associated with dull pain originating in the lower anterior abdomen that may radiate

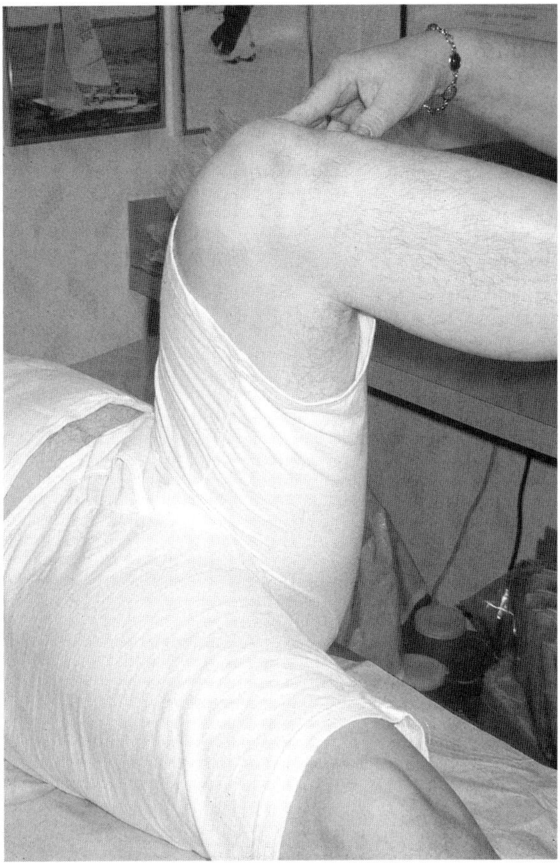

Figure 6.16. Internal rotation of the hip joint.

posteriorly. Previous surgery to the knees may make testing for the patellar reflexes unreliable. Diabetic polyneuropathy can likewise obscure detection of deep tendon reflexes in the lower extremities. Here there may be *stocking–glove* hypesthesia (Fig. 6.19) plus a history of diabetes, usually type I. Type II diabetes, if severe, can also produce neuropathy. Multiple sclerosis should also be kept in mind. Intermittent claudication caused by arterial insufficiency is characterized by pain in the calves on walking, with rapid relief on rest. A simple palpation of the dorsalis pedis or posterior tibial pulse can eliminate this diagnosis. Cauda equina tumors lead to the classical cauda equina syndrome and are outside of the parameters of this text.

With reference to thoracic discs (2% of all intervertebral disc disease), there is only the history of radicular pain affecting the dermatome served by the involved disc. In addition to pain, there may be numbness and tingling. The laser surgeon should depend on the pain diagram and the MRI findings

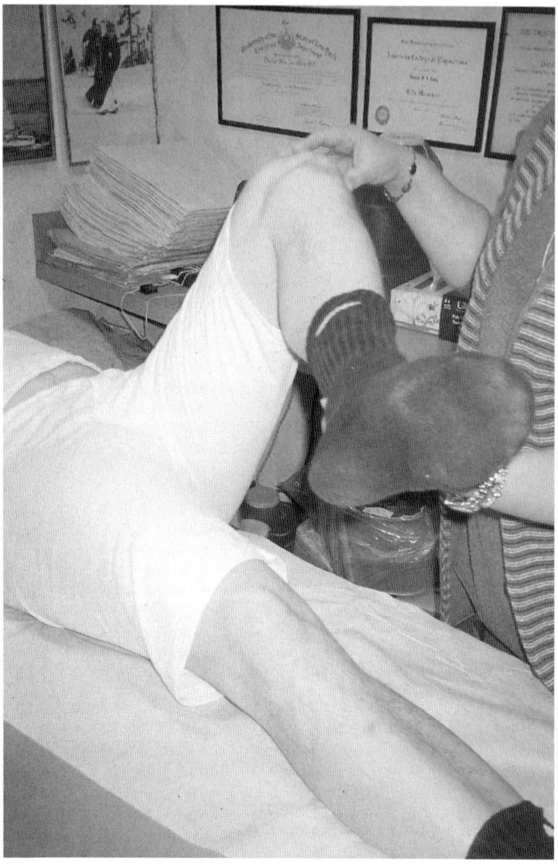

Figure 6.17. External rotation of the hip joint.

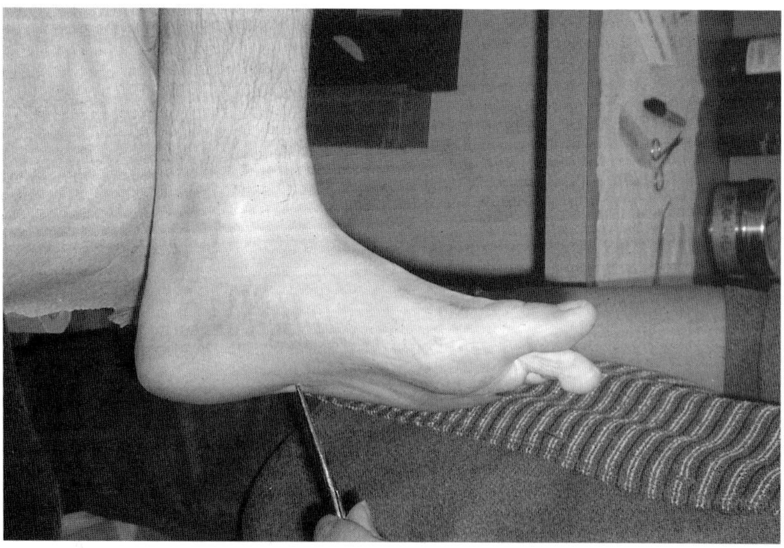

Figure 6.18. A positive Babinski's sign, indicating long-tract involvement.

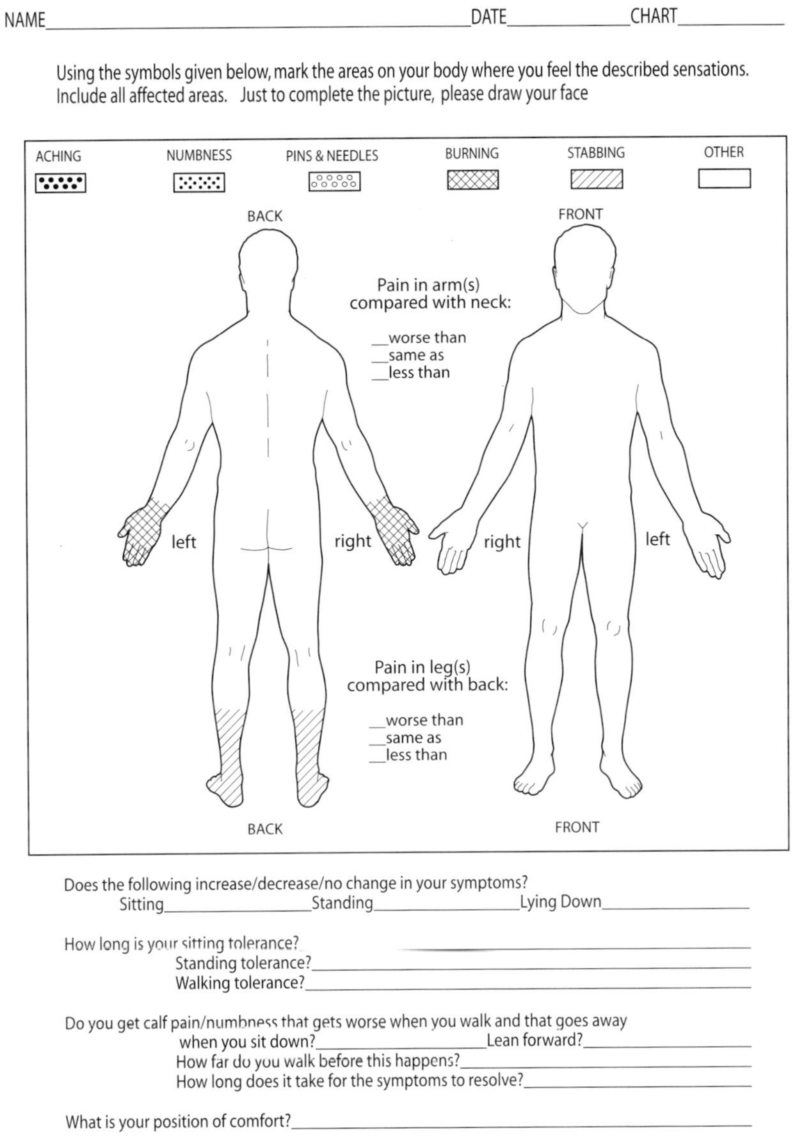

Figure 6.19. Stocking–glove hypesthesia, as indicated on a pain diagram.

The cervical discs, on the other hand, present a wealth of neurologic signs. In addition to the pain diagram, the patient may complain of pain radiating up to the occiput (even when C2 is not involved) and down the upper back to below the scapulae (even with no involvement of C6-7). These are the curiosities of referred pain that have no neuroanatomic basis. The laser surgeon just has to accept the patient's word that such pain exists and not try to ascribe every symptom to a specific anatomic abnormality.

The neurologic examination is divided into (1) muscle weakness and/or atrophy, (2) reflex abnormalities, and (3) limitations

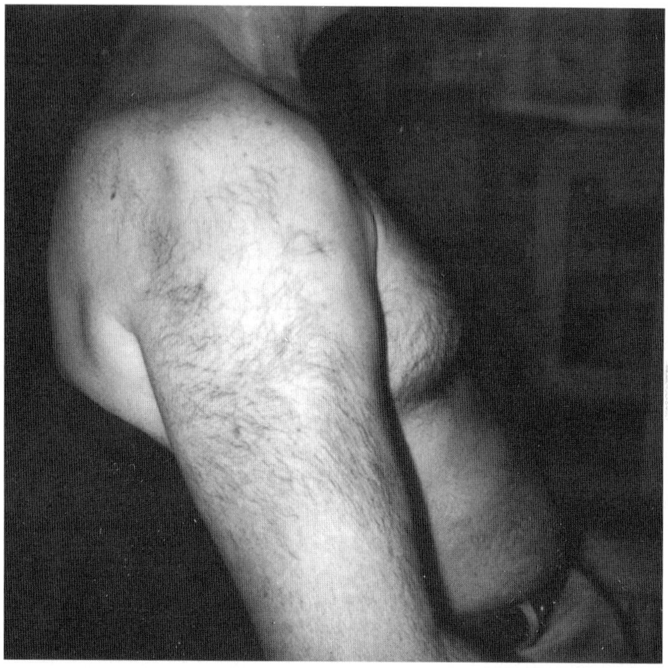

Figure 6.20. Severe supraspinatus muscle atrophy from a C5-6 lesion.

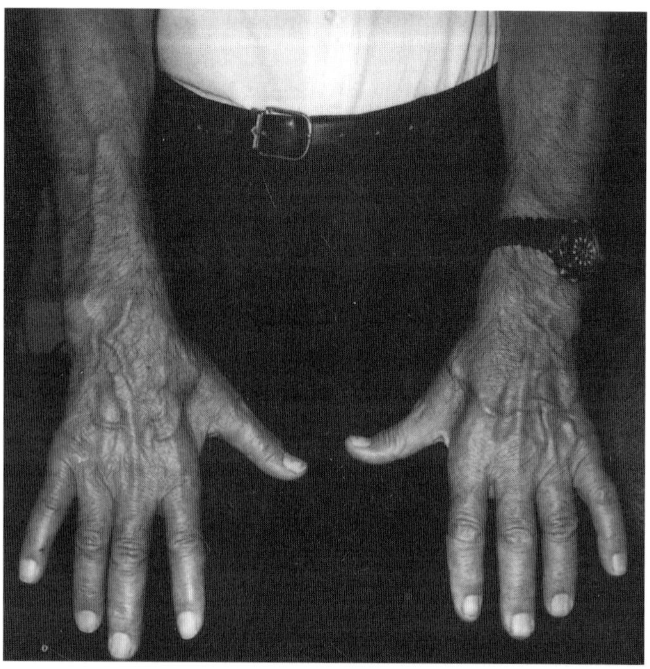

Figure 6.21. Severe atrophy of the interosseous muscles (C6-7).

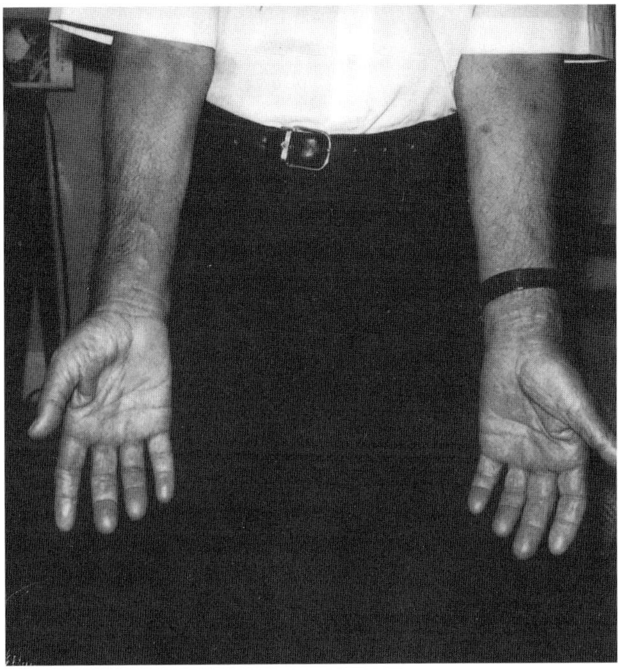

Figure 6.22. Thenar and hypothenar atrophy.

of motion of the head or the upper extremities. If the patient complains of weakness in the hand, and of dropping things, or being unable to perform skilled tasks such as threading a needle, the thumb is usually involved, pointing to a C5-6 lesion. Supraspinatus muscle atrophy (Fig. 6.20) spells C5-6. If there is interosseous muscle atrophy (Fig. 6.21), C6-7 is implicated. Thenar atrophy implies C5-6 (Fig. 6.22), and hypothenar atrophy, C6-7 (Fig. 6.22). Strength of hand grip, resistance of thumb abduction, digital extensors and flexors, and deltoid, biceps, and triceps power should be tested.

Rotation and flexion of the head toward the side of the disc protrusion can aggravate pain, while rotation and flexion to the opposite side generally relieves pain. A very stiff neck results from a body defense mechanism to immobilize the cervical spine to reduce pain. Sometimes direct tenderness can be elicited by pressure on the spinous process of the involved disc.

Absent or diminished biceps reflexes are caused by C5-6 lesions, while absent or diminished triceps reflexes point to C6-7 involvement.

It has been my experience that a good history and a careful neurologic asssessment can usually yield the diagnosis. Elsewhere I have stated that the usual MRI of the lumbar spine is unphysiologic, and that I like to treat the patient, and not the MRI. The patient feels pain; the MRI does not.

7

The Role of Radiology in Percutaneous Laser Disc Decompression

John A. Botsford

Diagnostic radiology is an integral part of percutaneous laser disc decompression (PLDD). To optimize results and avoid complications, all physicians involved in PLDD patient selection and treatment must be familiar with the radiologic concepts unique to this procedure. This chapter defines the role of diagnostic imaging in four areas of PLDD: preoperative patient selection, intraoperative imaging, postoperative evaluation, and the imaging of suspected operative complications. An earlier version of this chapter was published in 1993,[1] and updated and expanded in 1995.[2] This work is based on the cumulative experience gained since 1992 in performing over 350 PLDD procedures at the Deaconess Hospital in Cincinnati, Ohio, using Neodymium:YAG (Nd:YAG) and Holmium:YAG (Ho:YAG) lasers and the potassium triphosphide (KTP) laser systems (Nitek, 1992). The information should provide a better understanding of the radiology specific to PLDD for both the laser physician and the radiologist.

Preoperative Patient Selection

Choice of Imaging Techniques

Inadequate attention has been given to the major part that diagnostic radiology plays in the prospective selection of patients for

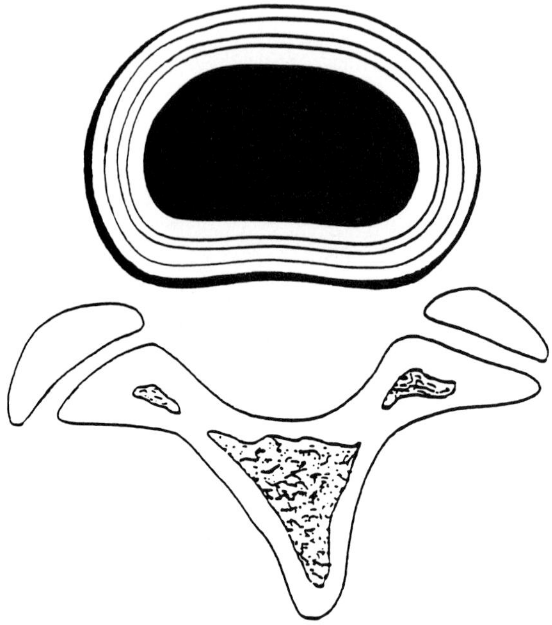

Figure 7.1. Diagrammatic representation of the axial appearance of the normal lumbar disc.

intradiscal therapy. The vocabulary specific to lumbar imaging can be confusing and demands clarification prior to any discussion of diagnostic testing.

"Degenerative disc disease" is a general term used to refer to the broad range of changes that occur with aging in the discovertebral unit (vertebral endplates, annulus fibrosis, and nucleus pulposus). The gelatinous central nucleus is circumferentially enclosed by the basket weave layers of the peripheral annulus. The thinner fibers of the axially oriented annulus merge with the thicker vertically configured posterior longitudinal ligament (PLL) at the level of the disc interspace. The PLL reinforces the annulus posteriorly and is diagrammatically represented by the thicker black line behind the thinner circular rings of the annulus (Fig. 7.1).

A disc *bulge* can best be described as a generalized extension of nuclear material beyond the expected posterior border of the *normal* annulus and sometimes beyond the posterior margin of the vertebral body. It is the result of stretching of the weakened annulus and implies the presence of internal annular tears. As commonly used, the term does not usually distinguish between the inner concentric or transverse tear and the full-thickness ra-

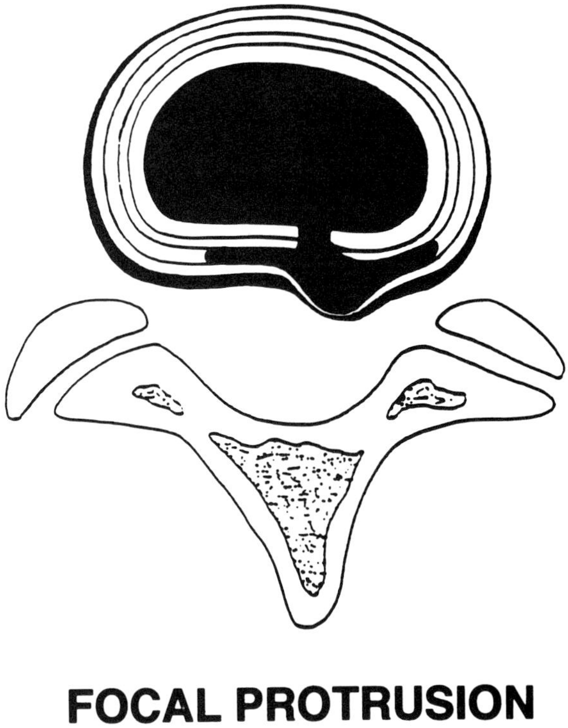

Figure 7.2. Diagrammatic representation of the contained focal disc herniation (protrusion).

dial tear. This may be more than a semantic distinction, since by definition the deeper radial tear extends into the innervated outer layers of the annulus. Therefore, a radial tear may be a cause of significant discogenic pain and its diagnosis an indication for provocative diagnostic discography without or with postdiscographic lumbar computed tomography discography (CT-D). However even with multiple tears and severe bulging, the majority of the annular fibers remain intact, and there is rarely imaging evidence of focal neural element compression.

A disc *herniation* occurs when the tear in the annulus fibrosis extends all the way to the nucleus. This allows the central gelatinous material to squeeze to varying degrees through the defect, constituting a true nuclear herniation. At best, the categorization of the stages of herniation is arbitrary.

A *disc protrusion* or *focal herniation* represents a localized extension of nuclear material into the annulus through the tear (Fig. 7.2). As discussed earlier, because the annular–PLL complex is focally weakened, the herniating disc can locally protrude posteriorly. This deforms the dural sac and may compress lumbar neural elements. Since by definition some portion of the outer annular fibers or the closely applied PLL remains intact, the her-

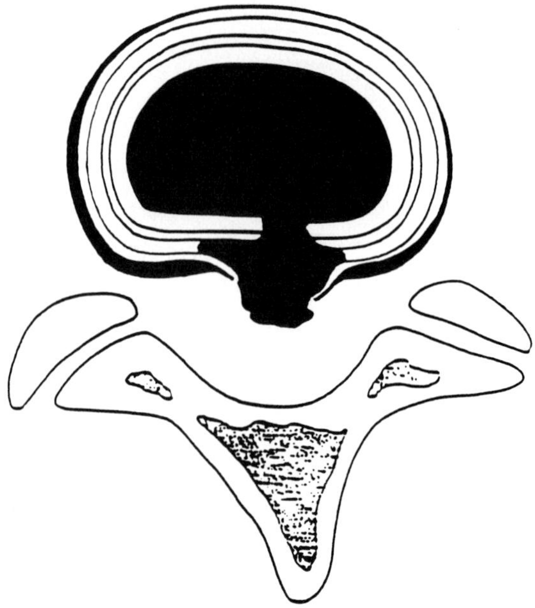

EXTRUSION

Figure 7.3. Diagrammatic representation of the noncontained disc extrusion.

niating nuclear material is said to be *contained*. A *disc extrusion* occurs when focally protruding nuclear material completely traverses the annular–PLL complex (Fig. 7.3). The herniated nuclear component is now in direct contact with the epidural space but remains connected to the parent disc of origin by a pedicle. Because all layers of restraining ligaments are ruptured, this transligamentous extrusion represents a *noncontained* herniation.

A *sequestered* or *free-fragment* herniation is also the result of a full-thickness tear and is therefore also noncontained. However, in this case the herniating fragment is no longer connected to the parent disc of origin (Fig. 7.4). Most of these dissociated disc fragments fully traverse both the annulus and the posterior longitudinal ligament and come to rest in the epidural fat, often adjacent to the vertebral pedicle. Sometimes they pass longitudinally through a complete tear in a severely bulging annulus and lie subligamentous in the potential space behind the vertebral body anterior to the displaced PLL. Movement of a sequestered or free fragment away from the interspace is termed *migration* and occurs with equal frequency in superior and inferior directions.

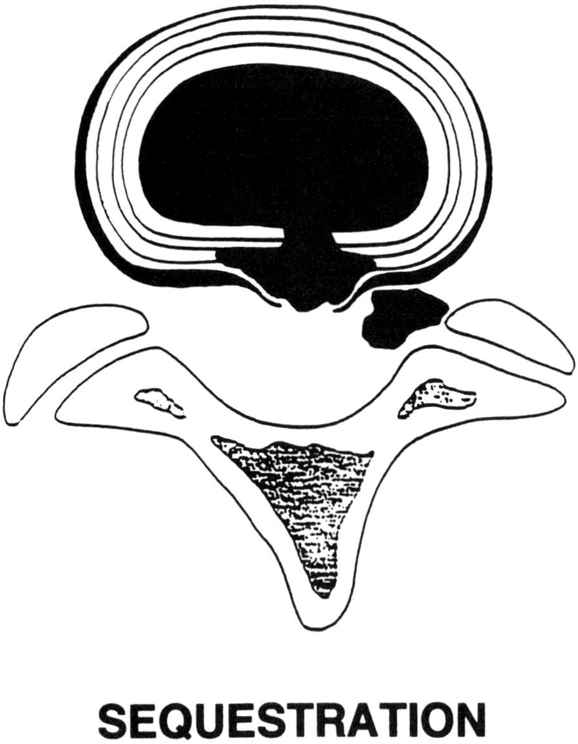

Figure 7.4. Diagrammatic representation of the noncontained disc sequestration.

An additional directional modifier is often added when one is describing the herniated nucleus pulposis (HNP). A *central* HNP refers to a direct midline dural sac compression that could conceivably cause bilateral symptoms. A paracentral or paramedian HNP describes an eccentric, off-midline disc herniation usually causing only unilateral symptoms. A posterolateral HNP occurs along the posterolateral or foraminal aspect of the vertebral body, compromising the exiting root as it enters the bony neural foramen. If sufficiently lateral, this herniation can be extraforaminal and the compression can directly affect the dorsal root ganglion. Finally, an anterior herniation occurs along the true anterior aspect of the vertebral body. Although it does not cause lumbar dural sac compression, it may still be a cause of low back pain, again best proven by provocative discography.

As discussed earlier, the lumbar discovertebral unit has been likened to a closed hydraulic space subject to the same pressure–volume relationship.[3–5] Other investigators have shown that a small reduction in central intradiscal volume by mechanical removal, chemical dissolution, or laser ablation results in a marked reduction in pressure within the enclosed space.[6–8] This pressure reduction will be transmitted to the posteriorly projecting disc material, provided the herniation remains connected to the parent disc of origin and the annular–PLL complex is intact. Theoretically the best candidate for PLDD has a freely communicating and contained lumbar disc herniation that is symptomatic, with familiar pain during a pressure challenge to the central disc. Connected but noncontained herniations that have ruptured through the annular–PLL complex (complete extrusions) as well as herniations that have broken free into the epidural space (sequestrations) violate the closed-space principle outlined earlier and are not suitable for PLDD.

In addition, any surgical therapy directed at the abnormal nucleus, including PLDD, may produce suboptimal results unless there is pretreatment confirmation that altered intradiscal pressure is related to the patient's pain. Failure to recognize the importance of both these factors in evaluating PLDD candidates will lower the treatment success rate entirely for reasons of poor patient selection. The radiographic study that most reliably provides both these pieces of information will be the best at predicting a successful outcome when the diagnostic test is abnormal.[9] Therefore, preoperative lumbar imaging studies in PLDD candidates must do more than merely diagnose a generic herniated disc. Diagnostic testing must be able to consistently characterize the herniation as contained (protruded or focally herniated) or noncontained (extruded or sequestered). Ideally, it should also confirm that the imaging abnormality is the cause of the presenting clinical pain complaint. Incorrect preoperative classification of a herniation as contained and/or symptomatic will lead to inappropriate application of the technique and a less than optimal success rate. Furthermore, diagnostic testing should reliably exclude patients with significant secondary conditions such as acquired bony spinal stenosis and vertebral compression fracture.

Multiple imaging modalities have been used alone or in combination to evaluate the lumbar spine in the symptomatic patient (Table 7.1). All these tests differ with respect to sensitivity and specificity in diagnosing the contained HNP and therefore are not equally useful in prospective selection patients for intradiscal therapy.[9,10] Routine lumbar x-ray radiographs cannot diagnose an HNP but are necessary to identify the correct level prior to PLDD, particularly if a transitional vertebral body is suggested on prior cross-sectional imaging [computed tomography (CT) or magnetic resonance imaging (MRI)]. At least once a week I review a lumbar imaging examination in which incorrect level nomenclature would have been assigned if conventional lumbar spine films had not been obtained. Lumbar radiographs can re-

Table 7.1 Lumber Imaging Modalities

Routine radiography
Myelography
Unenhanced computed tomography (CT)
Intravenous contrast-enhanced CT
Computed tomography (CT) myelography
Unenhanced magnetic resonance imaging
Intravenous contrast-enhanced magnetic resonance imaging
Discography
Computed tomography discography (CT-D)

liably show multilevel disease, facet arthropathy, or severe bony spinal stenosis, all of which are relative contraindications to PLDD. Finally, plain films can demonstrate intradiscal vacuum phenomena. Gas within the central disc can occur only with advanced disc dehydration and desiccation. It implies the presence of a relatively low or negative pressure state within the nucleus. Since PLDD's success depends on its ability to reduce nerve pressure from a hydrated, soft nuclear protrusion, the mere presence of an intradiscal vacuum phenomenon becomes a strict contraindication to PLDD.

Water-soluble myelography consistently but indirectly demonstrates dural sac/root sleeve compression and displacement, implying the presence of an underlying HNP. It rarely detects far paracentral and lateral disc herniations and cannot answer the critical question of containment even when combined with postmyelographic CT.[9] Furthermore, myelography is by definition an invasive procedure and continues to be relatively expensive. It is inadequate as the only diagnostic examination for the preoperative evaluation of the prospective PLDD patient. However, lumbar myelography performed with lateral flexion and extension plain films continues to have a role in evaluating stability and canal stenosis in patients with spondylolysis and spondylolisthesis (Fig. 7.5).

Unenhanced high-resolution computed tomography (HRCT or CT) directly diagnoses the lumbar HNP with a high degree of accuracy.[11] It is particularly useful in the assessment of secondary conditions such as spondylolysis, facet hypertrophy, and bony acquired spinal stenosis.[12] It remains an accurate and cost-efficient imaging modality in the initial evaluation of the patient with a suspected lumbar radiculopathy.[13] But even the best scanners cannot consistently distinguish the central nuclear material from the annular–PLL complex and therefore cannot reliably dif-

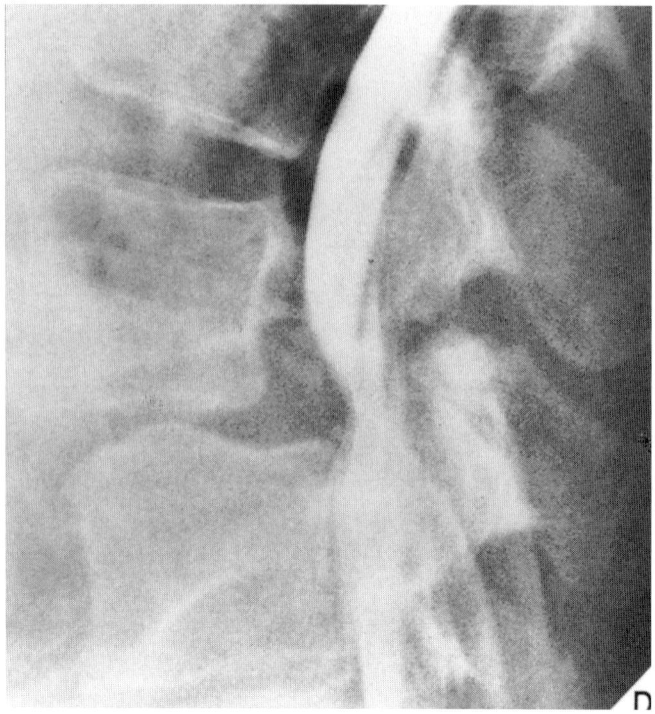

Figure 7.5. Lateral spot film from lumbar myelogram demonstrating spondolytic instability and dural sac compression.

ferentiate the contained subligamentous herniation (focal protrusion) from the transligamentous extrusion even with intravenous (IV) contrast enhancement (Fig. 7.6).[10,14]

Multiplanar unenhanced MRI is currently the most specific cross-sectional imaging modality performed in patients suspected of having an HNP.[15,16] Imaging of longitudinal (T1), transverse (T2), and effective transverse relaxation time equivalents (T2*) in the sagittal and axial planes can potentially separate the protruding intermediate (gray) and/or high (white) signal HNP from the bordering low-signal (black) annular/PLL complex.[17,18] A continuous hypointense ligament signal on all images in both planes suggests containment (Fig. 7.7). Focal interruption of this black line consistently implies extrusion and raises the question of sequestration (Fig. 7.8). Sagittal T2/T2* sequences primarily show continuity between the herniating, posteriorly projecting nuclear material and the central parent disc of origin. A well-defined separation of this disc signal indicates sequestration and the addition of T1 coronal imaging may confirm subtle free-fragment migration (Fig. 7.9). However, even high-quality noncontrast lumbar MRI will incorrectly categorize transligamentous ruptures as subligamentous herniations in more than one third

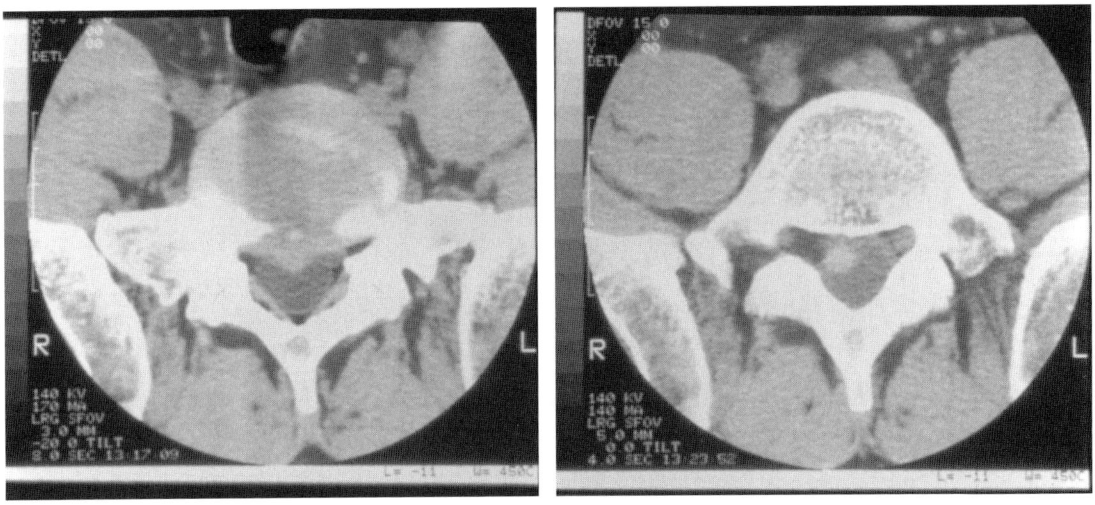

Figure 7.6. Sequential computed tomography (CT) images at L5-SI. The image on the left suggests a contained herniation. The image on the right suggests a noncontained free fragment.

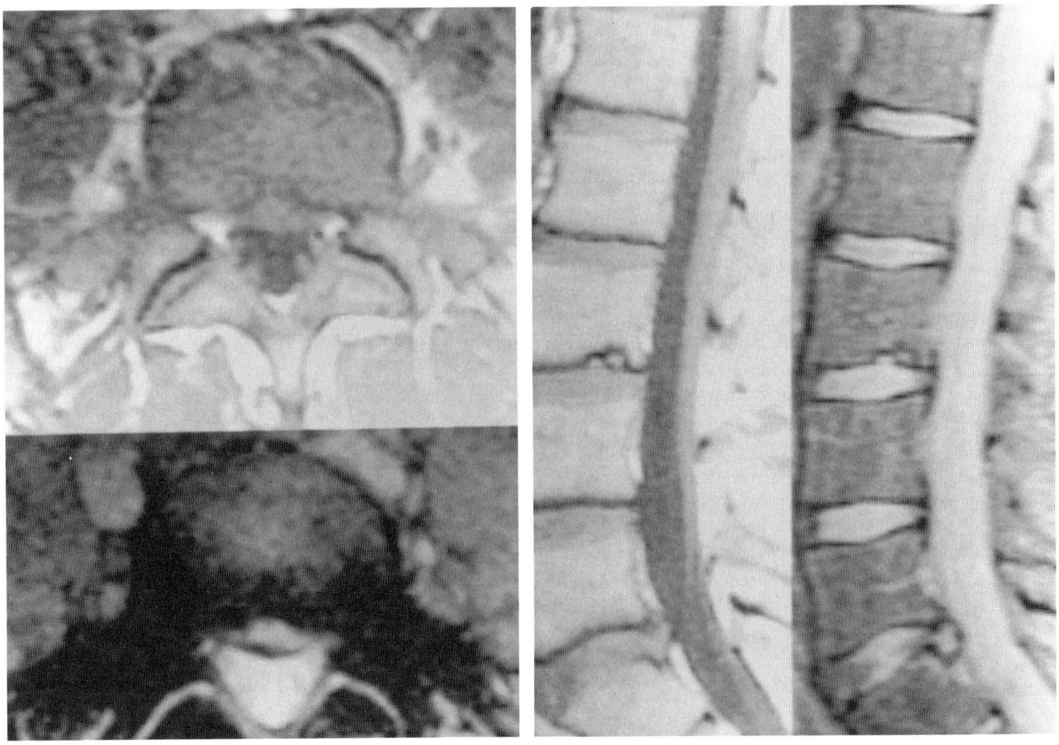

Figure 7.7. Sequential axial and sagittal magnetic resonance (MR) images of a contained L5-S1 herniation (focal protrusion). Note thin intact black line of the annular–posterior longitudinal ligament (PLL) complex best seen on the T2 sequences on the right.

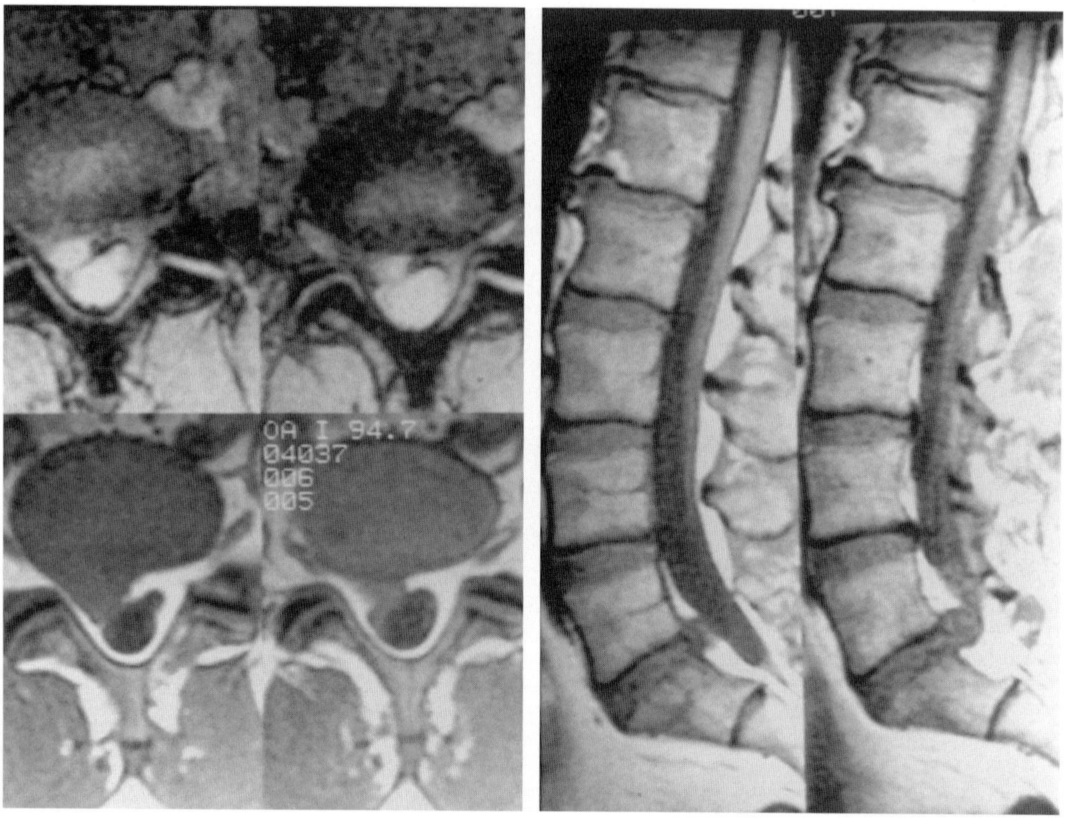

Figure 7.8. Sequential axial and sagittal magnetic resonance (MR) images of an extruded L5-S1 herniated nucleus pulposis (HNP). Note well-defined interruption of the black annular–posterior longitudinal ligament complex in both images on the right.

of patients imaged.[10,19,20] This imaging mistake classifies a noncontained herniation, best treated by open surgery, as contained and therefore suitable for PLDD. This *downstaging* error will doom a significant number of PLDD candidates identified by MRI findings alone to treatment failure based entirely on inaccurate preoperative patient selection. An MR image enhanced by intravenous gadolinium–diethylenetriamine pentaacetic acid (IV Gd-DTPA) may be useful to answer the critical question of containment prior to PLDD.[20] Contrast administration is also recommended for confirming suspected free-fragment sequestration and mandatory for evaluation of postoperative patients and infectious disciitis.[21–24] However, both sequestration and previous open surgery may be relative contraindications to PLDD at this time and the addition of IV enhancement in routine lumbar MRI may be unnecessary unless noncontrast images are abnormal and suggest a contained HNP.

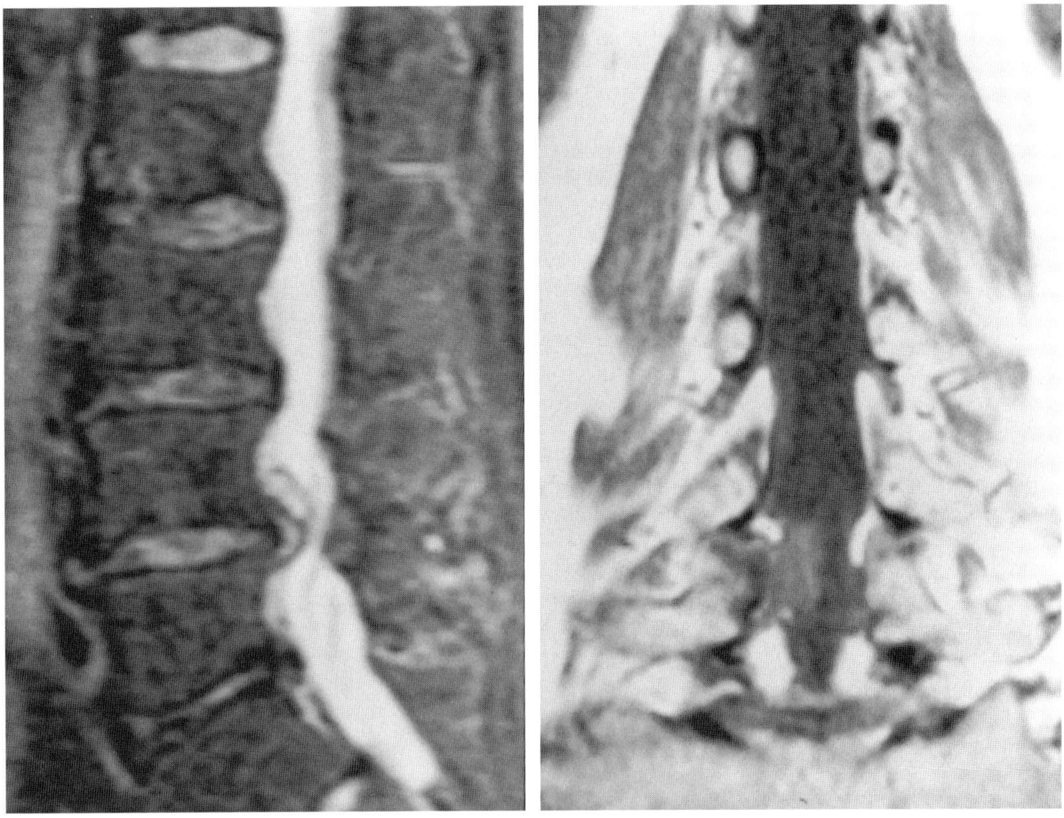

Figure 7.9. Sagittal and coronal magnetic resonance (MR) images of sequestered (free-fragment) disc herniation. Note white migrated fragment behind L4 body on the sagittal T2 image and adjacent to the right vertebral pedicle on the coronal T1 image.

But not all patients with abnormal lumbar disc morphology on MRI are symptomatic, and the mere presence of a contained HNP does not prove causality.[25,26] Any surgical therapy directed at the abnormal nucleus, including PLDD, will meet with suboptimal results unless there is preoperative confirmation of a discal origin of the patient's pain. Thin-needle nonionic water-soluble discography followed by thin-section CT of the injected disc (CT-D) is the most specific test prior to intradiscal therapy (Fig. 7.10).[27,28] It correctly predicts the type of disc herniation as contained or noncontained (extruded or sequestered) in the highest percentage of cases found in any radiologic study.[19,29] It is the only diagnostic examination that combines anatomic information with a physiologic pain provocation challenge to the lumbar disc[30,31] and should be considered positive only when there are both anatomic abnormality and familiar pain reproduction during injection.[32] Lumbar CT-D is more sensitive than CT or MRI

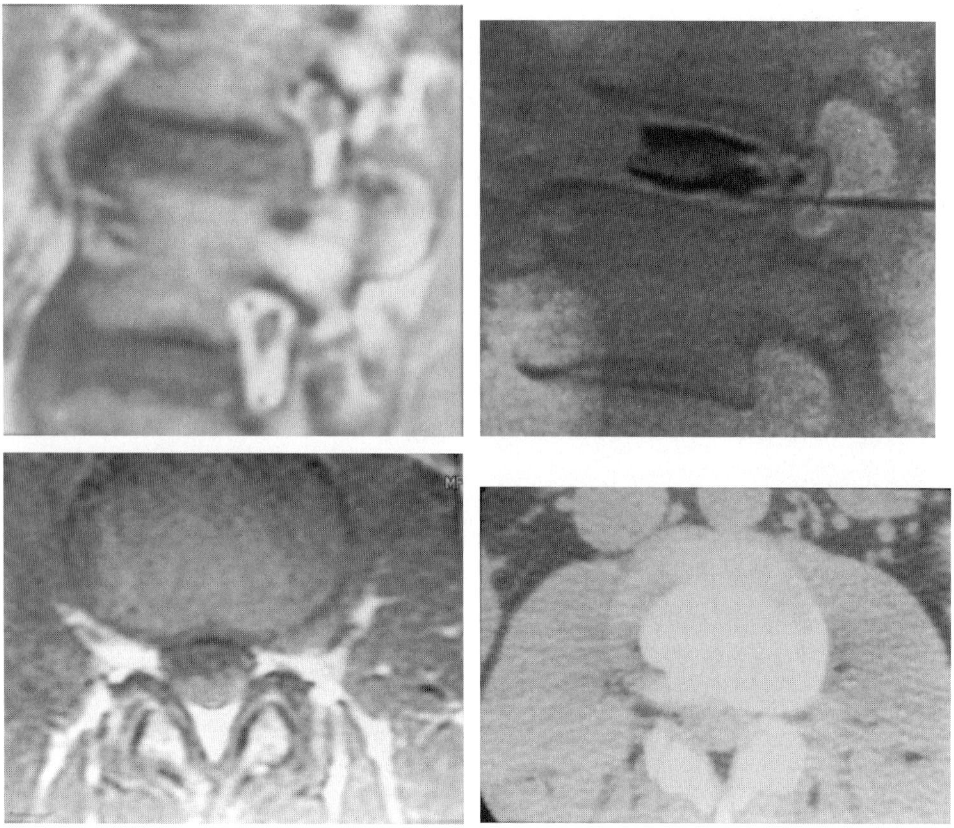

Figure 7.10. Multimodality images demonstrating a left posterolateral contained herniation. (A) Sagittal magnetic resonance (MR) image showing suspected contained herniation encroaching on neural foramen. (B) Lateral spot film from discogram showing contrast-filled disc fragment. (C) Axial MR image showing herniation compressing left root. (D) Axial computed tomography (CT) discogram showing contrast-filled herniation compressing root.

in the early stages of disc degeneration and annular disruption, both of which can cause discogenic back pain without radiculopathy.[33,34] This mode of discography may also be useful to identify the culprit disc in patients who would otherwise be candidates for PLDD because MRI has indicated multilevel involvement (Fig. 7.11).

Others have questioned the safety of discography, suggesting infection and premature disc degeneration as complications of the procedure. Careful attention to detail and a coaxial needle technique reduce the risk of induced bacterial disciitis to acceptable levels. A recent large CT-D study reported only one postprocedure infection in 725 levels examined (>0.15%).[29] There is no evidence to support iatrogenic disc damage from contrast injection in either human or animal studies.[35–37]

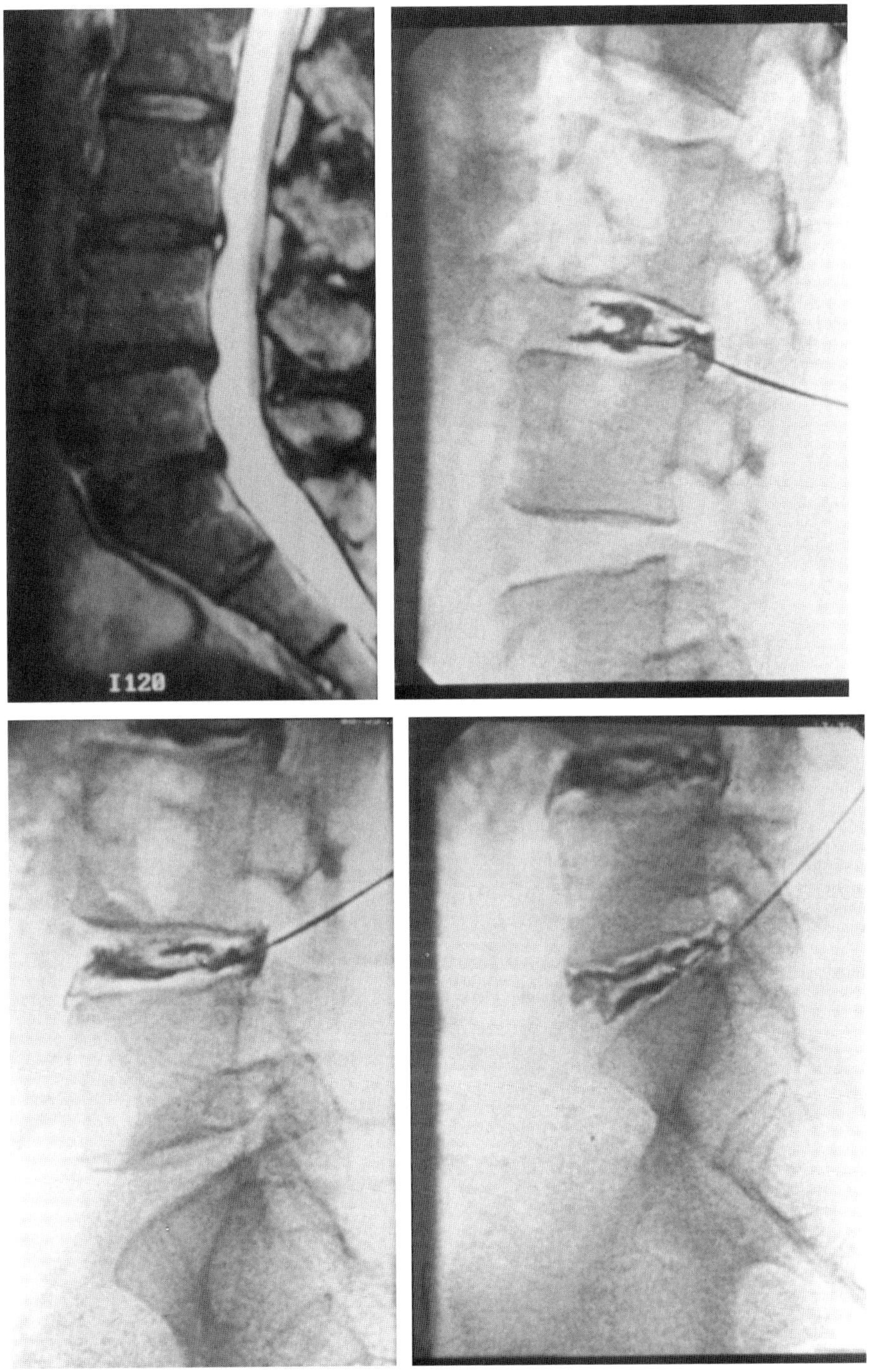

Figure 7.11. Multimodality images in multilevel lumbar disc disease with bilateral symptoms. (A) Sagittal magnetic resonance (MR) image demonstrating shallow three-level disc herniation. (B) Lateral spot film from L3-4 discogram showing contained herniation causing left leg symptoms. Symptoms improved following PLDD. (C) Lateral spot film from L4-5 discogram showing contained herniation causing right leg symptoms. Symptoms improved following percutaneous laser disc decompression (PLDD). (D) Lateral spot film from L5-S1 discogram showing internal disc degeneration and producing no symptoms. PLDD not performed.

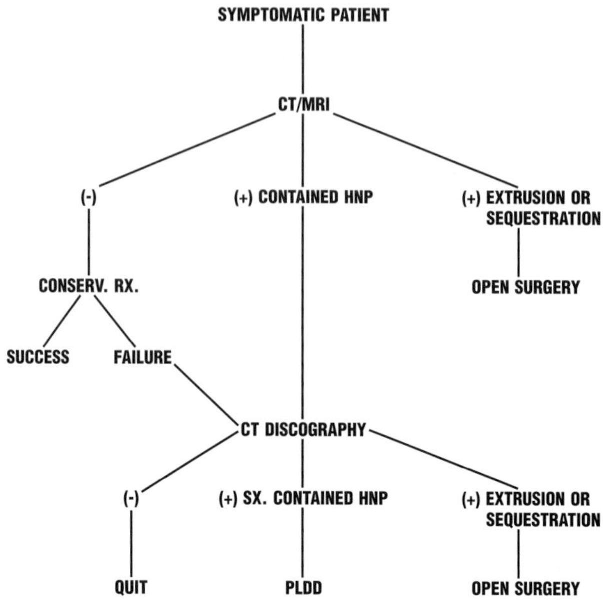

Figure 7.12. Percutaneous laser disc decompression (PLDD) diagnostic evaluation algorithm indicating path to PLDD for a patient with symptoms of contained herniated nucleus pulposis (HNP).

Despite its proven value in the PLDD candidate,[9,28] CT-D should *not* be used as the primary method of diagnosing a lumbar HNP. Studies indicate that CT and MRI are unquestionably superior in the initial evaluation of a suspected lumbar radiculopathy.[13,38] Instead CT-D should be performed only to confirm containment and causality where a cross-sectional imaging study has suggested that disc herniation and PLDD might be appropriate. The symptomatic patient who has both a contained HNP on preoperative cross-sectional imaging and a positive CT discogram will have a much higher chance of a successful PLDD outcome than one who has only abnormal results from a CT or MRI exam.[9] These principles have been integrated into an imaging strategy and a diagnostic algorithm developed for the evaluation of the PLDD candidate (Fig. 7.12).

Operative Technique

Others have discussed the basic surgical principles of the percutaneous approach to the lumbar intervertebral disc.[39,40] However, these discussions have not emphasized the crucial role of fluoroscopy in guiding intradiscal therapy. No matter how much care has been devoted to patient selection, PLDD can be successful only if the laser is correctly positioned within the central nuclear material of the abnormal disc. Clearly, a better understanding of the radiology specific to PLDD is needed by both the laser physician and the radiologist.

The radiological considerations in the operative imaging of PLDD can be arbitrarily separated into four areas for discussion: (1) imaging equipment selection, (2) puncture site identification, (3) disc entry monitoring, and (4) permanent image recording.

Imaging Equipment Selection

A high-quality, multiplanar, fixed-unit, power-assisted fluoroscopic device with at least a 9-inch image intensifier and with permanent image recording capability is the optimal system for PLDD. A cardiac catheterization lab or special radiologic procedures room is ideal and usually has an air filtration system similar to that of a traditional operating room. The portable unassisted C-arm found in most surgical suites usually provides images of lesser quality and has a limited ability to move into the complex planes needed for monitoring disc entry. However, a mobile C-arm is still preferable to a fixed unit that has its rotational capability restricted to one plane. In addition, the participation of an experienced special procedures technologist or interventional radiologist may be invaluable in guiding disc entry and/or confirming a central intradiscal location prior to lasing the nucleus.

Puncture Site Identification

Percutaneous laser disc decompression (PLDD) may be performed in the lateral decubitus or prone position. The prone position is personally preferred because it restricts the ability of a patient to move in response to any pain that may be experienced during needle entry. In addition, the relationship between the fluoroscopic image and the actual needle position is often better understood when the patient is prone, making positional adjustment of the needle easier. Once the patient has been positioned, a wide area should be prepped and both the patient and the radiographic unit draped with sterile covers. Although the habit is hard to break, the physical identification and marking of anatomic landmarks is unnecessary when adequate fluoroscopic monitoring is available.

Since the entire needle placement will radiologically guided, the x-ray tube–image intensifier (T-II) combination can and should be used to identify the correct skin puncture site. Initially the T-II should be angulated (skewed) cephalad from the direct posterior–anterior (PA) plane so that the front and back cortical margins of the vertebral bodies above and below the target disc level are perfectly superimposed. This maneuver is designed to

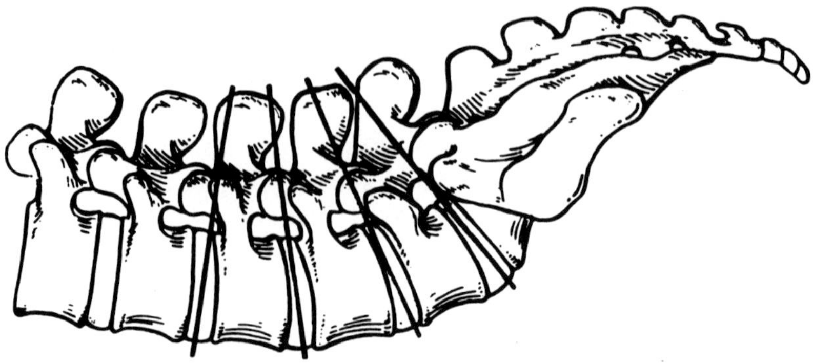

Figure 7.13. Solid lines indicate degree of angulation needed in A-PA plane to image parallel to disc interspace when patient is in the prone position.

eliminate radiographic parallax and establish a new angulated PA (A-PA) imaging plane directly parallel to the interspace to be punctured. The L5-S1 level will require significantly more T-II angulation than either L3-4 or L4-5 (Fig. 7.13). Once this A-PA plane parallel to the disc has been established, a line may be drawn across the back of the patient toward the operator and perpendicular to the long axis of the spine originating from the fluoroscopic image center of the target disc.

Maintaining the already established A-PA cephalad angulation or skewed position, the T-II is then rotated 40 to 45 degrees laterally (along the line) toward the operator into the oblique–angulated posterior–anterior (OA-PA) plane to establish the final puncture site. Once parallax has again been corrected by minor T-II adjustment, this site will ideally project just anterior to the facet joint at the selected interspace. It will be adjacent to the junction of the ear and nose of the so-called Scottie dog formed by the projected image of the posterior elements (Fig. 7.14). Often the best L5-S1 entry point will appear to be over the iliac crest in the PA plane, but will still be free of intervening bone when appropriately imaged in the OA-PA plane. It is often at or higher than the L4-5 entry point, particularly in obese patients. With careful attention to skew and rotation, virtually all L5-S1 interspaces can be entered without resorting to curved or directable needles that may not enter the interspace parallel to the long axis of the disc.

A paramedian angulated PA extrathecal approach can also be employed to gain access to the L5-S1 disc by using an off-midline puncture site. This technique, which has been described by Choy, takes advantage of the normal tapering of the dural sac

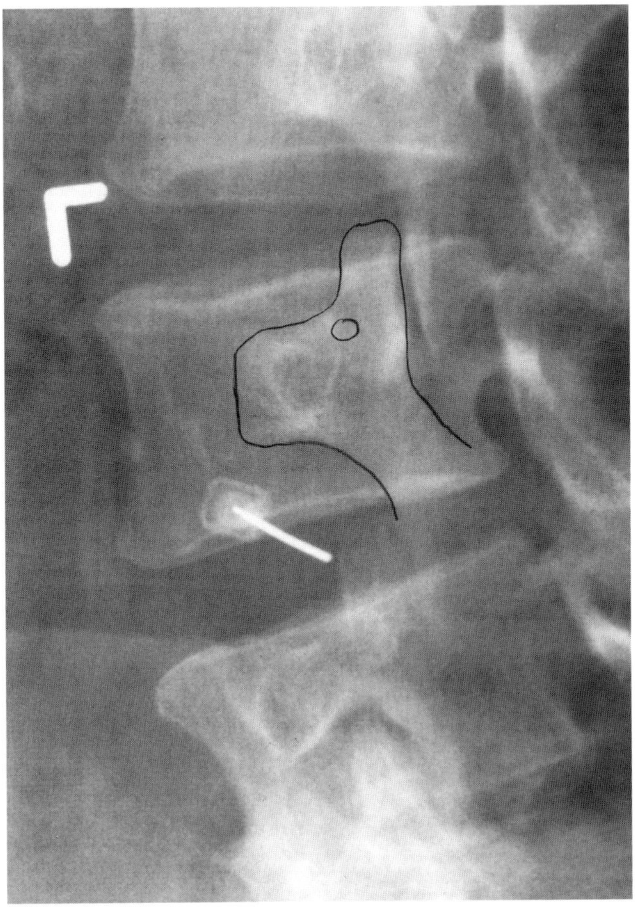

Figure 7.14. The 45-degree oblique–angulated posterior-anterior (OA-PA) view shows the needle just anterior to the L4-5 facet joint. Note line drawing of projected "Scottie Dog" image over the L3-4 elements.

at the lumbosacral junction.[41] Ideally, a needle advanced anterocentrally toward the L5-SI interspace, beginning posteriorly but several centimeters off the midline will miss the narrowing dural sac, passing only through the epidural fat avoiding the cerebrospinal fluid (CSF) (Fig. 7.15).

Local anesthesia is then infiltrated at the selected puncture site and the needle left beneath the skin to serve as a radiopaque marker. The punctured site is then reimaged in the A-PA and OA-PA projections, correcting the skew for parallax with each rotation to confirm that the best site has been selected. Continued T-II rotation to the full lateral position may be useful to confirm the needle angulation needed from the marked puncture site to the selected disc in a plane directly parallel to the adjacent vertebral endplates.

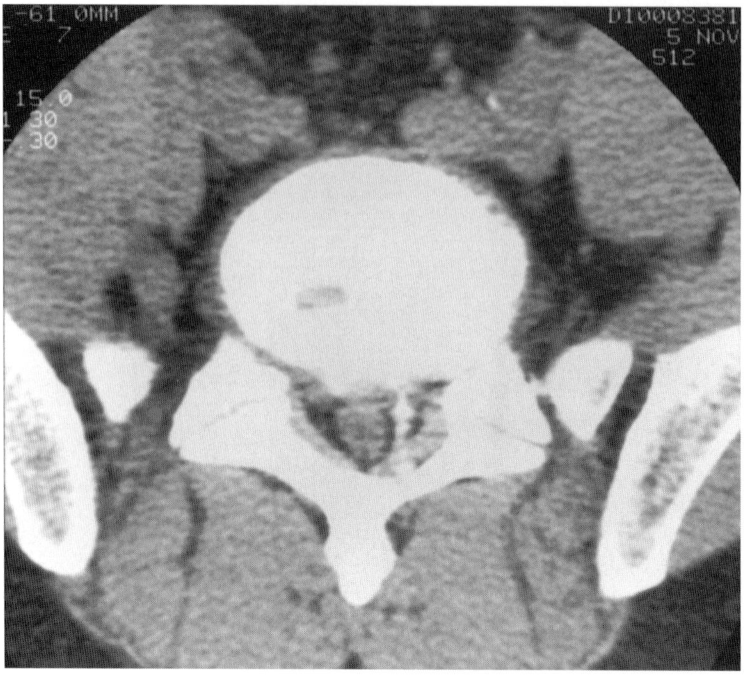

Figure 7.15. Axial computed tomography (CT) scan following extrathecal discography showing contrast material that has leaked into the epidural fat along the extradural puncture tract.

Disc Entry Monitoring

Once the optimal puncture site has been selected and local anesthesia infiltrated, the T-II should be realigned in the 45 degree OA-PA plane parallel to the interspace. When properly aligned, the T-II is now right along the ideal puncture line, ready to enter the interspace parallel to the endplates. Simple visual observation of the T-II alignment provides a rough guide for the beginning approach angle needed to enter the selected disc. This projection looks down the length of the puncture needle, resulting in its marked foreshortening on the fluoroscopic image (Fig. 7.16). When the needle is properly imaged in this view, the hub of the needle will superimpose on the tip and project over the disc interspace nearly free of surrounding bone. The resultant image of the needle on end constitutes what this author and others call the *gun barrel view*. Intermittent fluoroscopy in this OA-PA plane provides adequate monitoring as the skin is punctured and the disc space is initially approached. However, never advance the needle more than half-way to the expected depth of the disc without rechecking the needle position in two if not three orthogonal planes. Remember, parallax MUST be corrected each

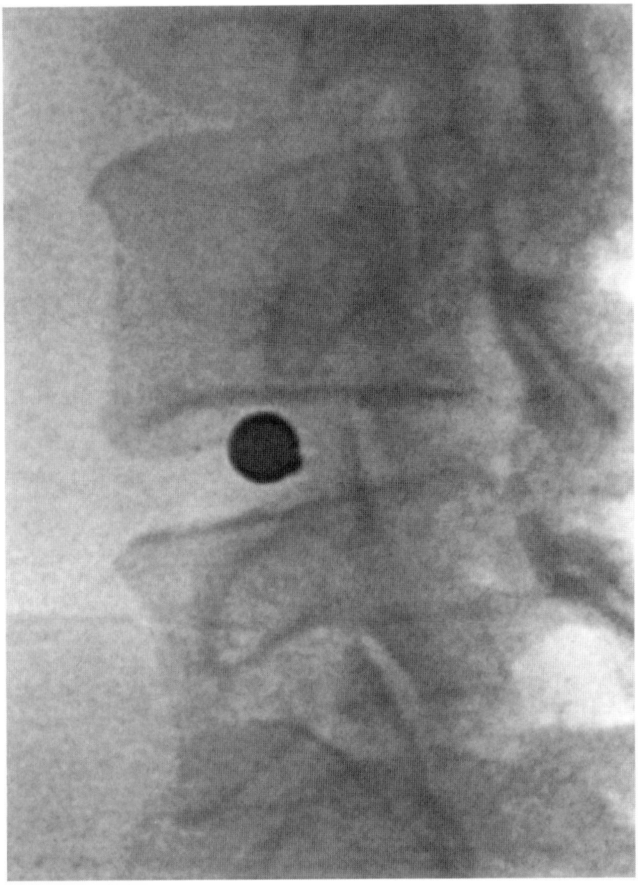

Figure 7.16. This 45-degree oblique–angulated posterior–anterior (OA-PA) view shows the relationship of the superimposed hub and tip of the needle in this "gun barrel" view and its projection over the disc interspace.

time the T-II is moved into a new position to maintain an optimal image.

It is critical to remember that the configuration of the lumbar vertebral body and disc in cross section is ovoid (NOT round). This means that the anatomic center of the disc will not be in the center of the fluoroscopic image in the oblique gun barrel projection (Fig. 7.17). Therefore, in this OA-PA view the needle should be aimed just behind the junction of the anterior third with the posterior two thirds of the disc space, not at the dead center. As indicated earlier, this point will be just anterior to the facet joint by the *ear of the dog* (Fig. 7.14). At all times the needle tip should be seen completely free of overlying bone, equidistant from endplates above and below the disc. Constant correction of tube angulation for parallax may necessary during this stage to

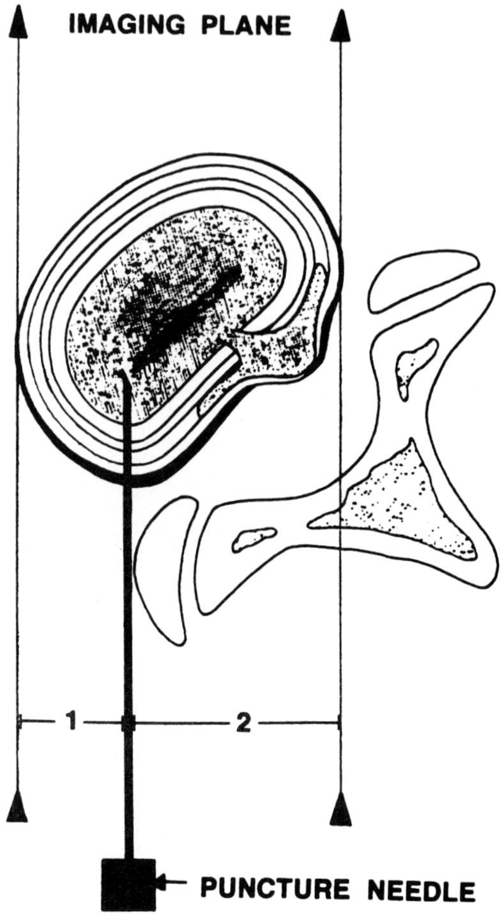

Figure 7.17. Diagrammatic representation of the relationship of the puncture needle to the projected anterior and posterior image of the vertebral body.

achieve this result and to assure an appropriate angle of approach parallel to the interspace. Once the solid feel of the annulus has been encountered, the T-II is rotated back through the A-PA plane into the opposite OA-PA projection to confirm its position just adjacent to the disc. Being roughly 90 degrees opposed to the initial entry plane and thus eliminating needle foreshortening, this projection accurately depicts the relationship of the needle to the border of the disc.

Then, with constant fluoroscopic monitoring in the opposite OA-PA plane, the annulus should be penetrated and the disc entered. The needle should be advanced no more than one third the width of the interspace in this projection until a satisfactory position is again confirmed by imaging in at least one additional orthogonal plane. Fluoroscopic monitoring of this entire process is critical no matter which laser system is to be used for the decompression procedure. Never fully insert the needle into the expected center of the disc without confirming the position in more than one plane. A puncture that is too horizontal can enter the dural sac, while an overly vertical insertion risks entry into paraspinal vasculature.

If a paramedian approach to L5-SI is being employed, then fluoroscopic monitoring can usually be limited to the A-PA and true lateral projections. However constant minor adjustments of T-II position with skewing will still be necessary to maintain an imaging plane parallel to the selected interspace. It should be cautioned that when this approach is used, the lamina of L5 often interferes with the ideal puncture plane. This forces the puncture site inferiorly on the patient and not infrequently results in a disc puncture that is angulated too cephalad (Fig. 7.18). Do *not* accept a nonparallel puncture even if there seems to be no other way to

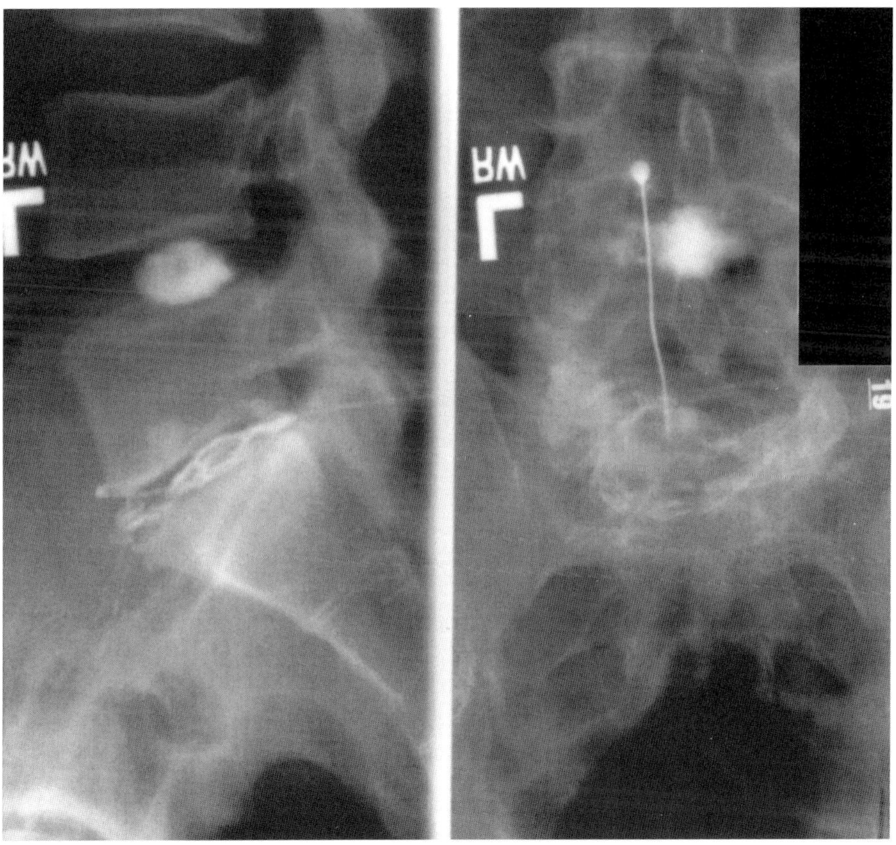

Figure 7.18. Lateral and frontal spot films from paramidline, extrathecal L5-S1 discogram showing puncture needle directed cephalad by low left lamina of L5. The position is acceptable for discography but NOT for percutaneous laser disc decompression (PLDD).

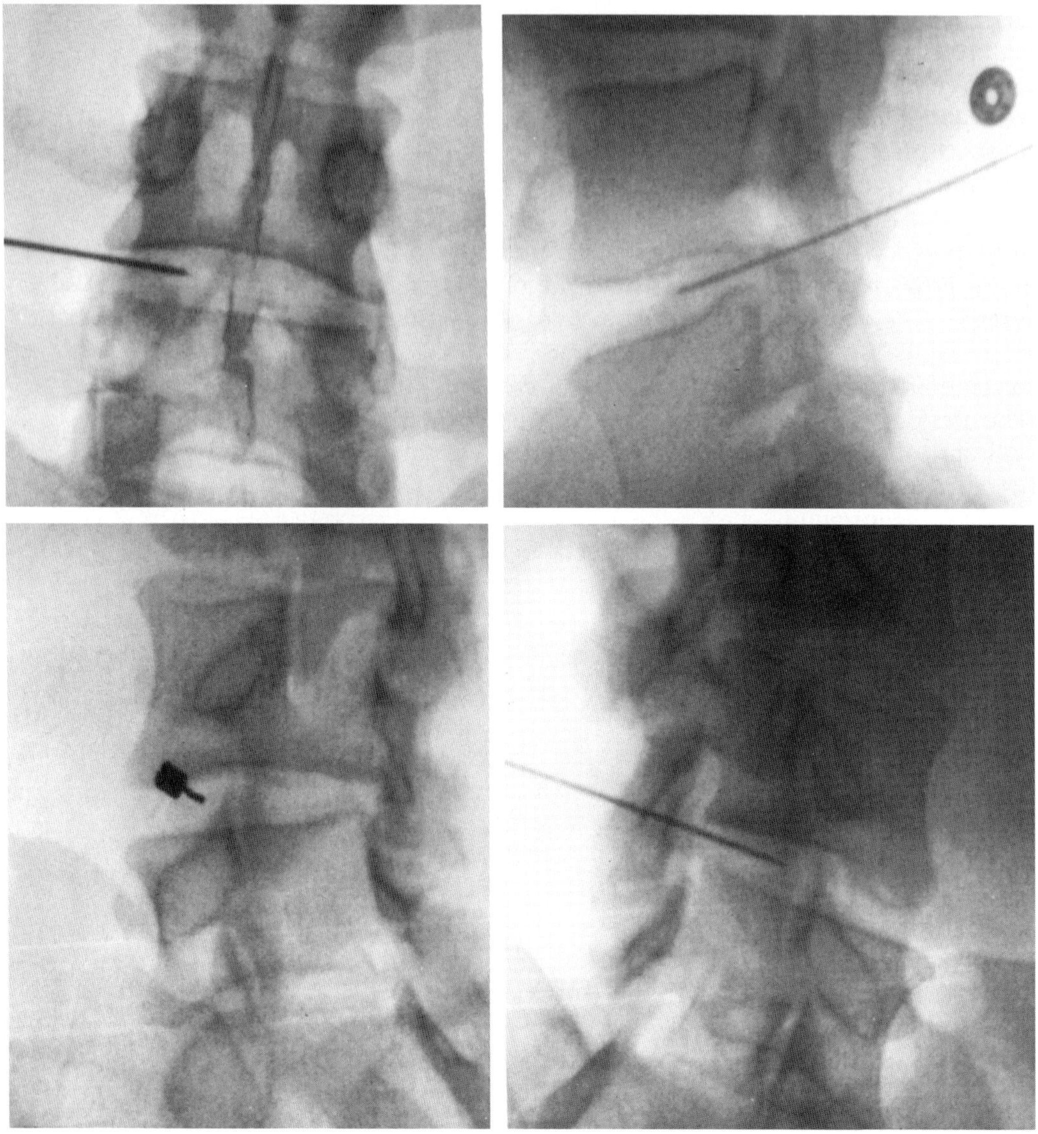

Figure 7.19. Images of appropriate needle position in posterior-anterior (PA), lateral, and both 45-degree oblique–angulated posterior–anterior (OA-PA).

enter the interspace. Most all significant complications of PLDD are related to lasing when the needle is not positioned completely parallel to the interspace and not centrally seated within the nucleus, as will be discussed later.

Permanent Imaging Recording

Once the needle has been fully seated into the desired position, images in four orthogonal planes must be recorded if a single puncture system (Percudisc) is being used. If a multistep system is used (Coherent, Santa Cruz, CA; Laserscope, San Jose, CA; Trimedyne, Irvine, CA), images should be obtained after the last phase of the laser sheath insertion process. Only a portion of the components of any of these lasing systems is radiopaque. *Invisible* laser fibers and catheters will be advanced through the devices that can be *seen* under the fluoroscope. Be sure all personnel involved with imaging the insertion understand in advance the correct radiologic appearance of the ideal final position of the system being employed. Four kinds of film (PA, lateral, and both OA-PA 45-degree oblique: Fig. 7.19) are critical for medicolegal documentation of appropriate final positioning within the central aspect of the interspace prior to lasing. The author has already participated in legal actions that resulted when patients claimed sustained damages due to laser malposition; in each of two cases there is no permanent record of the final laser position and therefore no proof it was correct. There is no substitute for hard copy evidence that optimal technique was employed. The addition of intermittent fluoroscopy during lasing is suggested to exclude needle or sheath migration, particularly if the lasing device is removed or if the patient develops postprocedural pain.

Postprocedure Evaluation

Contrast-enhanced MRI is the preferred method of imaging the postoperative lumbar spine in patients with failed back syndrome.[23,42] The MR appearance of infectious disciitis, epidural scar, and recurrent disc herniation have been thoroughly reviewed elsewhere.[21,22,43,44] Little attention has been paid to the postoperative MR appearance of the lumbar disc herniation successfully treated by surgery. In some cases, the herniating disc signal material seen on MRI is reduced in volume by open discectomy. However, recent investigations of now asymptomatic open surgical patients demonstrated persistent anterior epidural mass at the site of the original HNP despite the complete relief of leg pain.[45,46] This intermediate signal intensity tissue was present in all patients imaged and was contiguous with the disc space, mimicking a recurrent disc. The residual mass of this tissue despite relief of symptoms may support the work of others who believe it is disc pressure, not mass effect, that induces clinical symptoms.[8] In the majority of patients this nondiscal residual epidural tissue resolved over a 6-month period as part of an orderly regression of other imaging abnormalities.

No comprehensive discussion of the MR appearance of the patient successfully treated by PLDD has been published. Over 30 now asymptomatic PLDD-treated patients have undergone routine postoperative contrast-enhanced MRI at the Deaconess Hospital in Cincinnati. Based on a review of these examinations, the expected postoperative appearance of the treated central nucleus, the contained herniated fragment, and the peridiscal bone and soft tissues can be described.

The Treated Nucleus

Magnetic resonance imaging (MRI) of the cadaveric lumbar spine has been performed at the Deaconess Hospital both before and after laser energy application via Nd:YAG and Ho:YAG systems. Both produce a distinctive MR defect in the cadaveric nucleus after delivery of 1000 joules, which corresponds to the laser tract upon histologic examination of the treated disc (Fig. 7.20). There is little change in the size of the defect with increasing energy until one surpasses about 1800 joules. However, no similar MR defect has yet been identified in the central nucleus of the PLDD-treated patient, even when imaged within 2 hours of the therapy. No successfully treated PLDD patient has demonstrated a significant focal or generalized change in the T1 signal originating from the nucleus. No abnormal T1 nuclear enhancement has been noted after Gd-DTPA administration, although a thin line of enhancement sometimes appears along the peripheral aspect of the disc just adjacent to the bony endplates. A few patients have shown a uniform decrease in T2 signal throughout the entire disc by 2 weeks post-PLDD, possibly related to an overall decrease in

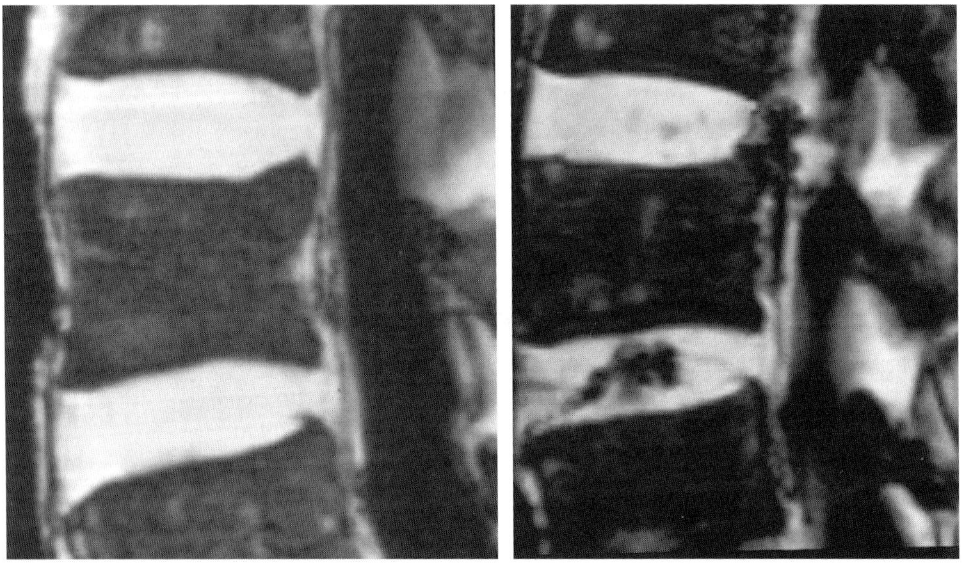

Figure 7.20. Sagittal magnetic resonance (MR) images of cadaver spine before and after application of 1000 joules of Neodymium:YAG (Nd:YAG) energy to central nucleus via laser fiber.

intradiscal water content. One in the group has shown a new focal area of markedly diminished T1 and T2 signal, suggesting an intradiscal vacuum phenomenum.

The Herniated Fragment

No characteristic or consistent change in T1 or T2 signal was reported within the herniating fragment in any of the PLDD-treated patients even with complete resolution of symptoms. However, unlike the open surgical patient, a definite decrease in epidural mass from the herniating fragment has been identified on the MR image in the many of the patients successfully treated with PLDD. The majority show at least a 50% reduction in the volume of posteriorly projecting disc signal material, while a few have shown complete resolution (Fig. 7.21). A significant minority have shown no definite change on MRI in the size of the fragment or the degree of dural sac compression post-PLDD despite symptomatic improvement (Fig. 7.22). Two factors may combine to at least partially explain this lack of MR image change in now

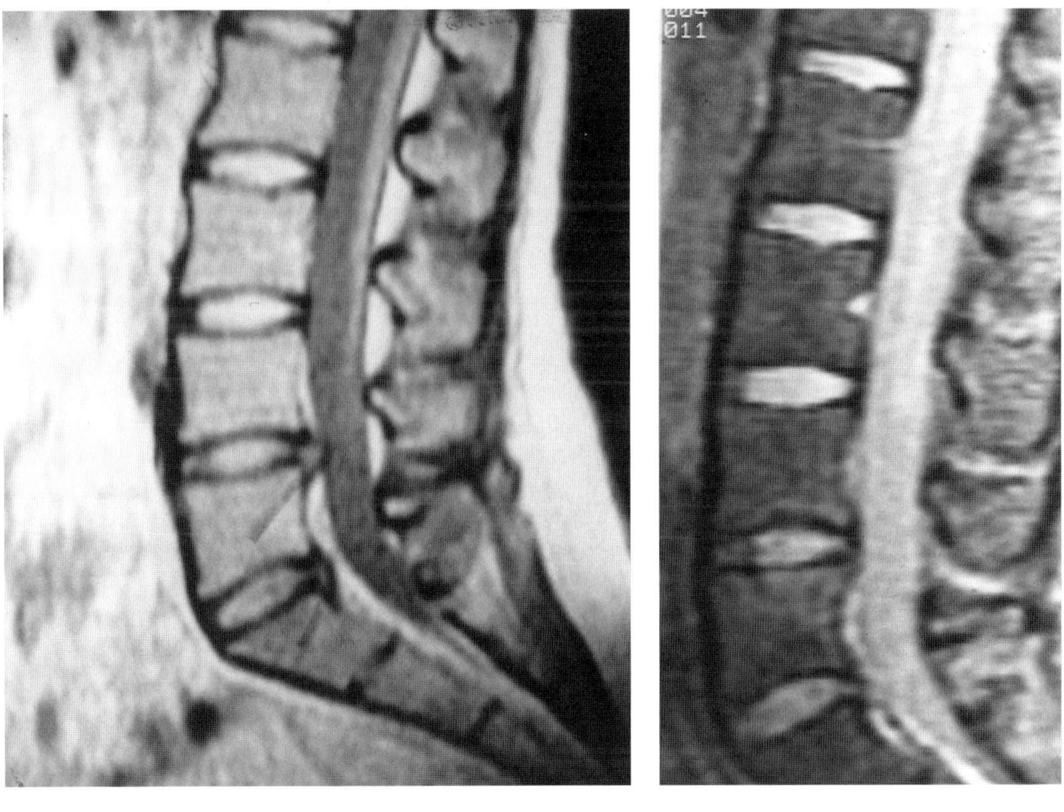

Figure 7.21. Sagittal magnetic resonance (MR) images before (left) and after (right) percutaneous laser disc decompression (PLDD) showing regression of the contained herniating disc fragment with only minor end-plate change. This patient is now asymptomatic.

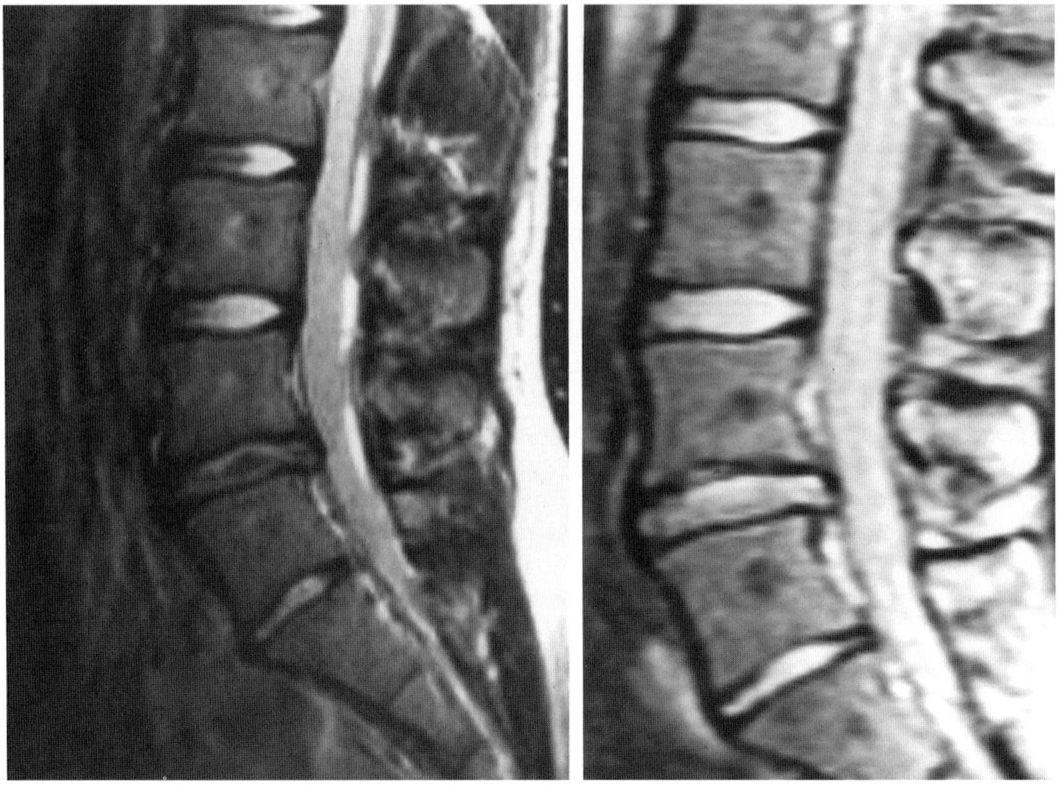

Figure 7.22. Sagittal magnetic resonance (MR) images before (left) and after (right) percutaneous laser disc decompression (PLDD) with no definite change in size of contained herniated nucleus pulposis (HNP) or central nucleus. This patient, too, is now asymptomatic.

asymptomatic individuals. As already discussed, Choy and Altman have shown that there need be only a small change in intradiscal volume to effect a marked decrease in intradiscal pressure.[8] Second, most high-field (1.0 and 1.5 tesla), closed MR scanners performing routine lumbar imaging have T1 spatial resolution potential between 0.8 and 1.0 mm in the axial and sagittal planes (GE Medical Systems; personal communication). Low- and midfield closed and open systems will be not be as good. Therefore, the actual physical retraction of the treated HNP sufficient to alleviate pressure on the affected nerve root may well be less than the resolution of even the best MR imager.

Although not a normal postoperative finding, several patients who were successfully treated by PLDD experienced recurrent symptoms more than 3 but less than 6 months after their initial improvement. Two developed a transligamentous disc extrusion with new contralateral symptoms at the treated level (Fig. 7.23), and both improved following open laminotomy and discectomy. Two more developed a new symptomatic, contained herniation

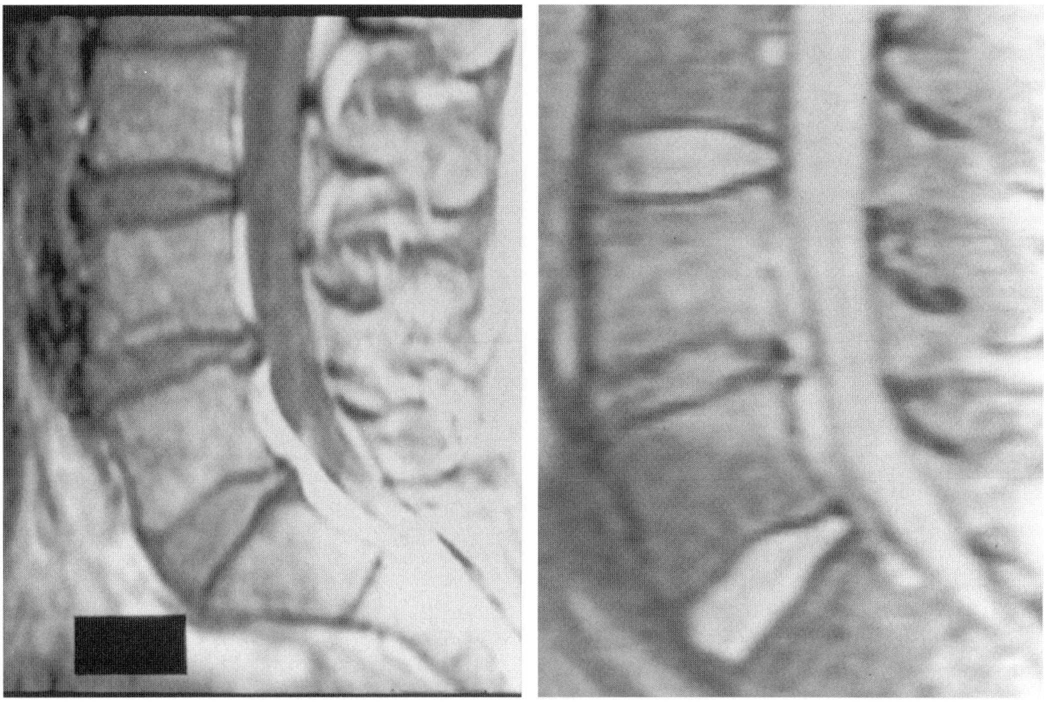

Figure 7.23. Sagittal magnetic resonance (MR) images before (left) and after (right) recurrent symptoms following initially successful percutaneous laser disc decompression (PLDD). The residual asymptomatic contained protrusion (left) converts to a symptomatic transligamentous herniation with extrusion (right) following reinjury.

on CT-D at a different untreated level and improved following PLDD. Finally, two additional patients developed a recurrent symptomatic, contained herniation on CT-D at the same level and improved following repeat PLDD.

Peridiscal Bone and Soft Tissues

Although little change occurs within the disc itself, MR bone marrow signal alterations have been identified adjacent to the vertebral endplates in the majority of patients. Slightly decreased T1 and increased T2/T2* signal bands can be seen in the vertebral bodies above and below the treated interspace for 3 to 9 months after intradiscal therapy (Fig. 7.24). There appears to be no constant relationship between the width of this stripe and the amount of energy delivered to the disc. Some investigators as well this author have seen this finding more frequently in patients treated with the Ho:YAG and those treated with the Nd:YAG laser system. There may be mild T1 enhancement of this stripe with Gd-DTPA administration. Unlike the diffuse bone, disc, and epidural enhancement in patients with discitis, this en-

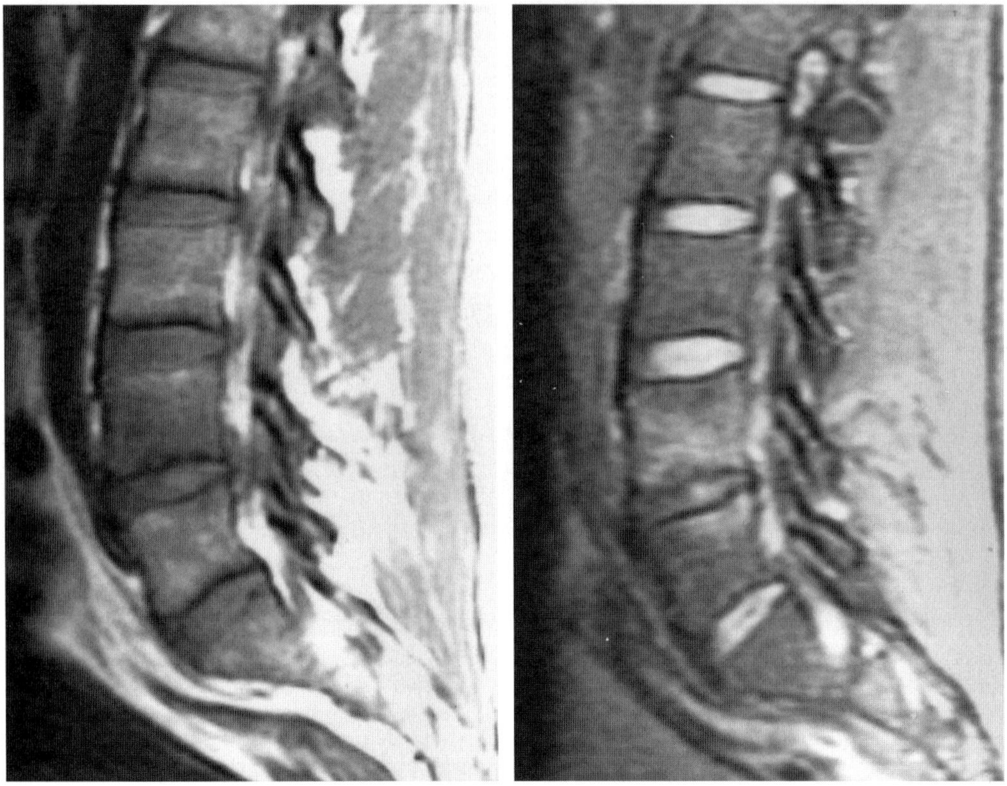

Figure 7.24. Sagittal T1 and T2 magnetic resonance (MR) images post–percutaneous laser disc decompression (PLDD) with pronounced typical marrow signal changes adjacent to the L4-5 vertebral end plate. Patient now asymptomatic despite magnetic resonance (MR) findings.

hancement is completely confined to the vertebral marrow beneath the endplates. Successfully treated asymptomatic patients may show the same marrow signal changes as those whose radiculopathy persists or even those who develop postprocedural back pain. However, when the same signal changes involve only a localized area of one endplate and are associated with cortical interruption, a laser thermal injury to the vertebra should be suspected (Fig. 7.25).[47]

No consistent pattern of MR signal alteration within the soft tissues of the successfully treated PLDD patient has yet been identified. No patients have shown any epidural soft tissue signal change unless they present with symptoms of a sterile or infectious postoperative discitis or a new/recurrent disc herniation. As we will discuss later, paravertebral or posterior soft tissue signal alterations have occurred only when there has been suspected thermal trauma from laser malposition, needle displacement, or needle heating.

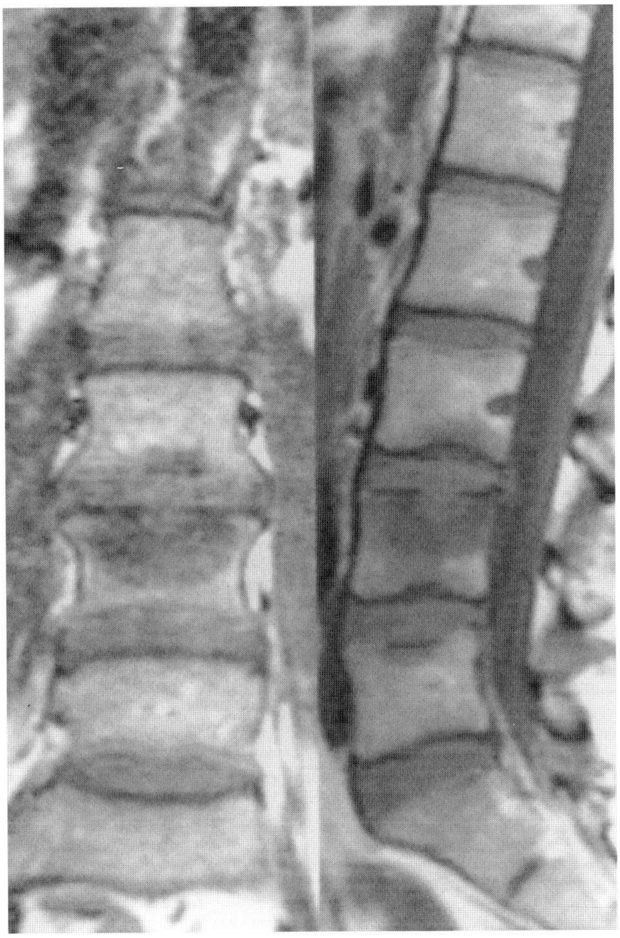

Figure 7.25. Coronal and sagittal T1 magnetic resonance (MR) images post-percutaneous laser disc decompression (PLDD) showing triangle of abnormal marrow signal (edema) within the L4 vertebral body beneath focal defect in the overlying cortical bone end plate.

Imaging Operative Complications

For ease of discussion, the complications of PLDD can arbitrarily be divided into generic and specific groups.[48] Generic complications can occur whenever a disc space is entered and are the same as those described for lumbar discography. They include sterile or infectious discitis, retroperitoneal or epidural hemorrhage, and direct needle trauma to the nerve root or dural sac. Specific complications are unique to PLDD and include thermal trauma to adjacent bone and soft tissues, thermal and/or trephine injury to the annulus or dural sac, and laser fiber or catheter vaporization, fracture, or dissociation. While both routine radiography and computerized tomography are useful in some of these conditions, MR is the primary tool in evaluating patients thought to have experienced complications due to a PLDD procedure.

Disciitis in the PLDD patient may be sterile or infectious. Sterile disciitis is probably related to an inflammatory response to the thermal trauma that normally accompanies laser vaporization. Pyogenic disciitis is a bacterial infection that is likely related to operative contamination. The patient with postoperative disciitis classically presents with new back pain and fever. However, the pain pattern can be confusing and the fever low grade or absent. The erythrocyte sedimentation rate is usually normal with sterile thermal injury and elevated with true infection. Magnetic resonance imaging (MRI) is the procedure of choice to diagnose postoperative sterile or infectious disciitis. As cited earlier, the early MR findings in disciitis have been well described[21] and apply to patients treated by PLDD. When disciitis is suspected by imaging, fluoroscopic or CT-guided thin-needle disc aspiration for bacterial culture becomes mandatory to separate aseptic from pyogenic inflammation.

Hemorrhage into the retroperitoneum or paraspinal musculature is usually the result of aggressive puncture with large-caliber laser systems. Although MR and CT are equally reliable examinations for the diagnosis of retroperitoneal hemorrhage, MR may be more sensitive for the diagnosis of epidural bleeding.[49] Despite frequent citation as a complication in the discography literature,[29] no documented case of abnormal bleeding has occurred in my practice in literally thousands of disc entry procedures for discography and PLDD. Careful attention to technique, constant monitoring of needle position, and the use of smaller caliber needles appear to be effective in preventing hemorrhagic complications.

Direct nerve root trauma usually results in new radicular symptoms including paresthesias. It is most likely to occur in the oversedated patient whose response to nerve root irritation during disc entry is diminished. Imaging plays a lesser role when direct nerve root trauma is suspected. A slow, cautious constantly monitored approach to the interspace adjusting needle position when new radicular and/or dermatomal pain is elicited will avoid trouble.

Dural sac laceration results in leakage of cerebrospinal fluid (CSF) and a typical spinal headache. It usually occurs if the puncture needle, trephine, or laser system is directed too far posteriorly or in patients with congenital nerve root cysts or dural ectasia. Water-soluble CT myelography can be used to demonstrate a CSF leak from an inadvertent dural sac puncture.

Direct thermal trauma to an adjacent vertebral endplate and the underlying bone marrow has been identified in eight patients

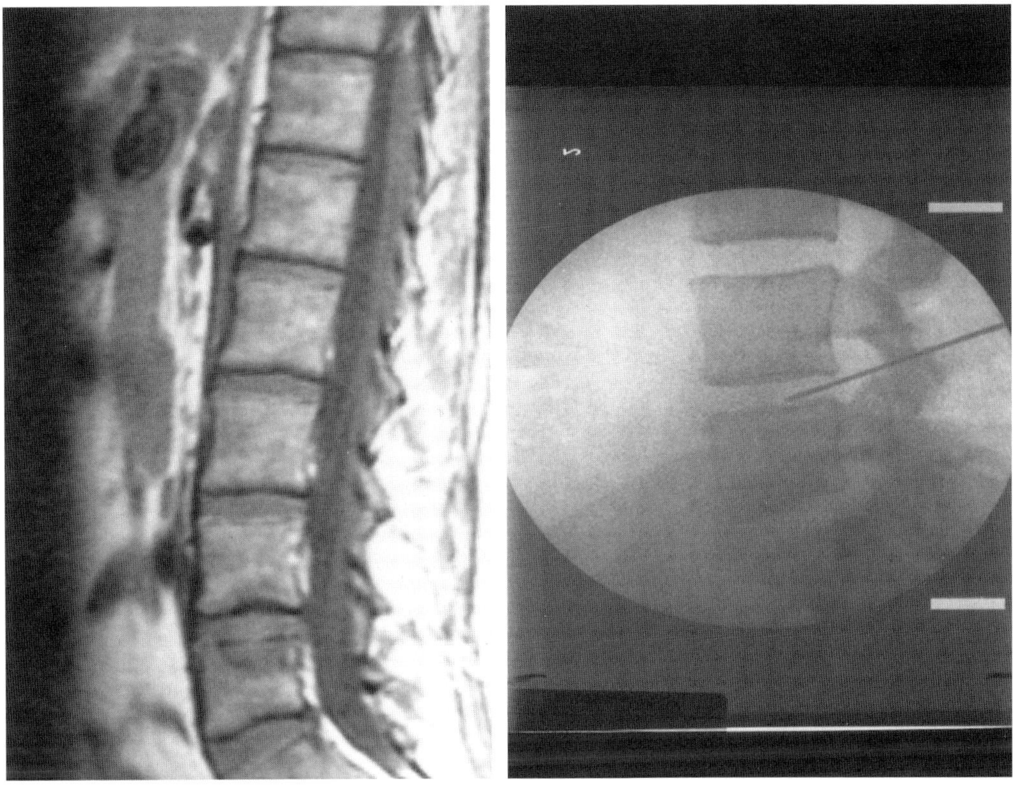

Figure 7.26. Postoperative sagittal magnetic resonance (MR) image and intraoperative spot film. Note the inappropriate angle of side-firing laser cannula toward the resultant cortical defect in the L5 vertebral endplate. This patient developed new back pain despite resolution of the presenting radiculopathy.

and has been the most common PLDD-specific complication. The resulting bone necrosis presents a characteristic MR appearance as described earlier in this chapter. With two exceptions, it has been confined to patients for whom a side-firing laser system was used. Retrospective review of the intraoperative spot films on these patients has consistently shown inappropriate angulation of the laser cannula toward the injured endplates (Fig. 7.26). The importance of disc entry directly parallel to the interspace, no matter what approach or laser system is used, cannot be overemphasized.

Thermal injury to the soft tissues or paraspinal muscles has been seen in four patients and again has been more frequent in those treated with a multistep system. It is the result of direct laser energy deposition in the affected area. It has occurred both from unrecognized malpositioning of the laser system (Fig. 7.27) and after sheath dislodgement away from the annulus during laser catheter removal and reinsertion. Theoretically, these iatro-

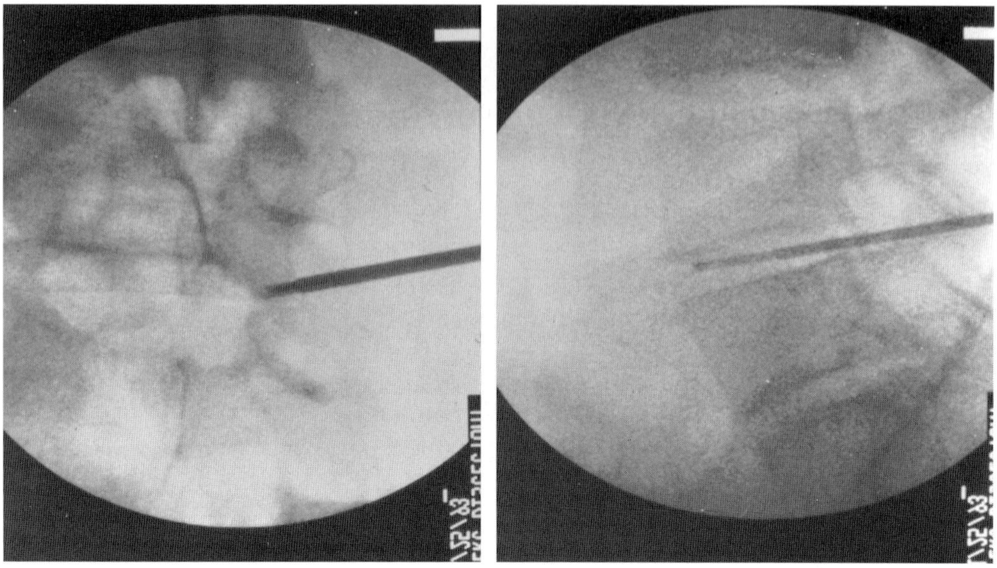

Figure 7.27. Intraoperative spot films from percutaneous laser disc decompression (PLDD) procedure retrospectively noted to show holmium laser cannula in left paravertebral soft tissues. Laser energy was applied despite the malposition.

genic soft tissue laser injuries could have been avoided if the imaging guidelines outlined earlier had been strictly followed. One additional patient experienced heat-related soft tissue damage from inadvertent needle heating, an injury unpreventable by imaging. In all these patients, MRI shows a loss of normal T1 soft tissue/fat planes and increased T2/T2* signal in the damaged region probably secondary to reactive tissue edema from a thermal burn. The T1 contrast enhancement is dramatic and parallels the laser entry tract. It continues for at least 6 weeks in the injured tissues and theoretically may persist even longer.[47,48]

Although Nd:YAG laser fiber vaporization with foreshortening and resultant abnormal needle heating has been visually recognized, it cannot be *seen* fluoroscopically. Intermittent direct inspection of fiber length after application of each 200 joules should be employed to prevent the soft tissue thermal injury that could result with a "hot" needle or guiding sheath. Laser catheter tip dissociation from "meltdown" has also been identified with a multistep system, most likely related to inadequate fluid cooling from inflow or outflow obstruction (Fig. 7.28). Although the laser tip left in the disc space is a Food and Drug Administration (FDA)–approved biocompatible device (personal communication, Coherent Laser Systems), its long-term effect on the nucleus is unknown. Routine radiography or fluoroscopic spot films ad-

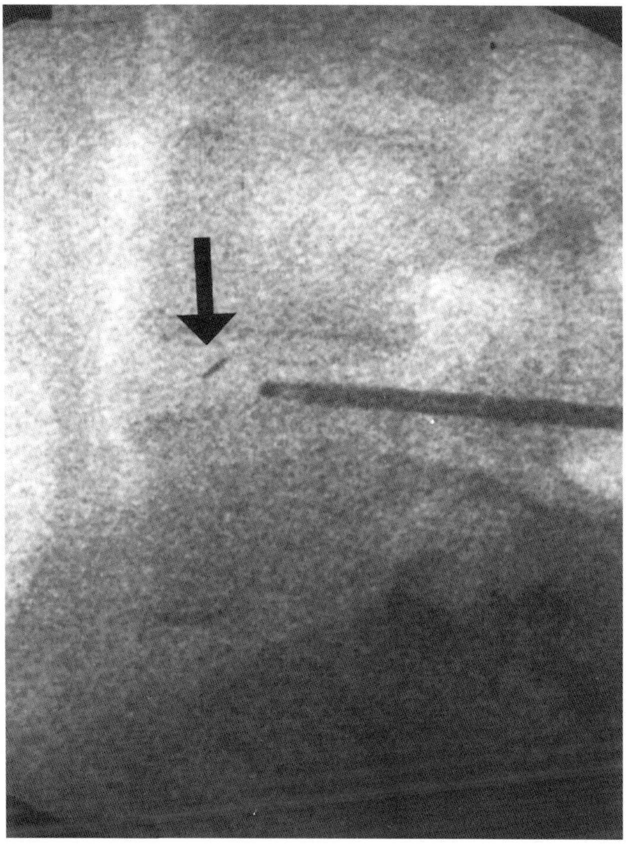

Figure 7.28. Lateral intraoperative spot film showing metallic component of dissociated tip of laser cannula (arrow). The majority of the retained fragment is radiolucent.

equately demonstrate the radiopaque portion of the separated catheter fragment, as long as one realizes that the majority of the catheter tip is radiolucent.

Conclusion

Diagnostic radiology plays a major but formerly underemphasized role in the diagnosis and treatment of the PLDD patient. Laser treatment success rates can be improved when patient selection is based on preoperative diagnostic imaging performed by physicians knowledgeable in the specific needs of the PLDD candidate. A clear understanding of fundamental radiologic principles combined with state of the art intraoperative imaging will result in rapid, accurate positioning of the laser of choice within the central nucleus, optimizing the chances for symptomatic improvement by PLDD. When treatment fails, diagnostic imaging modalities can usually identify the reason for failure or uncover a postoperative complication.

References

1. Botsford JA. Radiological considerations: percutaneous laser disc decompression. *J Clin Laser Med Surg* 1993;11(5):223–231.
2. Botsford JA. The role of radiology in percutaneous laser disc decompression. *J Clin Laser Med Surg* 1995;13(3):173–186.
3. Adams MA, Hutton WC. Mechanics of the intervertebral disc. In: Ghosh P, ed. *The Biology of the Intervertebral Disc.* Boca Raton, FL: CRC Press; 1989.
4. Nachemson, A. Disc pressure measurement. *Spine* 1981;6:93–97.
5. Choy DSJ. Intervertebral disc pressure as a function of fluid volume infused. *Spine* 1993;7(1) (state-of-the-art review: laser discectomy): 11–15.
6. Onik G, Helms CA, Ginsberg L, Hoaglund FT, Morris J. Percutaneous lumbar discectomy using a new aspiration probe. *AJR Am J Roentgenol* 1985;144:1137–1140.
7. Brock M, Gorge H, Curio G. Intradiskal pressure volume response: a methodological contribution to chemonucleolysis. *J Neurosurg* 1984;60:1029–1032.
8. Choy DSJ, Altman P. Fall of intradiscal pressure with laser ablation. *Spine* 1993;7(1)(state-of-the-art review: laser discectomy):23–29.
9. Botsford JA. Radiological considerations: patient selection for percutaneous laser disc decompression. *J Clin Laser Med Surg* 1994;12(5): 255–259.
10. Thornbury JR, Fryback DG, Turski PA, et al. Disk-caused nerve compression in patients with acute low back pain. Diagnosis with MR, CT myelography, and plain CT. *Radiology* 1993;186:731–738.
11. Firooznia H, Benjamin V, Kricheff II, et al. CT of the lumbar spine disc herniation: correlation with surgical findings. *AJR Am J Roentgenol* 1984;142:587–592.
12. Modic MT, Masaryk TJ, Boumphrey F, et al. Lumbar herniated disc disease and canal stenosis: prospective evaluation by surface coil MR, CT, and myelography. *AJR Am J Roentgenol* 1986;147:757–765.
13. Thornbury JR, Fryback DG, Lawrence WF, et al. Reply: diagnostic accuracy, patient outcome, and economic factors in lumbar radiculopathy. *Radiology* 1994;190:21–30.
14. Schellinger D, Manz HJ, Vidic B, et al. Disc fragment migration. *Radiology* 1990;175:831–836.
15. Haughton VM. MR imaging of the spine. *Radiology* 1988;166:297–301.
16. Modic MT, Masaryk TJ, Ross JS, Carter JS. Imaging of degenerative disc disease. *Radiology* 1988;168:177–186.
17. Ross JS, Tkach J, VanDyke C, Modic MT. Clinical MR imaging of degenerative spinal disease: pulse sequences, gradient-echo techniques, and contrast agents. *J Magn Reson Imaging* 1991;1:29.
18. Ross JS, Modic MT. Current assessment of spinal degenerative dis-

ease with magnetic resonance imaging. *Clin Orthop Rel Res* 1992;279: 68–81.

19. Greenspan, A. CT discography vs MRI in intervertebral disk herniation. *Appl Radiol* March 1993:34–40.
20. Joubert JM, Laredo JD, Ziza JM, et al. Gadolinium-enhanced MR imaging in the preoperative evaluation of lumbar disc herniations. Presented at the 78th Scientific Assembly and Meeting of the Radiological Society of North America; November 29–December 4, 1992; Chicago. Abstract 304.
21. Boden SD, David DO, Dina TS, et al. Postoperative diskitis: distinguishing early MR imaging findings from normal postoperative disc space changes. *Radiology* 1992;184:767–771.
22. Georgy BA, Hesselink JR. Gadolinium-enhanced fat suppression MR imaging of the postoperative back. Presented at the 78th Scientific Assembly and Meeting of the Radiological Society of North America; November 29–December 4, 1992; Chicago. Abstract 303.
23. Ross JS, Delamarter R, Hueftle MG, et al. Gadolinium-DTPA enhanced MR imaging of the post-operative lumbar spine: time course and mechanism of enhancement. *Am J Neuroradiol* 1989;10:37–46.
24. Schellinger D, Manz HJ, Vidic B, et al. Disc fragment migration. *Radiology* 1990;175:831–836.
25. Modic MT, Ross JS. Morphology, symptoms, and causality. *Radiology* 1990;175:619–620.
26. Bozzao A, Gallucci M, Masciocchi C, et al. Lumbar disk herniation: MR imaging assessment of the natural history in patients treated without surgery. *Radiology* 1992;185:135–141.
27. Edwards WC, Orme TJ, Orr-Edwards G. CT discography: prognostic value in the selection of patients for chemonucleolysis. *Spine* 1987;12:792–795.
28. Botsford JA. CT discography: prognostic value in patient selection for percutaneous laser disc decompression (PLDD). Presented at the 94th Annual Meeting of the American Roentgen Ray Society; April 24–29, 1994; New Orleans. Abstract 265.
29. Bernard TN. Lumbar discography followed by computed tomography. *Spine* 1990;15:690–707.
30. Milette PC, Melanson D. Lumbar discography. *Radiology* 1987;163: 828–829.
31. Vanharanta H, Ska BE, Spivey MA, et al. The relationship of pain provocation to lumbar disc deterioration seen by CT discography. *Spine* 1987;12:295–298.
32. Walsh TR, Weinstein JN, Spratt KF, et al. Lumbar discography in normal subjects. *J Bone Joint Surg Am* 1990;72(7):1081–1088.
33. Collins CD, Stack JP, O'Connell DJ, et al. The role of discography in lumbar disc disease: a comparative study of magnetic resonance imaging and discography. *Clin Radiol* 1990;42:252–257.
34. Kornberg, M. Discography and magnetic resonance in the diagnosis of lumbar disc disruption. *Spine* 1989;14:1368–1372.
35. Collis JS Jr, Gardner WJ. Lumbar discography: analysis of 600 degenerated discs and diagnosis of degenerative disc disease. *JAMA* 1961;178:167–170.

36. Collis JS Jr, Gardner WJ. Lumbar discography: an analysis of one thousand cases. *J Neurosurg* 1962;19:452–461.
37. Goldie I. Changes observed in the intervertebral disc after discography. *Acta Pathol* 1958;42:193–197.
38. Seidenwurm D, Russel EJ, Hambly M. Diagnostic accuracy, patient outcome, and economic factors in lumbar radiculopathy. *Radiology* 1994;190:21–30.
39. Choy DSJ, Ascher PW, Saddekni S, et al. Percutaneous laser disc decompression. *Spine* 1992;17:949–956.
40. Hijikata S, Yamagishi M, Nakayama T, Oomori K. Percutaneous diskectomy: a new treatment for lumbar disc herniation. *J Toden Hosp* 1975;5:5–13.
41. Choy DSJ. The problem of the L5-S1 disc solved by needle entry with an extrathecal approach. *J Clin Laser Med Surg* 1994;12(6): 321–324.
42. Hueftle MG, Modic MT, Ross JS, et al. Lumbar spine: postoperative MR imaging with Gd-DTPA. *Radiology* 1988;167:817–824.
43. Soitropoulos S, Chafetz NI, Lang P, et al. Differentiation between postoperative scar and recurrent disc herniation: prospective comparison of MR, CT, and contrast enhanced CT. *Am J Neuroradiol* 1989;10:639–643.
44. Bundschuh CV, Modic MT, Ross JS, Masaryk TJ, Bohlman H. Epidural fibrosis and recurrent disc herniation in the lumbar spine: MR imaging assessment. *Am J Neuroradiol* 1988;9:169–178.
45. Boden SD, Davis DO, Dina TS, et al. Contrast enhanced MR imaging performed after successful lumbar disk surgery: prospective study. *Radiology* 1992;182:59–64.
46. Dina TS, Boden SD, David DO. Lumbar spine after surgery for herniated disk: imaging findings in the early postoperative period. *AJR Am J Roentgenol* 1995;164:665–671.
47. Kosaka R, Abe M, Yonezawa T, Ichimura Y, Onomura T. Bone necrosis adjacent to the disc after percutaneous laser disc decompression—an analysis of magnetic resonance imaging. In: Gerber BE, Knight M, Siebert WE, eds. *Lasers in the Musculoskeletal System.* Berlin: Springer-Verlag; 2001:345–350.
48. Botsford JA. Potential operative complications of percutaneous laser discectomy. In: Gerber BE, Knight M, Siebert WE, eds. *Lasers in the Musculoskeletal System* Berlin: Springer-Verlag; 2001:351–356.
49. Gundry CR, Heithoff KB. Epidural hematoma of the lumbar spine: 18 surgically confirmed cases. *Radiology* 1993;187:427–431.

8

Magnetic Resonance Imaging of the Lumbothoracic Spine Under Compression

Daniel S.J. Choy

Central to the diagnosis of herniated intervertebral disc disease is magnetic resonance imaging (MRI). Yet every MR image of the spine is unphysiologic. The most comfortable position for a patient with a herniated disc is the supine one. It is the position in which Nachemson and Morris[1] in 1964 found intradiscal pressure to be 15 to 25 kPa. Standing pressures were 100 kPa, while sitting pressures were 150 to 200 kPa. Equivalents in other units are 112.5 to 187.5 mmHg, 0.15 to 0.25 atm, and 1.69 to 2.22 psi supine. A sitting intradiscal pressure of 200 kPa = 1500 mmHg = 1.97 atm = 29.6 psi. The highest intradiscal pressures naturally produce the most symtoms, and therefore it made sense to suggest that a *sitting* MRI would be the best MRI for diagnosing herniated disc disease.

The Compression Frame

A *sitting* MRI would indeed be the best MRI. At the 1995 Laser Association of Neurosurgeons International (LANSI) meeting in Salzburg, the author stated that it is not uncommon to find dissociation between severity of clinical pain and MRI findings: for some patients who suffer from severe pain, the MRI reveals a minor change, whereas others exhibit marked disc protrusions in the MRI and suffer few if any symptoms. A hand went up in the

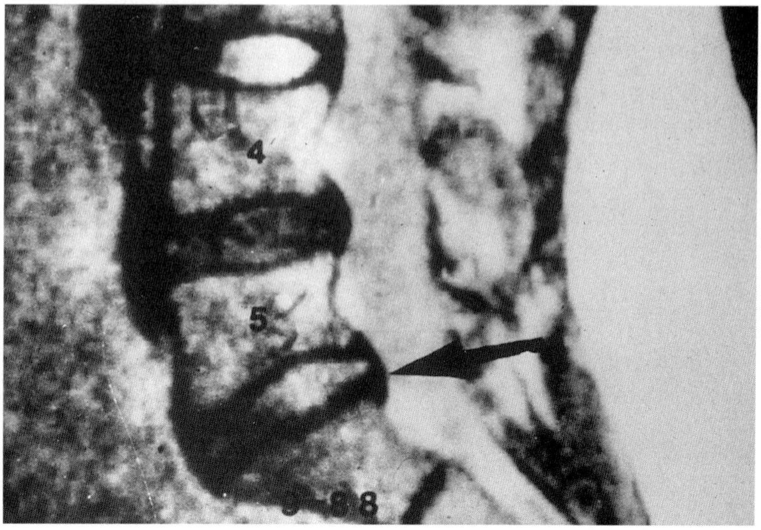

Figure 8.1. Magnetic resonance (MR) image of L5-S1 showing a mild bulge. (Reprinted with permission from Choy DSJ. Magnetic resonance imaging (MRI) of the lumbosacral spine under compression. *J Clin Laser Med Surg* 1997;15:71–73.)

audience: it was Professor Ferenc Jolecz, chief of MRI at the Beth Israel Hospital, Harvard University. "Yes, Frank," I acknowledged. "When it is time for my lecture," he said, "I will show three slides that will show that what you just said is absolutely true." "I can't wait that long," I replied, "I'm leaving the podium. Please come up and show us your three slides."

The first slide (Fig. 8.1) was a sagittal section of the lumbar spine showing a mild bulge of the L5-S1 disc. The second slide (Fig. 8.2) was of the same patient, taken 5 minutes later. Note that large protrusion of the L5-S1 disc. The collective gasp in the audience was followed by the third slide (Fig. 8.3) showing that the slide in Figure 8.2 was taken in a sitting MRI. While sitting, the patient also had an increase in symptoms.

At the time there were only two sitting MRIs in the world, one in Zurich and the other at Harvard. On my return to New York I called Dr. Morris Blumenfeld, head of MRI at General Electric, to inquire about the price of a sitting MRI machine. "Five million dollars," was the reply.

"How much is one for me?" I pursued.

"Five million dollars."

"But Morrie, I'm your doctor."

"Dan," he replied, "I don't set the prices, GE does."

"All right, you'll be sorry. I'm going to invent something that will make your five-million dollar machine obsolete!"

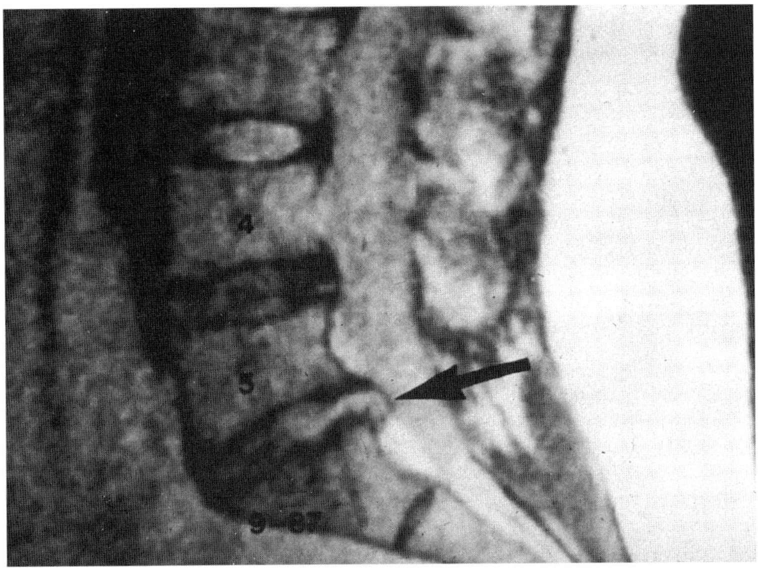

Figure 8.2. Magnetic resonance (MR) image of the same patient, 5 minutes later. Note the marked protrusion of the L5-S1 disc. (Reprinted with permission from Choy DSJ. Magnetic resonance imaging (MRI) under compression. *J Clin Laser Med Surg* 1997;15:71–73.)

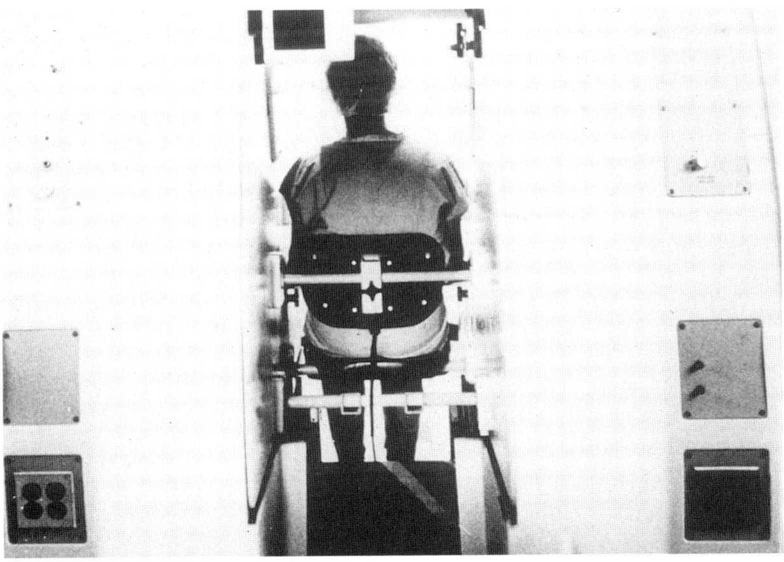

Figure 8.3. The patient in the *sitting* magnetic resonance imaging (MRI) machine, where the image in Fig. 8.2 was taken. (Reprinted with permission from Choy DSJ. MRI of the lumbosacral spine under compression. *J Clin Laser Med Surg* 1997;15:71–73.)

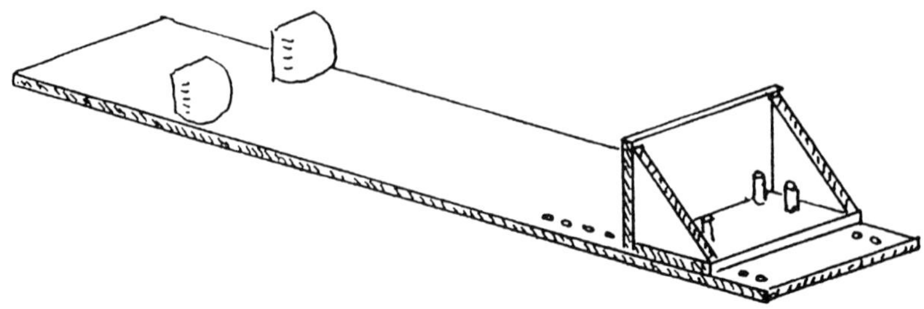

Figure 8.4. The first prototype plywood frame built in 1996, and still in use at the Computerized Diagnostic Scanning Associates, New York.

With $75 worth of three-quarter-inch marine-grade plywood, I designed and built a simple compression frame (Fig. 8.4) consisting of a baseboard 8 feet 6 inches long, 16 inches wide (to fit into a standard MR tube), two fixed padded shoulder restraints, and a sliding, movable foot board that could be secured in place with hardwood dowel pegs. In use, a patient is positioned supine on the frame, with the shoulders abutting the fixed shoulder pads and the knees bent so that the shoulder-to-foot distance is 4 to 5 inches shorter than the fully extended length. The footboard is fixed in position with the four hardwood dowels. The patient and frame are slid into the MR tube, and the patient is imaged in the usual manner. Then the patient is asked to forcibly extend both knees, which compresses the thoracolumbar spine. The early prototype model had no pressure gauge.

Experience

Since 1996 all my lumbosacral MRIs have been performed with the compression frame. In 1997 a report of this frame was published in the *Journal of Clinical Laser Medicine and Surgery*,[2] and a paper was presented to the International Musculoskeletal Laser Society (IMLAS) at the University of Kassel, Germany. Mr. Martin Knight was in the audience and thought enough of the idea to have his carpenters construct a copy on his return to the Spinal Foundation in Manchester, U.K. One year later, at the IMLAS meeting in Kyoto, Japan, Mr. Knight reported on the "Choy MRI compression frame." He reported that approximately one third of his patients experienced increased pain reproducing the presenting complaints. There was also augmentation of the disc herniation by MRI. I had been obtaining increased pain and image augmentation in approximately half of the patients.

Three physicists from General Electric visited the Laser Spine Center and the Computerized Diagnostic Associates (to whom I had given my compression frame) in 2000 and were suitably im-

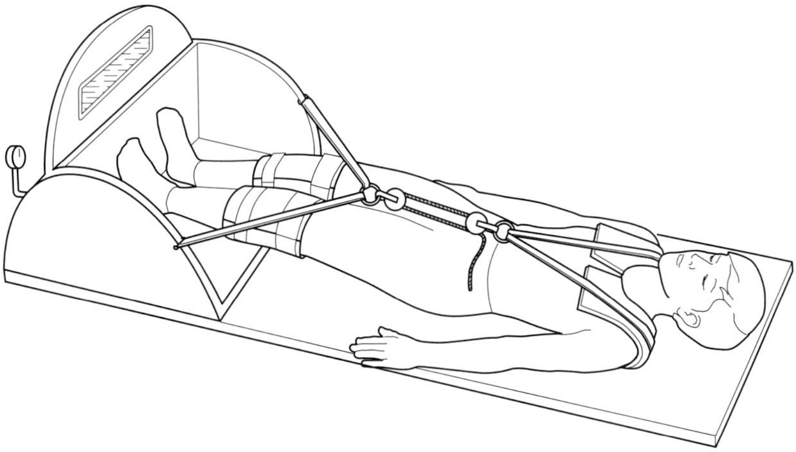

Figure 8.5. The latest compression frame, being built with a pressure meter.

pressed. However, they discovered that a group of scientists in Sweden had thought of the same idea and actually formed a company to market their compression frame, which was professionally engineered and had a pressure gauge. Accompanying their brochure were three impressive references.[3–5] The Scandinavian entrepreneurs, however, overcharged for their machine and promptly went bankrupt. In any event, my patent preceded theirs by 5 weeks. Our group has now designed and is in the process of building a second-generation compression frame (Fig. 8.5). We are negotiating with a major university to use it in a prospective, double-blind, crossover study.

Discussion

In equivocal cases, concordance between MRI findings and the clinical picture often does not exist. It would be helpful to the clinician if his or her findings were confirmed by a positive MRI. In such instances I believe MRI with compression of the thoracolumbar spine should be employed, because the study is then performed under more physiologic conditions.

Some laser spine surgeons still prefer to perform discography before percutaneous laser disc decompression (PLDD). Elsewhere in this book I have set out my reasons for opposing this approach in general. The compression frame is a form of noninvasive discography with no morbidity. The intradiscal pressure is increased, and in our experience, exacerbation of presenting symptoms occurs in 50% of patients. Additionally, there is the extra benefit of image augmentation.

With the new compression frame equipped with a pressure meter, we will be able to obtain more standardization of image acquisition. Intuitively I do not believe that 200 kPa registered at the footboard will produce 200 kPa at the lower lumbar discs. The intervening knees, hips, and sacroiliac joints probably exert a dampening effect on pressure transmission. A colleague in Europe will be conducting in vivo studies of intradiscal pressure as a function of foot-plate pressure. The pressure relationship data he will develop will be an invaluable guide for future use of the new compression frame.

I close with a plea to spine surgeons: please pay more attention to the clinical picture and less to the MRI, unless such imaging is one performed with the spine under compression.

References

1. Nachemson A., Morris J. In vivo measurements of intradiscal pressure. Discometry, a method for determination of pressure in the lower lumbar discs. *J Bone Joint Surg Am* 1964;46(5):1077–1092.
2. Choy DSJ. Magnetic resonance imaging of the lumbosacral spine under compression. *J Clin Laser Med Surg* 1997;15(2):71–73.
3. Willen J, Danielson B, Gaulitz A, Niklasson T, Schonstrom N, Hansson T. Dynamic effects on the lumbar spinal canal. *Spine* 1997;22: 2968–2976.
4. Hargens, AR, Hutchinson KJ, Ballard RE, Fechner KP, Murthy G. Intervertebral disc: loaded on earth and unloaded in space. In: *Connectivity Tissue Biology*; vol 7; *Integration and Reductionism*; London: Portland Press; 1998; ch. 10.
5. Danielsson BI, Willen J, Gaulitz A, Nidlason T, Hansson TH. Axial loading of the spine during CT and MR in patients with suspected lumbar spinal stenosis. *Acta Radiol* 1998;39:604–611.

9

Initial Consultation and First Interview

Daniel S.J. Choy

Before the interview, the patient has been provided with a pain diagram (see Figs. 6.1 and 6.19) to mark and a list of questions (Table 9.1) to answer.

Listening to the Patient

The prospective patient and family first meet the laser surgeon at the initial consultation and interview. The first impression is all important. The doctor should not act distracted, and the staff should be instructed not to allow intrusive telephone calls except for emergencies.

The doctor's focus should be on the patient and reinforced with eye contact. This generates a sense of caring and compassion on the part of the doctor, and the patient tends to respond with trust and faith in the doctor. These may seem like obvious caveats, but I have seen these basic principles more often violated than not. Too often the patient leaves the office feeling like a "number" and that the doctor is "running a factory."

Everything the patient says should be listened to with attention and respect, and the patient should never be made to feel foolish in reciting his or her history, no matter how immaterial some items of information may sound.

Table 9.1. Questions for the Patient

1. Does the following increase/decrease/or cause no change in your symptoms?
   Sitting   Standing   Lying down   Coughing/sneezing
2. How long is your
   Sitting tolerance?
   Standing tolerance?
   Walking tolerance?
3. Do you get calf pain/numbness that gets worse when you walk and that goes away when you stop? Lean forward?
4. How far do you walk before this happens?
5. How long does it take for the symptoms to disappear?
6. What is your position of greatest comfort?
   Lying down   Standing   Sitting

Questioning the Patient

Only when the patient has ended the recitation should the doctor begin to ask questions. These are my questions.

1. (Pointing to the pain diagram) Is this where the pain is?
2. Is this where the numbness is?
3. Have you left out anything?
4. How long have you had these symptoms?
5. Was there a precipitating cause, such as an accident, lifting something heavy, falling, or twisting your body?
6. Are you currently engaged in a lawsuit?
7. Is this pain or numbness constant or on and off?
8. On a scale of 1 to 10, 10 being the worst, how would you rate your symptoms?
9. What aggravates these symptoms?
   a. Lying down, standing, sitting, changing positions?
   b. Walking?
   c. Reaching for something high up?
   d. Coughing or sneezing?
   e. Straining during bowel movements?
10. Are you taking any pain medications? Any muscle relaxants? Any anti-inflammatories?
11. What has been done for you so far?
    a. Physiotherapy?
    b. Chiropractic?
    c. Acupuncture?
    d. Epidural blocks?
    e. Nerve blocks?
    f. Trigger point injections?
    g. Surgery?

h. Vax-D?
i. Intradiscal electrothermoplasty (IDET)?
j. Anything else?

12. Have you seen a neurosurgeon or orthopedic surgeon?
13. What advice did he or she give you?
14. How did you hear about percutaneous laser disc decompression? Naturally, patient referrals are the best; second best are Internet referrals, since these patients have usually done considerable research on the different therapeutic modalities being offered for herniated disc disease and are thus fairly well informed. If the patient was referred by a physician, and if geography is not a factor, it is my practice to have the patient invite the referring physician to observe the procedure. To see that the laser surgeon has enough self-assurance to invite a professional observer greatly enhances patient confidence.

My next step is to explain the dynamics of disc herniation with the aid of a plastic model of a spine and a disk. I point out that a disc hernia occurs much like an inguinal hernia: there must be an increase in pressure of the herniating anatomic part, coupled with a weakness of the restraining wall—the posterior longitudinal ligament and posterior annulus in the case of the intervertebral disc, and the anterior abdominal wall in case of the inguinal hernia. I then explain that the nucleus pulposus is 55 to 80% water, depending on the age of the patient. And since water is noncompressible, a small reduction in volume results in a sharp and disproportionate decrease in intradiscal pressure. This is further illustrated with a small toy balloon filled with water and connected to a syringe. Pulling back on the plunger shrinks the balloon, and pushing in causes the balloon to expand. The laser vaporizes water, so the intradiscal pressure decreases.

These maneuvers may seem simplistic to a sophisticated spine surgeon, but they are remarkably well received by patients. A concrete demonstration is supremely effective in enlightening a patient. As a famous TV commercial in the United States states, "An educated consumer is the best customer!"

The magnetic resonance imaging (MRI) which should be less than 6 months old, is then read by the laser surgeon, without referring to the official written report. This is because approximately 20% of MRIs that cross my desk have been incorrectly read. Upon deciding which discs are protruded, the surgeon should demonstrate them to the patient and family. Only then should the doctor read the official report.

At this point I emphasize to the patient that I do not treat MRIs, I treat only patients (see Chapter 8). The decision of which discs to treat is deferred until the patient has been examined. Every spine surgeon has had the experience of seeing multiple protruded discs on the MRI of a patient who has no or few symptoms. The reverse is also true: the MRI of a patient who has severe symptoms may show a minimally protruding disc. If the MRI reveals, for instance, five protruding lumbar discs, and the patient's pain diagram and history, and the physical examination, point to only L5-S1 involvement, that is the only disc that should be treated. The converse is also true: if the MRI shows only a single protruding disc, but the signs and symptoms point to another disc as well, I then treat both discs. This requires courage on the part of the laser surgeon, and a trusting relationship between doctor and patient.

Prognosis Form

In over 17 years of clinical experience with PLDD, first at St. Luke's–Roosevelt Hospital (200 procedures over a 2-year period), there was a success rate according to the MacNab criteria of 75% and a complication rate of 1%. When I began to perform PLDD at an outpatient surgical facility (New York Laser Spine Center), the success rate increased to 89% and the complication rate fell to 0.4% (complications are the subject of Chapter 11). I believe that the higher rate of nosocomial infections in a hospital setting is the reason for the higher complication rate of the first 2 years. The higher success rate subsequently is not due to passing the *learning curve* of the earlier experience. I attribute it to better equipment and better patient education, as described in the next chapter. Also in the entire period there have been no instances of nerve damage, cord damage, or deaths.

I also indicate that approximately 10% of the responding group may take 1 week to 11 months to obtain total pain relief, since in my experience, the disc may continue to shrink for up to 11 months.

Patients who have had previous surgery, or those over the age of 65, are offered a lower chance of improvement, in the range of 70 to 75%.

This information is summarized in a "prognosis form," dated, and given to the patient. A copy is retained for the chart. Care is taken to point out that although the incidence of infectious discitis is only 0.4%, in the patient who develops this complication, it becomes 100%. However, every patient with discitis was cured with appropriate antibiotics.

The prognosis form incorporates a written statement that the surgeon has not promised a 100% result, that some patients may take longer to respond, and that there is a complication rate. If the patient understands this, the chances of a malpractice suit are minimized.

All candidates are screened by their internists or general practitioners for *medical clearance.* The objective is to detect systemic infection or other clinical states that may be contraindications to even a relatively noninvasive procedure such as PLDD. The intervertebral disc is poorly vascularized and is therefore more susceptible to infection than tissues that are well supplied with blood vessels. In over 17 years, I have discovered one patient with unsuspected ascending colon cancer, one case of osteomyelitis next to the offending disc, and one case of compensated hemolytic anemia. The medical clearance includes a medical history, a complete physical examination, a blood survey with special attention to bleeding indices, a chest roentgenogram, and in those over age 40 or those with cardiac symptoms, an electrocardiogram. The medical clearance also provides protection for both the patient and the laser surgeon.

To all patients, PLDD is an unknown territory. A certain degree of fear is natural. It is important for the laser surgeon to establish first of all solid rapport with the patient and the family. I will not insult you by suggesting how to do this; I am sure you know how.

During the intravenous administration of prophylactic vancomycin (500 mg in 250 mL of saline), I like to tell the patient that he or she is among friends, and that we are there not to hurt him or her, but to help. I tell the patient that the amount of pain during the procedure will be minimal, about as much as that caused by a tooth cleaning, and that there will be no surprises during the procedure. Each step will be explained before it is done. The patient is told not to move and not to talk unless it is necessary to answer a question, in which case it is essential not to turn the head, since that will result in the body following and make for a moving target. To help ensure that the patient remains as still as possible 3 to 7 mg of midazolam (Versed) is given intramuscularly as a tranquilizer.

I do not know if it is being spoken to that soothes the patient or the content of what is said that is reassuring. I have had patients tell me afterward that this little speech did wonders to allay their fears.

10

The Percutaneous Laser Disc Decompression Procedure

Daniel S.J. Choy

The major component of percutaneous laser disc decompression is needle placement. Needle placement is guided by biplane fluoroscopy. When I initially performed PLDD at St. Luke's–Roosevelt Hospital in New York City, I used a fixed table in a radiographic suite equipped with a GE C-arm fluoroscope. The device weighed perhaps 1 to 2 tons and had an electric motor. This meant that to move the C-arm I had to press a button to activate the motor. Because of the inertia of the C-arm, the fluoroscope did not move immediately, nor did it stop immediately. The images obtained were therefore suboptimal. The success rate of the PLDD procedure using this equipment was approximately 75%.

When I moved the procedure to the Laser Spine Center, a standalone outpatient laser surgical suite, I installed a new invention, a radiolucent table on casters, which could be moved by hand (Fig. 10.1). This table made it possible to move the patient as well as the C-arm, so that precise views of the needle position could be obtained, millimeter by millimeter. It was also much faster than the cumbersome motor-driven C-arm. I believe I am the only one in the world with this equipment. Very soon, the success rate went from 75 to 89%. It was not a matter of mastering a learning curve, since I had already performed 200 procedures at St. Luke's–Roosevelt. I attribute the increased success rate to the improved imaging provided by the movable radiolucent table. I urge those who are about to embark on PLDD to obtain or build such a table. When I had one made in 1992 in New York it cost

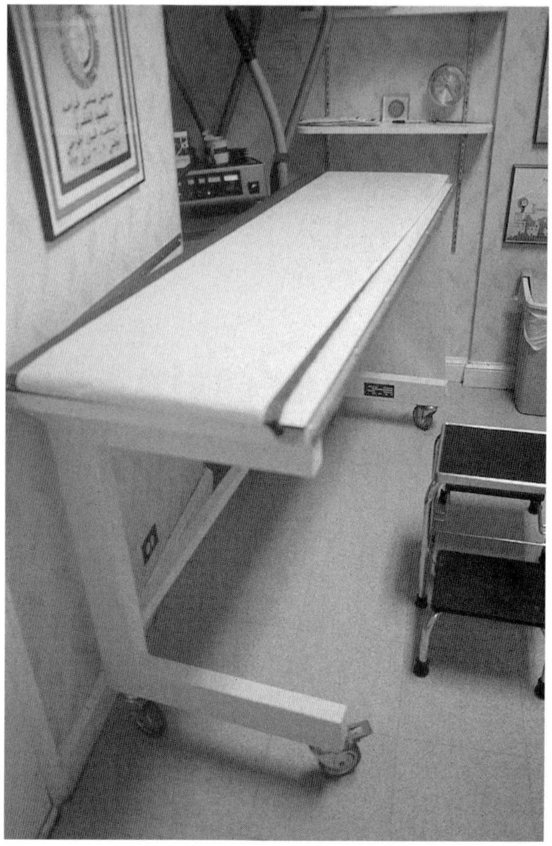

Figure 10.1. Radiolucent table on casters allows maximal movement of the patient and permits millimeter-by-millimeter adjustment in relation to the x-ray tube for optimal imaging.

$2000. Probably prices in or after 2003 will be slightly higher, but the convenience of being able to move the patient by hand so that the imaging is optimal cannot be overestimated.

The incidence of disc herniation in my experience is lumbar, 90%; cervical, 8%; and thoracic, 2%.

The step-by-step instructions for the PLDD procedure in lumbar discs are followed by briefer remarks on PLDD for thoracic and cervical discs.

Lumbar Discs

1. The patient is placed in the lateral recumbent position, with the head either to the right or the left (Fig. 10.2). The side chosen does not matter, since the reduction in pressure occurs throughout the disc.
2. The patient is told that he or she can follow the action on one of the radiologic screens.

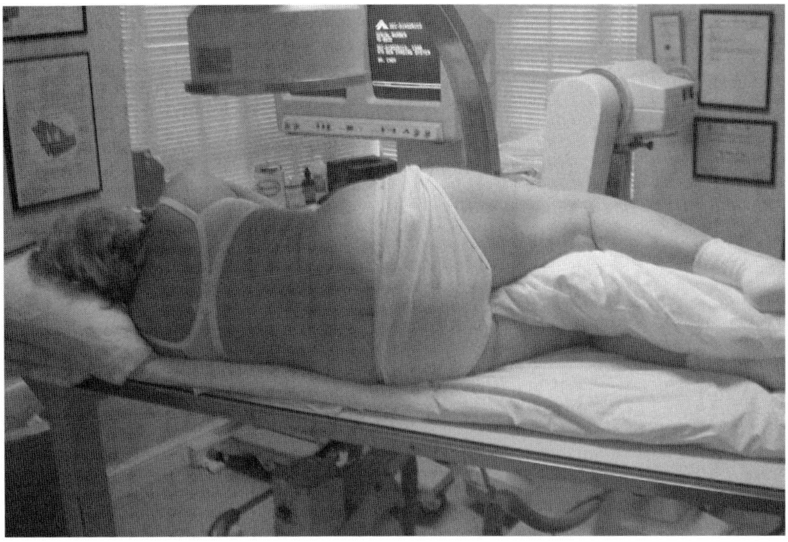

Figure 10.2. The patient is placed in the lateral recumbent position. The head may be to the right or the left, since pressure reduction occurs throughout the disc.

3. The outline of the pelvic crest is drawn with an indelible ink pen, and the needle must not enter south of this line (Fig. 10.3).
4. The middle of the spine (using the spinous processes as landmarks) is outlined with the same pen (Fig. 10.3).
5. A line parallel to and 10 cm above the midline is drawn (Fig. 10.3). A quick way to do this is to measure the combined width of four fingers of your nondominant hand. In my case it is 8 cm; then placing the hand on the patient's back, I can estimate the extra 2 cm. The entry point of the needle will be somewhere on this line.
6. The C-arm is turned on.
7. The appropriate disc is imaged.
8. A long radiopaque needle is placed on the trunk of the patient to overlie the target disc (Fig. 10.4).
9. A line is drawn along the needle (Fig. 10.4).
10. The point of needle entry is the intersection of the line drawn along the needle with the 10 cm horizontal line.
11. The surgeon dons sterile gloves.
12. The patient is prepped with soap, alcohol, and Betadine, being careful to wipe from center to periphery, and never to return to the center.
13. The patient is draped with a large drape, with the opening over the point of entry (Fig. 10.5).
14. The C-arm is sterile draped (Fig. 10.6).
15. The delivery kit (Percudisc, New York) (Fig. 10.7) is opened.

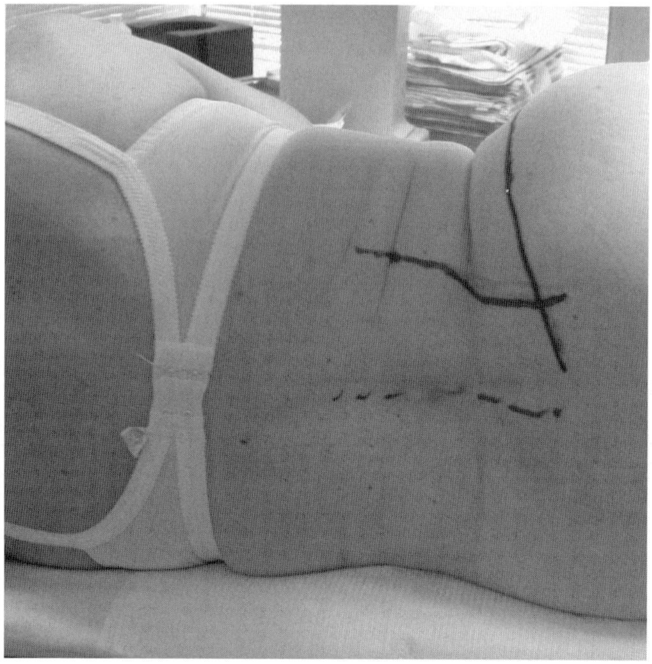

Figure 10.3. The iliac crest is outlined with a felt-tipped pen. Similarly, the midline is outlined by connecting the points over the spinous processes. A line parallel to and 10 cm above the midline is drawn. The needle entry point will be somewhere on this line.

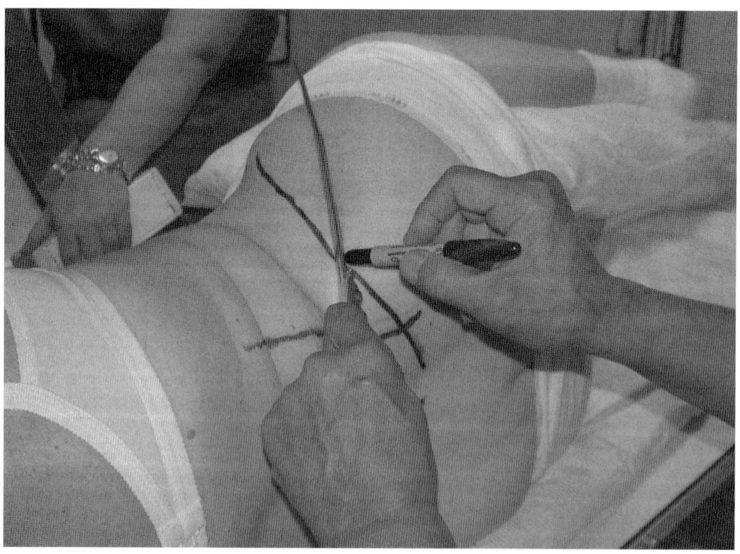

Figure 10.4. A radiopaque needle is placed on the trunk of the patient to overlie the target disc. A line is drawn along this needle. The intersection of this line with the horizontal line is the point of needle entry.

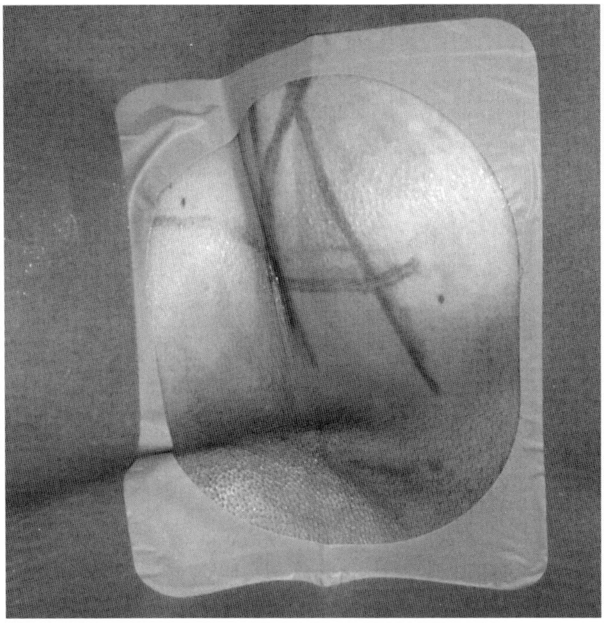

Figure 10.5. The patient is covered with a sterile drape.

16. The trochars are inserted into the two 18-gauge, 9-inch-long needles (Fig. 10.7).
17. The 5-inch-long spinal tap needle is prepared by withdrawing the trochar (Fig. 10.8).
18. The two long needles, the spinal tap needle, and the 24-gauge needle and the 10 mL syringe are brought to the operating

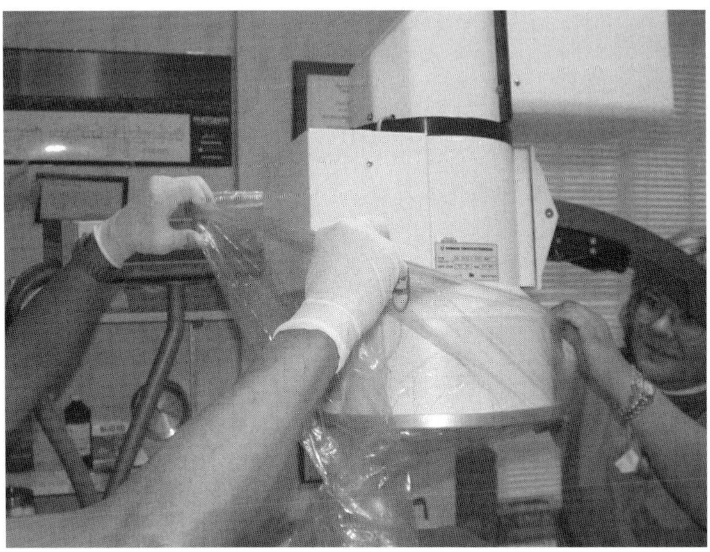

Figure 10.6. A sterile drape is placed over the C-arm.

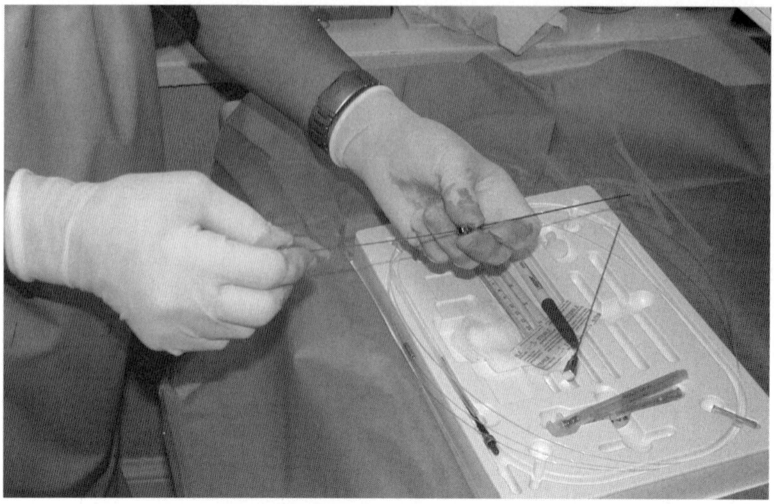

Figure 10.7. The Percudisc delivery kit is opened. Trochars are inserted into the two 18-gauge, 9-inch-long needles.

area and placed on a sterile part of the patient drape (Fig. 10.9).

19. One or two 10 mL syringes are filled with 1% lidocaine (Xylocaine) (Fig. 10.10).
20. The skin over the entry site (Fig. 10.11) is infiltrated with the anesthetic, using one of the syringes and the 24-gauge needle.
21. The anesthetized skin is then entered with the spinal tap needle, which is connected to the syringe bearing the Xylocaine

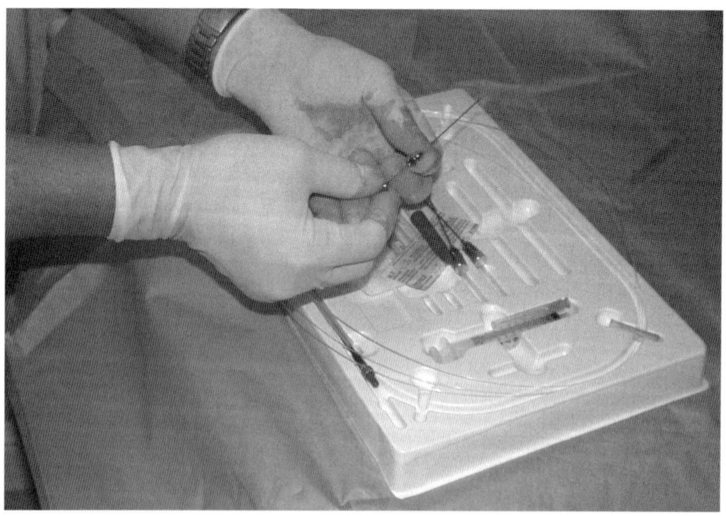

Figure 10.8. The trochar is withdrawn from the 5-inch-long spinal tap needle.

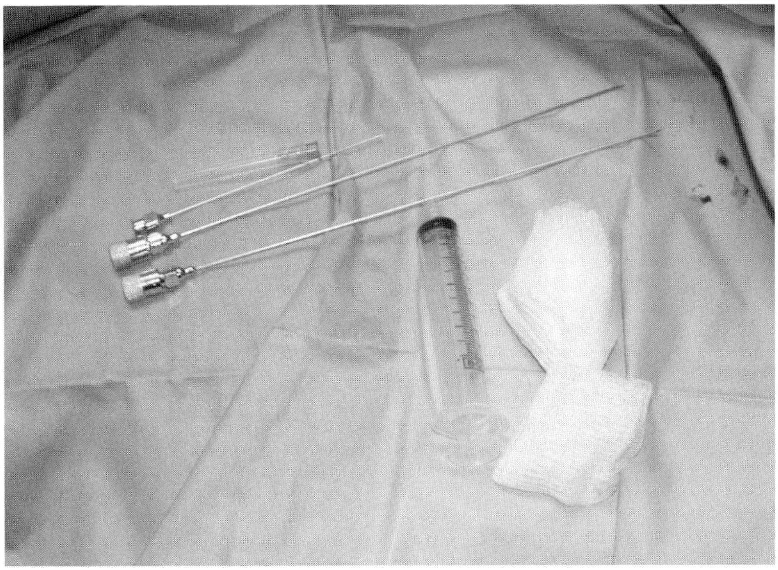

Figure 10.9. The 9-inch needles, the 27-gauge needle, and the 10 mL syringe, are brought to the operating area and placed on a sterile part of the patient drape.

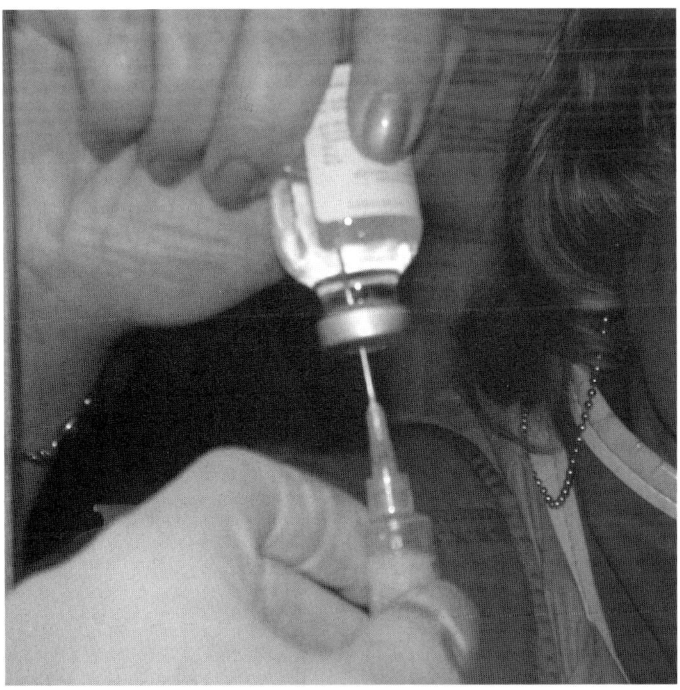

Figure 10.10. One or two 10 mL syringes are filled with 1% Xylocaine.

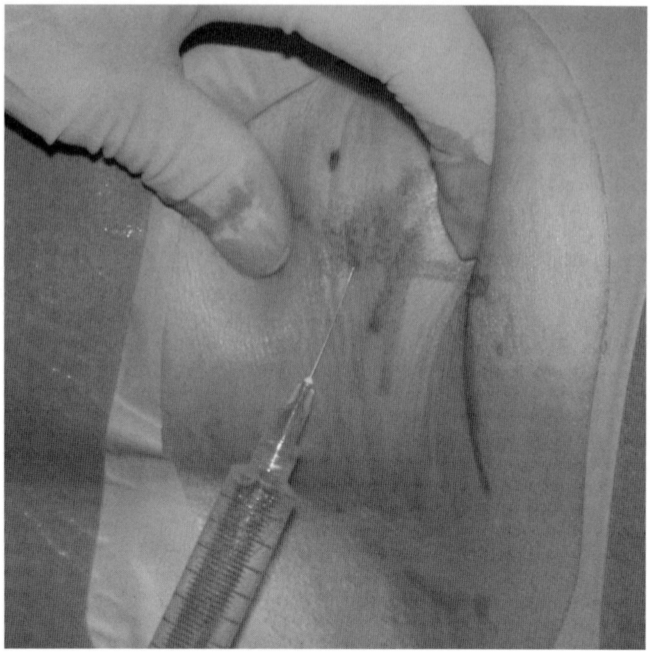

Figure 10.11. The skin over the entry site is infiltrated with Xylocaine.

and inserted at a 45-degree angle to the horizontal in the direction of the needle line drawn in step 9 (Fig. 10.12).

22. Xylocaine is injected, and the needle advanced 2 seconds later; more Xylocaine is injected, and the needle is further advanced until the needle tip is 2 to 3 cm from the spine (Fig. 10.13).
23. No Xylocaine is injected beyond this point, since one does not want to anesthetize the nerve root. This is to be left "live" so that the patient can feel sciatic pain if the needle touches the nerve root. If sciatic pain occurs, the needle is withdrawn and aimed at the "safe triangle" (Fig. 10.14), that is, caudad and posterior, to avoid the nerve root. In over 2000 procedures the author has observed these steps scrupulously, and no nerve root damage has occurred.
24. The 9-inch-long, 18-gauge needle with trochar is then inserted into the patient at a 45-degree angle in the direction of the line drawn in step 9 (Fig. 10.15). The patient is asked to report leg pain. If there is no leg pain, the needle is inserted until the tip appears to abut the edge of the spine (Fig. 10.16). An anteroposterior (AP) view is then obtained. If the tip appears to be some distance from the edge of the spine (Fig. 10.17), the needle is too far anterior, and must be redirected medially. The needle must be withdrawn at least

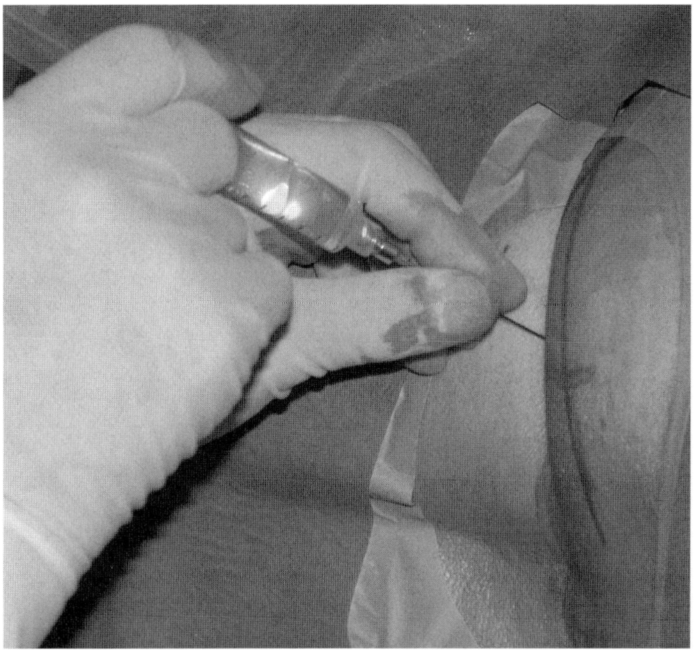

Figure 10.12. The syringe with Xylocaine is connected to the 5-inch spinal tap needle, which is inserted at a 45-degree angle to the horizontal in the direction of the needle shown in Figure 10.4.

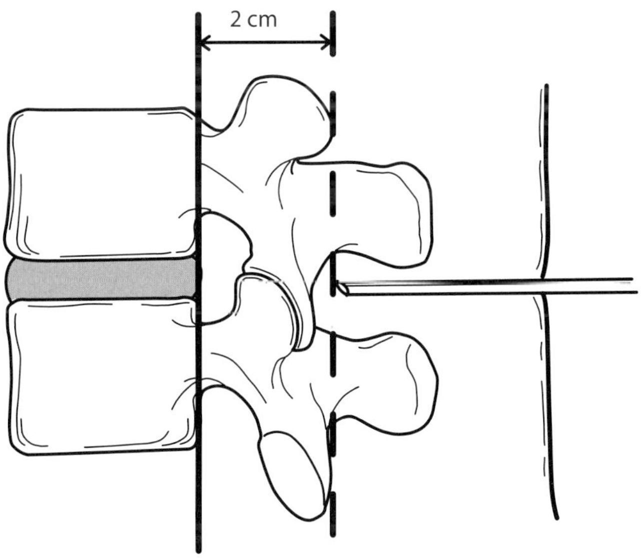

Figure 10.13. Xylocaine is injected as the needle is advanced until the tip is 2 to 3 cm from the spine.

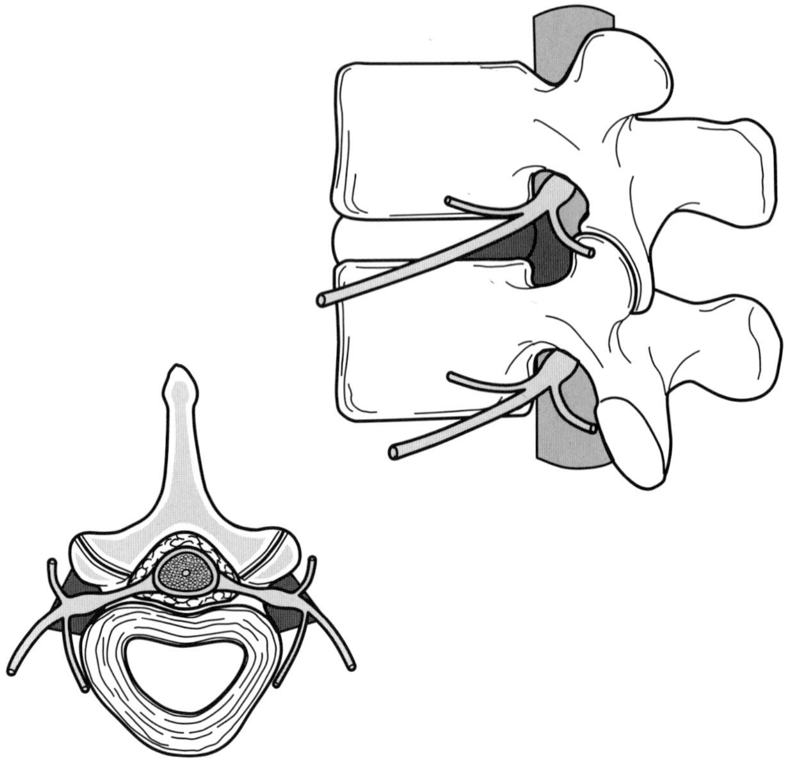

Figure 10.14. The *safe triangle* that avoids the nerve root: aim toward the apex caudally and inferiorly.

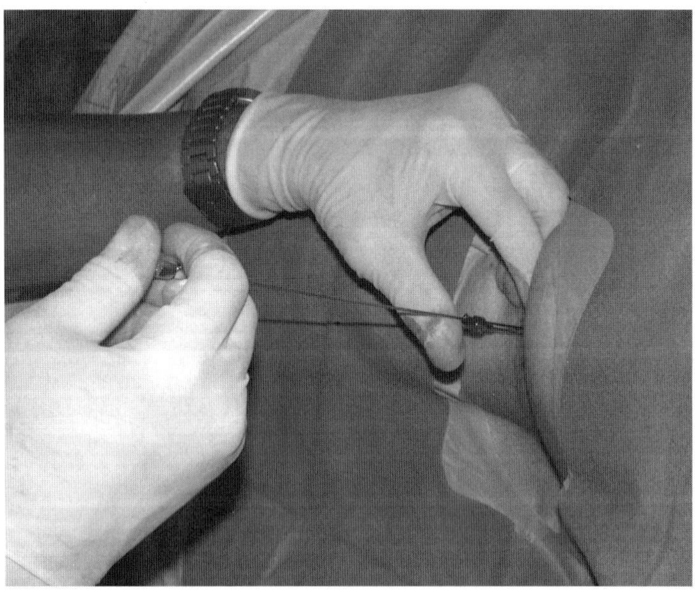

Figure 10.15. The 9-inch, 18-gauge needle is then inserted using the infiltration needle as a guide.

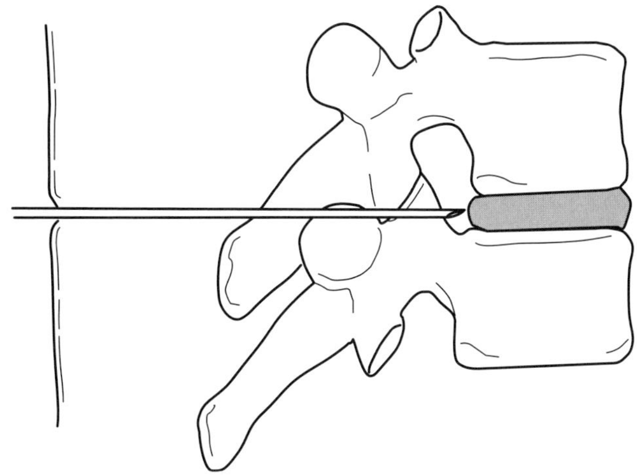

Figure 10.16. The needle tip now abuts the edge of the spine.

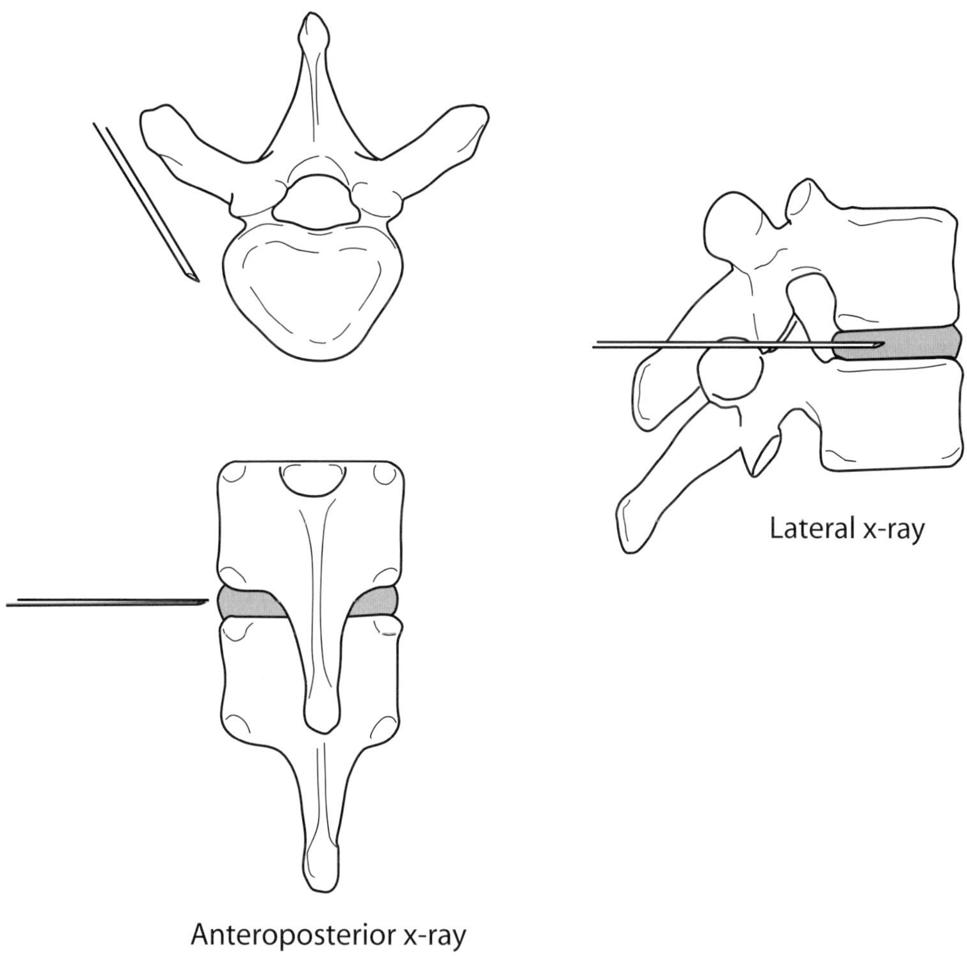

Figure 10.17. This needle tip is too far anterior and must be directed medially.

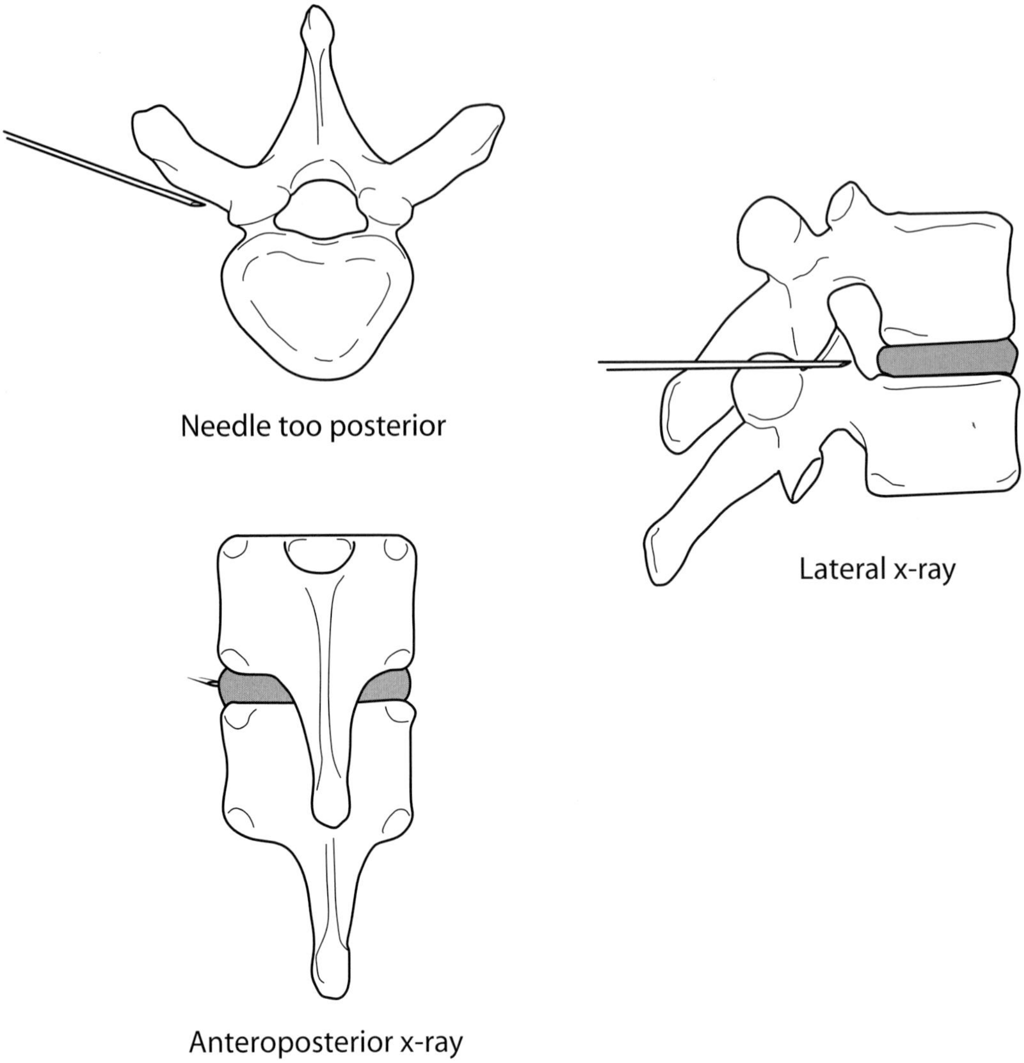

Figure 10.18. This needle tip is too medial and must be redirected anteriorly.

3 to 4 cm before it can be redirected. Now on reinsertion, if the tip is too medial to the edge of the spine in the AP view (Fig. 10.18), the needle must be redirected so that in both AP and lateral views, the tip just abuts the edge of the spine (Fig. 10.19). This, then, is the correct position of the needle, and it may be advanced past the annulus. Before this is done, the patient is told to expect a brief (half-second) moment of pain. On entry past the annulus, the pain will subside because only the surface layers of the annulus have pain fibers. At this point the needle tip is just past the annulus and should be left in place. Spot films are taken in both AP and lateral projections. The needle should also be parallel and midway be-

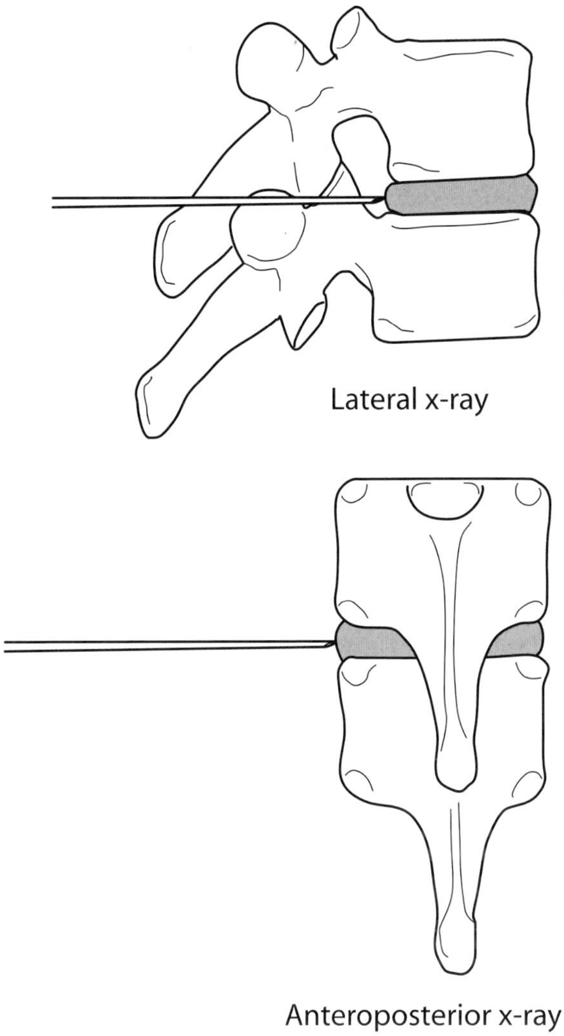

Figure 10.19. The anteroposterior and lateral views of correct needle tip position. In both views, the tip just abuts the edge of the spine.

tween the endplates (Fig. 10.20). With correct needle position, the laser can cause no damage because the tip is just past the annulus and is directed away from the endplates. The laser tract is elliptical and olive shaped, is 2.0 cm long and 5 to 6 mm in diameter, and will be confined to the nucleus pulposus. There will be no damage to any adjacent structures such as the opposite annulus, the intestines beyond, the nerve roots, or the spinal cord or nerves, depending on whether the level is above or below L-1.

Incorrect needle placement is illustrated in Figure 10.21: The needle has been inserted too far into the disc; there will be danger of the laser burning through the opposite annulus

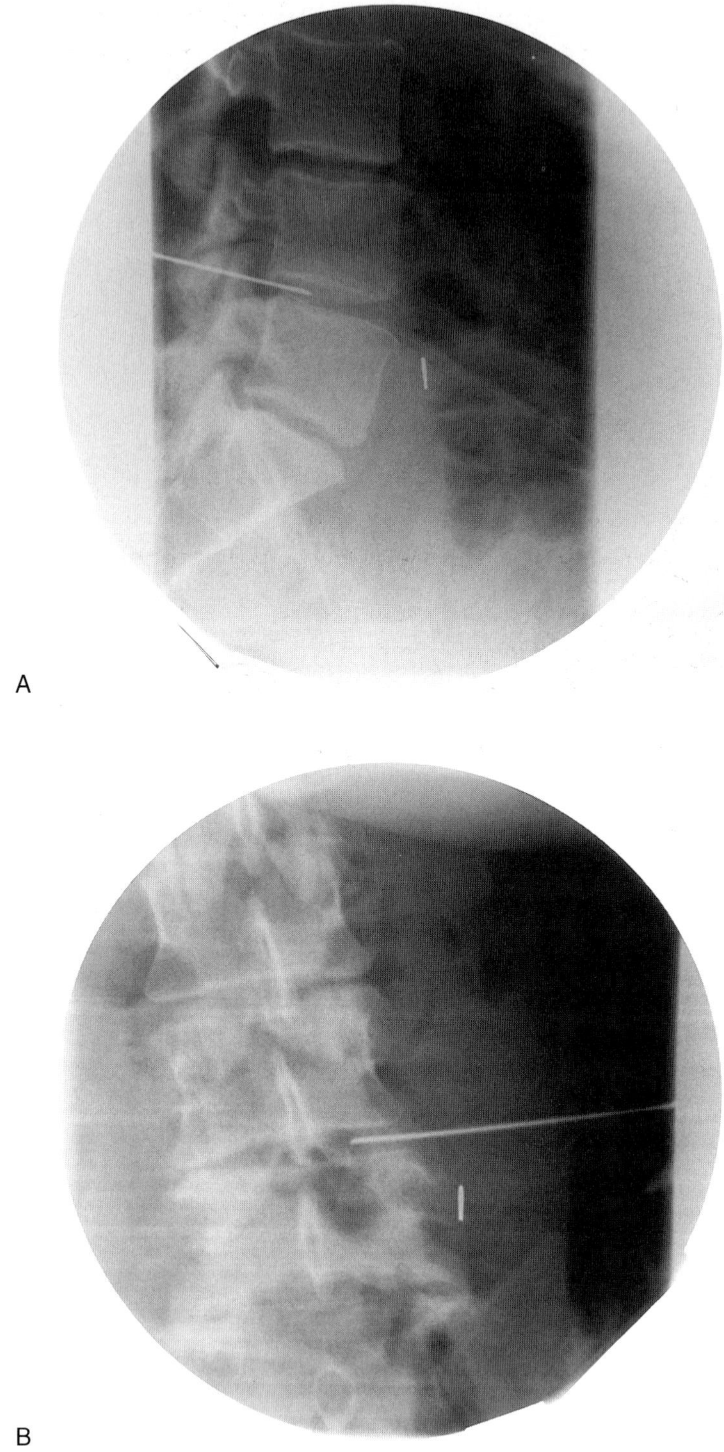

Figure 10.20. The needle is parallel and midway between the endplates.

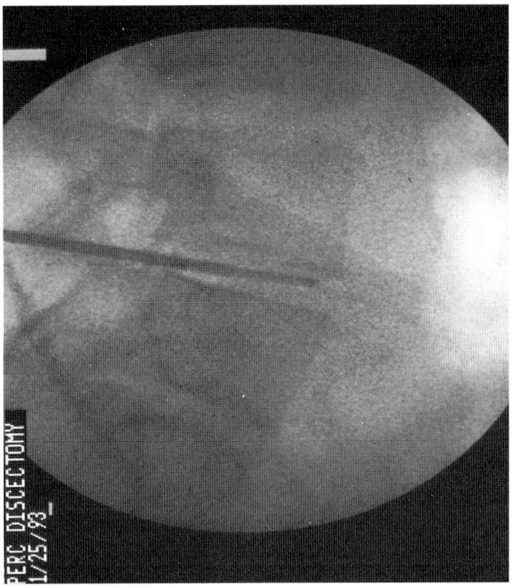

Figure 10.21. The needle has been inserted too far into the disc.

and perforating bowel (there are a few reports of this complication). The needle in Figure 10.22 also is angled incorrectly, being aimed at the endplate. The laser will inflict thermal injury on the endplate and the vertebral bone behind it.

When the needle is incorrectly placed, or if bony obstruction occurs, the needle should be partially withdrawn im-

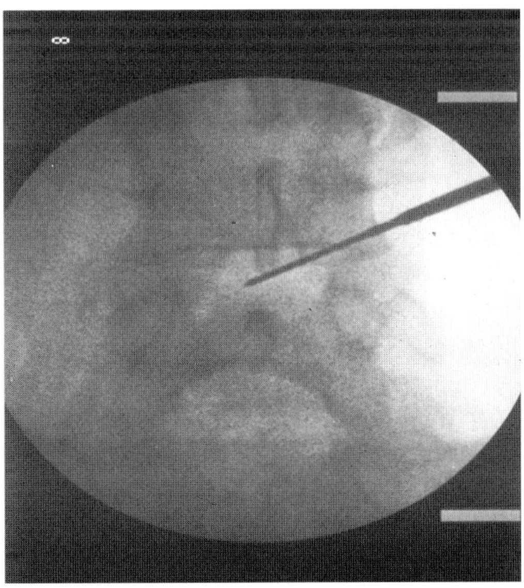

Figure 10.22. The needle is incorrectly placed, being aimed at the endplate.

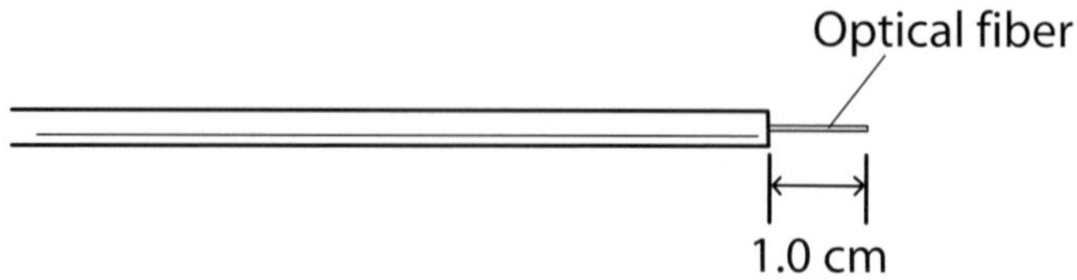

Figure 10.23. The laser fiber correctly protrudes 1.0 cm from the needle tip.

mediately and redirected. If in spite of the new direction, bony obstruction is again encountered, the laser surgeon should not waste time with repeated and fruitless attempts at reinsertion. The needle should be completely withdrawn, and a new entry point tried. This new point may be more medial or more lateral to the 10 cm horizontal line. One must experiment.

25. The optical fiber is carefully removed from the delivery kit and attached to the Neodymium:YAG (Nd:YAG) laser.
26. The laser is turned on and the fiber calibrated, with the fiber turned toward the floor and never toward the face of anyone in the room. (It is not necessary to provide patient or personnel with protective glasses, since the laser will be turned on only when the fiber is in the patient.)
27. The laser fiber is inserted into one of the 9-inch 18-gauge needles and observed to protrude 1.0 cm from the tip of the needle (Fig. 10.23).
28. Laser dosage is at 20 w with shots of 1.0-second duration separated by 5-second pauses. This equals 20 joules per firing. The patient is told to expect pressure and/or warmth. Low-grade pain may occur; if this exceeds 4 on a scale of 1 to 10, the pauses are lengthened appropriately to reduce pain to a more tolerable level. The cause of pain is inadequate heat dissipation, since the disc is poorly vascularized. Slowing down the laser applications will allow for better heat dissipation.
29. In extreme cases I allow the patient to control the firings. I will turn on the laser only when the pain is gone. This adds to patient confidence.
30. If the fiber lights up (turns incandescent), I withdraw the fiber to inspect it for "burnback," which means that the heat of the laser has burned the fiber so that the tip is now less than 1.0 cm from the needle tip. If this happens, a second fiber is obtained from another delivery kit. Because of the cost of the kits, it is helpful that this does not happen very often.
31. In most cases, the full dose of laser energy can be delivered with no problems. The total laser dose varies according to the height of the patient and the volume of the disc. If there

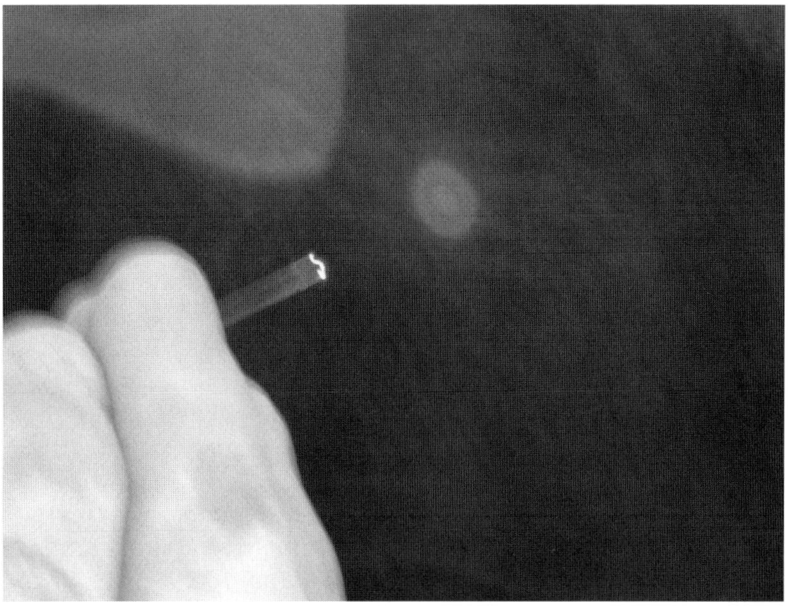

Figure 10.24. A sharp, round laser spot indicating good focus. (See color insert)

is no loss of disc height, the usual dose is 1000 joules (Nd:YAG) for a patient 152 to 165 cm tall, and 1500 joules for one 165 to 183 cm tall or taller. If the disc height is half of that of the other discs, the disc volume will be halved, and I will reduce the number of joules by 25%.

32. At 500 joules I routinely pull the fiber to inspect the tip. Usually the tip has been somewhat degraded; I then refresh the tip by breaking off a tiny portion with thumb and forefinger. This usually results in a sharper round laser spot (Fig. 10.24, see color plate). The laser must then be recalibrated, and the fiber measured against a spare 18-gauge needle to ensure protrusion of the fiber tip to be at least 1 cm beyond the needle tip. At the same time I will smell the proximal end of the needle to try to detect the characteristic odor of burning protein. One must use all one's senses to ascertain that laser vaporization is taking place. If there is no characteristic smell, one should check the laser to see that it is producing full power. If it is not, a backup laser is introduced online. At any rate, a backup laser is good insurance, since a laser that fails when a patient is on the table, draped, with a needle inserted, is a situation to avoid.
33. During the lasing it is important to engage the patient in (one-way) conversation, since it is very reassuring, and much useful information can be imparted. I tell the patient to expect back pain from the needling for about 5 days. If this does not

occur, and it often does not, the patient feels he or she is "ahead of the game." Also, the patient is informed that on day 3 or 4, 10% of patients experience muscle spasm on either the right or the left side, and if that happens, there is nothing to worry about, since it usually subsides in about 3 days. Treatment for this is discussed in Chapter 11, on complications of PLDD.

34. The patient is also informed that although the chance of developing infectious disciitis is only 0.4%, to the patient who does experience this complication, it is 100%. I point out that fever, together with severe midline pain, may be due to infectious disciitis. If these symptoms occur, the patient is to call me and the family doctor immediately. Blood tests will be done, usually a repeat magnetic resonance imaging (MRI), and needle aspiration for bacteriologic studies. All fever is not necessarily infectious disciitis: I had one patient whose post-PLDD fever turned out to be due to a viral pneumonia, one who had bronchitis, and one who had a fever of unknown origin (F.U.O.). If, however, infectious disciitis is found, intravenous (IV) access will be provided, together with appropriate IV antibiotics for a minimum of 6 weeks. The patient is also informed that such rare infections are not due to a fault in aseptic technique—if so, the incidence would be considerably higher. More likely there has been an unsuspected focus of infection, such as a skin, urologic, or dental infection that seeded such as the disc, a vulnerable, relatively avascular target.
35. Now the procedure is completed; the needle is withdrawn, and a dry sterile dressing is applied.
36. The drapes are removed, and the patient is positioned on his or her back.
37. The patient is asked if the pain in the back and leg is gone, or if reduced, by how much.
38. A repeat neurologic examination is performed and recorded.
39. The patient is now assisted to a sitting position.
40. The radial pulse is checked for adequate systolic pressure, and the face and temple are observed for good cerebral perfusion.
41. If both these observations are normal, the patient is allowed to get off the table and walk to the recovery room.
42. An Acubelt (Camp International, MI) is fitted on the patient (Fig. 10.25) and the patient is instructed to wear it during waking hours for 7 days.
43. The patient is sent home or to a nearby hotel and put to bed rest for 24 hours.
44. A methylprednisolone (Medrol) dose pack (4 mg) is prescribed, as well as Percocet (acetaminophen in combination with oxycodone), 5 mg four times a day, as needed, for pain.

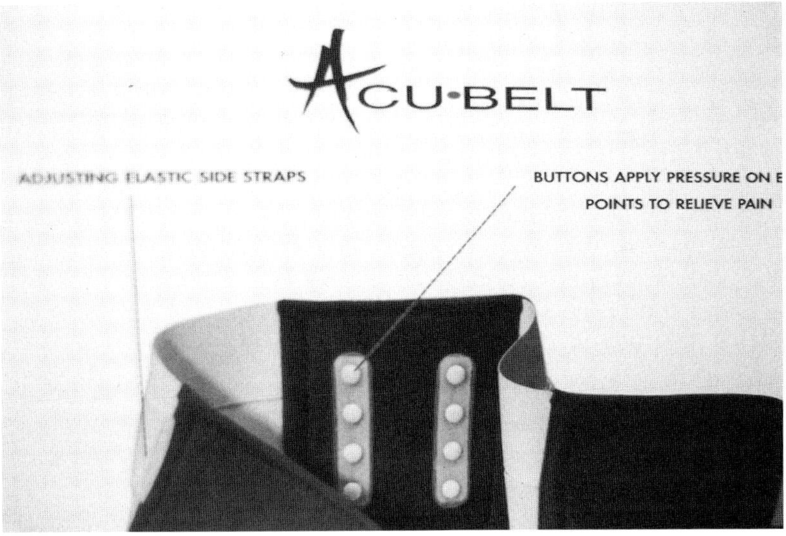

Figure 10.25. An Acubelt is a belt based on acupressure principles. There are eight buttons that press on acupuncture points in the back.

45. The patient is seen in follow-up the next day.
46. If the patient is in the 89% success group, he or she is encouraged to walk one mile in half-mile increments that day.
47. On day 3, the patient can walk more, up to pain limitations.
48. On day 5, the patient who is a white collar worker can return to work for a half-day.
49. If that is well tolerated, on day 6, the patient can resume a full work schedule.
50. The patient is not to drive a car for 7 days.
51. Patients whose work demands lifting or pulling heavy loads are encouraged to become supervisors or teachers or to seek other employment.

Thoracic Discs

Needle entry in the thoracic disc situation is much like that described for lumbar discs. However, the chief danger here is inadvertent creation of pneuomothorax. If the needle is placed too laterally (Fig. 10.26), the tip may enter the thorax and puncture lung tissue. I therefore draw the horizontal line 8 cm from the midline instead of the 10 cm as for the lumbar discs. Since the intercostal vessels and nerves are adjacent to the inferior rib surface (Fig. 10.27), every effort is made to enter the disc with the needle over the superior border of the rib.

At the end of the procedure, the trachea should be examined to ensure that it is not deviated; auscultation of the lungs should be performed to ensure the presence of good breath sounds; and

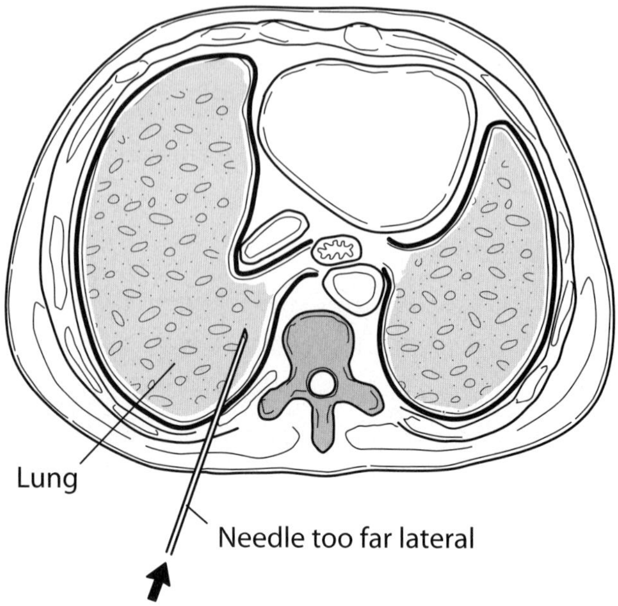

Figure 10.26. A needle placed too far laterally may enter the thoracic cavity and puncture lung tissue, causing pneumothorax.

the pulse is checked for tachycardia. If these signs are all normal, there is no pneumothorax.

When I first began performing PLDD on thoracic discs I had a nearby emergency room standing by with a chest surgeon ready with a chest tube, and a car outside my surgical suite with engine running. I have been lucky; there have been no cases of pneumothorax.

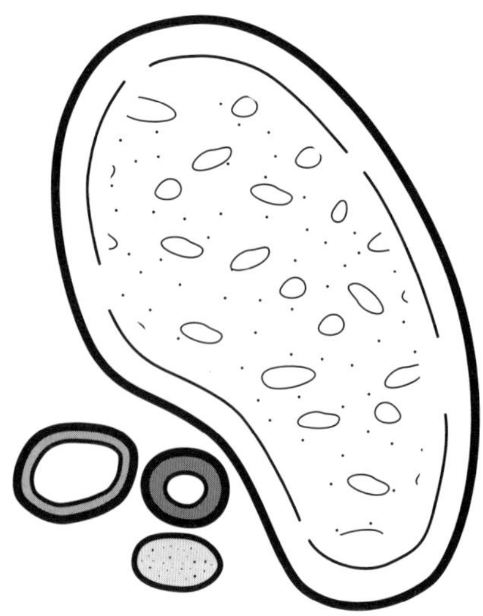

Figure 10.27. Cross-sectional view of a rib showing the position of intercostal artery, vein, and nerve just inferior to the rib.

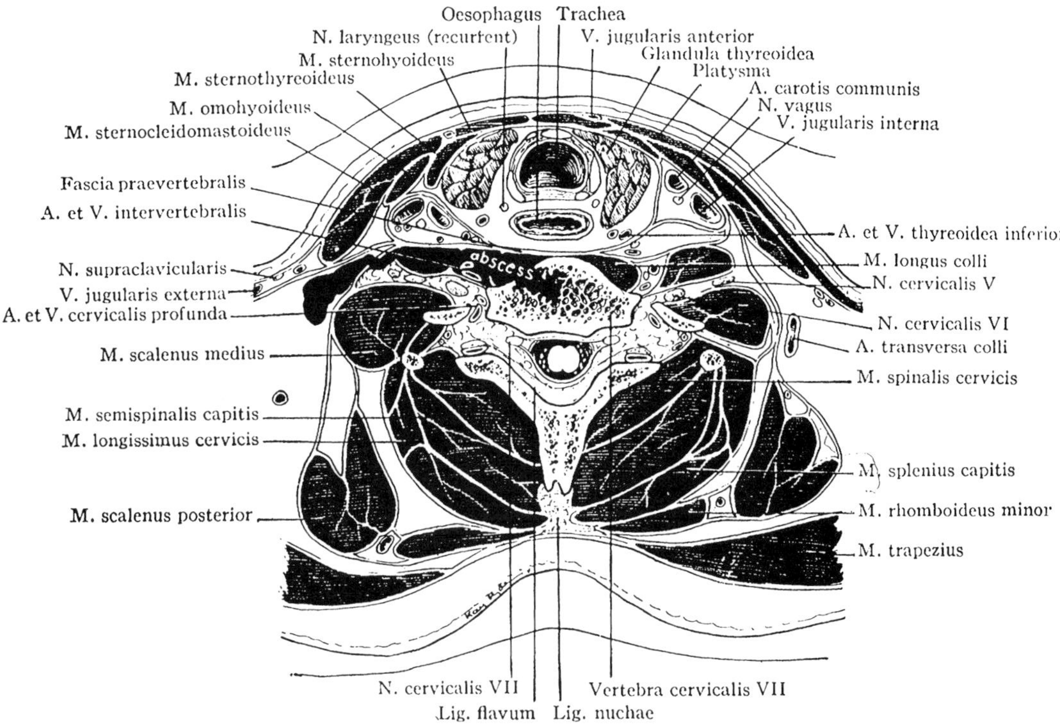

Figure 10.28. Cross-sectional view of the cervical area showing the many vital structures nearby: carotid sheath, vertebral arteries, esophagus, trachea, nerve roots, and spinal cord.

Cervical Discs

A brief outline of the procedure for cervical discs is included for completeness; it is not intended as detailed instructions for the novice laser surgeon. I wish to emphasize that because of the many vital nearby structures (Fig. 10.28) (carotid sheath, vertebral arteries, esophagus, trachea, nerve roots, spinal cord), and the much smaller size of cervical discs, and their angles, it is best not to attempt PLDD of these discs without a one-on-one intensive tutorial from an experienced user of this procedure. The risks are just too high and potentially too serious for the novice laser surgeon to attempt percutaneous decompression of a cervical disc without expert advice.

1. The patient is placed in the supine position.
2. For the C6-7 disc, the patient has been fluoroscoped or has had a single lateral radiograph taken to ensure that the disc can be seen (i.e., is not obscured by a short neck or high shoulders).
3. With thumb pressure to push the trachea and esophagus medially, a line is drawn along the anterior border of the sternocleidomastoid muscle (Fig. 10.29).

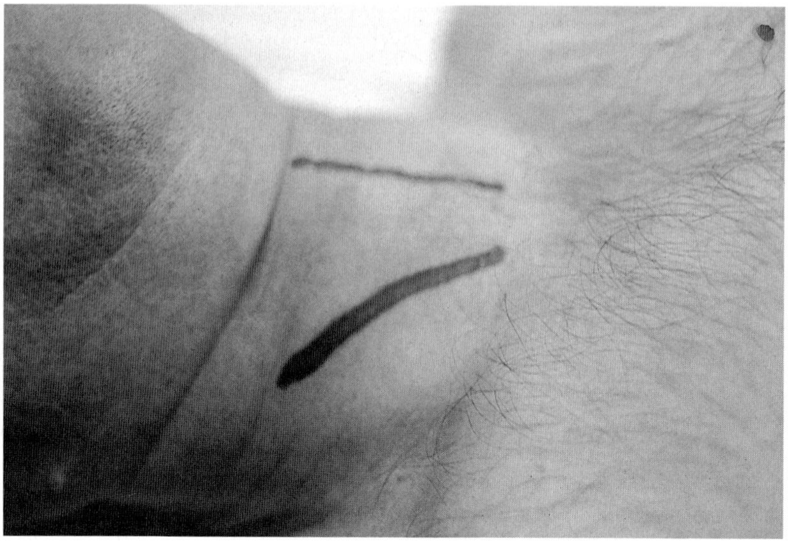

Figure 10.29. A line is drawn along the anterior border of the sternocleidomastoid muscle.

4. With the C-arm placed for a lateral view, a 20-gauge needle is lined up laterally so that it overlies the disc to be treated.
5. A line is drawn alongside this needle. Where it intersects the first line is the point of insertion.
6. A wheal is raised in the skin at this point with 1% Xylocaine.
7. Again, with pressure against the esophagus and trachea, a 21-gauge needle with syringe is used to anesthetize a tract at a 45-degree angle directly onto the disc under continuous fluoroscopic control. When the needle tip just touches the annulus, there is a distinct feel of a slight increase of resistance not unlike piercing a stiff sponge. There is no *give* if the needle hits bone. Anesthetic (1 mL) is injected into the outer surface of the annulus.

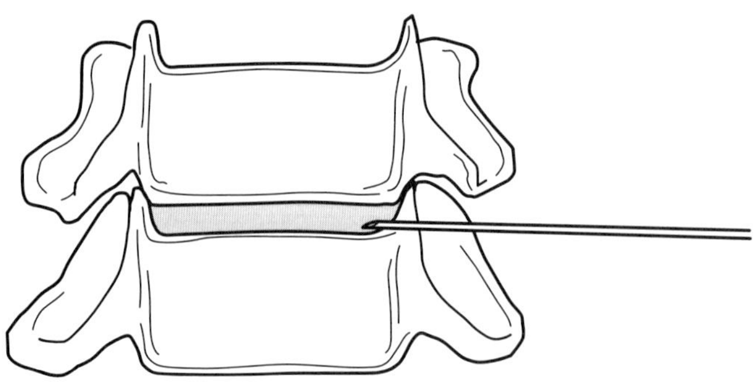

Figure 10.30. Correct needle position in the anteroposterior view.

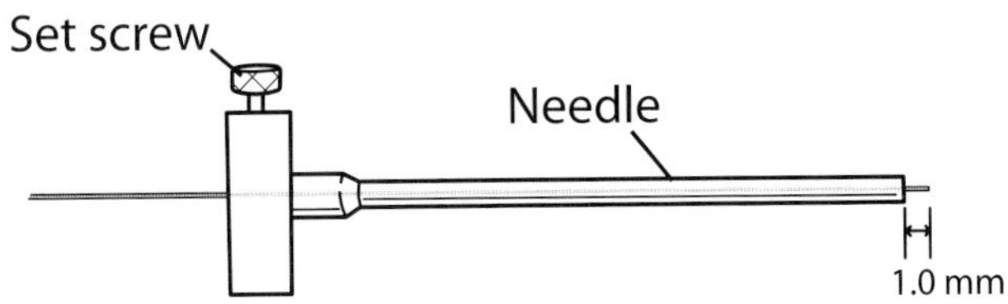

Figure 10.31. The fiber tip protrudes exactly 1.0 mm from the needle tip, and the fiber has been secured proximally by a plastic screw-on stopper.

8. The needle is withdrawn and an 18-gauge Seldinger needle inserted along the anesthetized tract, advanced until it touches the annulus and inserted 5 to 6 mm past the annulus. Anteroposterior and lateral views are obtained to verify correct needle position (Fig. 10.30). Spot films are taken. It is vital not to insert the needle too far.
9. The trochar is withdrawn and the optical fiber, previously measured against another Seldinger needle so that the tip protrudes exactly 1 mm from the needle tip and fitted proximally with a plastic screw-on stopper to maintain this geometry (Fig. 10.31), is inserted into the needle as far as the stopper will allow.
10. The fiber is connected to the laser.
11. The laser, previously calibrated to fire at 1 second × 10 watts, is now turned on with 2- to 3-second pauses until 300 joules has been delivered.
12. The fiber is withdrawn, then the needle.
13. A pressure dressing is applied.
14. In the first 24 hours the patient wears a soft cervical collar. Other than this, there are no restrictions. All my patients returned to work on the first postoperative day.

The Problem of the L5-S1 Disc

In the anterior–posterior view, the L5-S1 disc sits at the bottom of a valley flanked by the two hills of the iliac crest. It is difficult to draw a straight line from the apex of each hill to the disc and expect it to run into the disc such that it is midway between the two endplates and also be parallel to the disc axis.

In the past, this anatomic relationship made it impossible, 25% of the time, for spine surgeons to enter the L5-S1 disc. This was especially true in male patients because of the android shape of the pelvis, with its high crest.

Kambin introduced the curved needle (Fig. 10.32), but even Kambin had difficulty directing it some of the time. In less experienced hands this task is even more difficult.

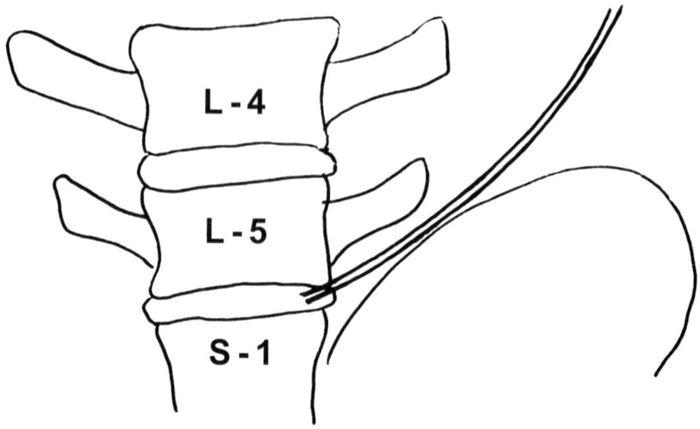

Figure 10.32. The Kambin curved needle.

In the 41 PLDDs of the L5-S1 disc performed by our group until October 1993, the disc was entered with either a straight or curved needle using a dorsolateral approach. Both approaches failed in case 42, so a direct, transthecal midline posterior insertion was used. This approach was used in 20 subsequent cases. *Spinal tap headache* occurred in only seven patients (33%). The design of the needle tip, with a rounded, conical point without a cutting beveled edge, permitted the nerve fibers of the cauda equina to be pushed apart without damage, with minimal radicular pain. There were no neurologic sequelae.

In case 63 (1993) we encountered a low-lying spinous process making the transthecal approach impossible, since the needle would have been pointed at the cephalad endplate. Therefore, entry was attempted 10 degrees away from the midline to bypass the spinous process and still maintain the position midway between the endplates and parallel to the disc axis. Thereafter we began to use this extrathecal route whenever the 45-degree dorsolateral approach was not possible; there have been no complications.

The entry point is determined by fluoroscopy. An AP view, with the radiographic beam directed in a gun barrel fashion so that the disc is viewed without parallax, is obtained. Where this line crosses the midline is marked. The entry point is 10 degrees on either side of the X. For a transthecal entry, the X is the point of entry.

The anatomic relationships are seen in Figure 10.33. The thecal sac is seen in a myelographic study (Fig. 10.34) to terminate between S1 and S2. The X is the entry point of the needle.

In practice, the midline is marked by palpation of the spinous processes of L3 through L5. The needle entry is monitored by lat-

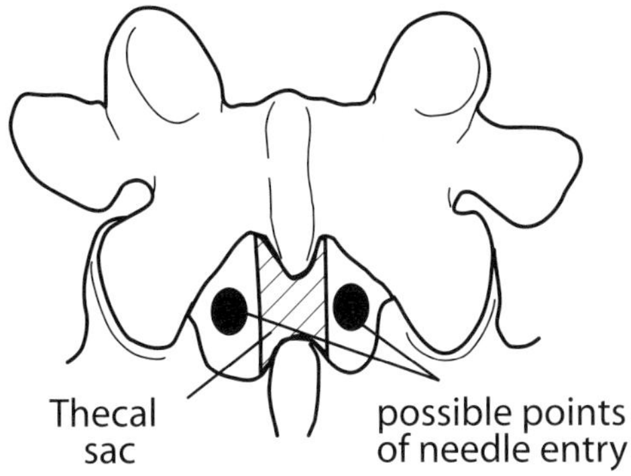

Figure 10.33. The anatomic relationships of the arch formed by the pedicles, cauda equina, and thecal sac.

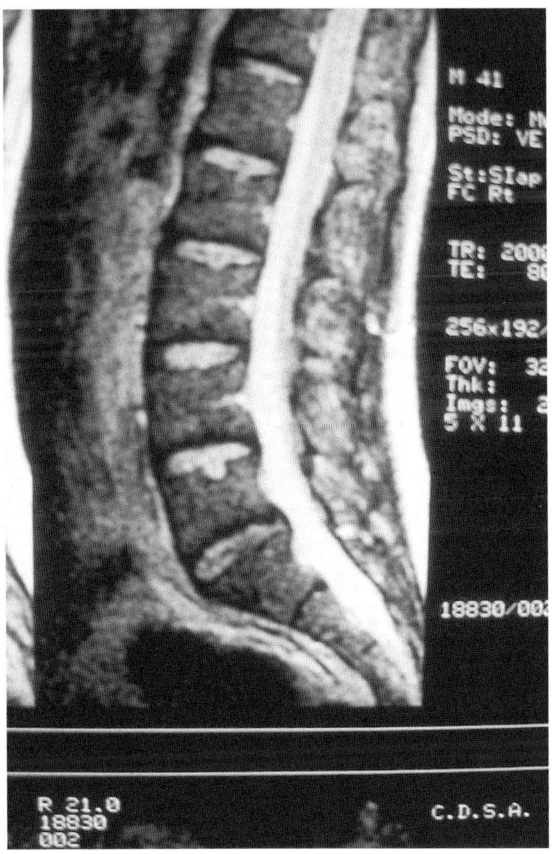

Figure 10.34. Myelographic study showing the termination of the thecal sac between S1 and S2.

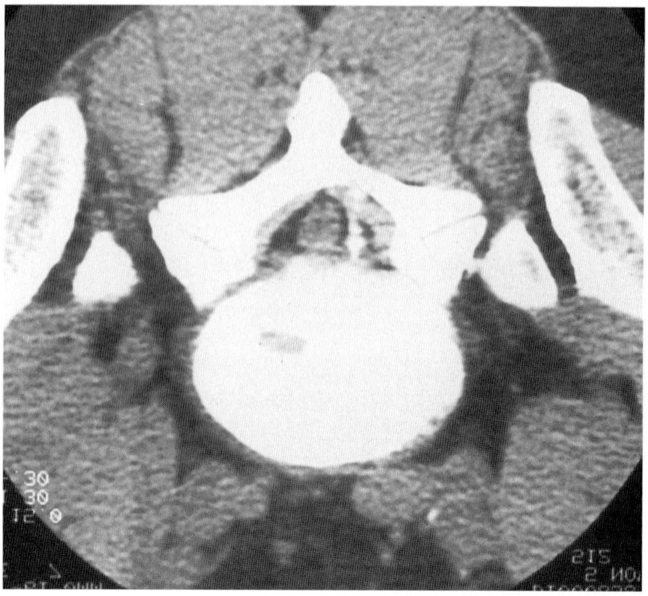

Figure 10.35. Axial view of a computed tomographic scan showing the needle lateral to the thecal sac.

eral fluoroscopy to ensure that the needle is parallel to the disc axis and midway between the two endplates. If the L5-S1 nerve root is touched, the needle is withdrawn and repositioned. I try to aim for the edge of the arch formed by the inferior margin of the L5 vertebral body. When the needle point touches bone, it is *walked* medially until it enters at point O. Further insertion permits entry into the disc while avoiding the thecal sac. In an axial cut of a computed tomography (CT) scan (Fig. 10.35), the needle can be seen to be lateral to the thecal sac. A lateral view is then obtained to ensure that the needle has not been advanced beyond the annulus. This is an extremely important point, since the needle is now aimed at the anterior border of the disc, and excessively deep penetraton risks perforaton of the anterior annulus and damage to pelvic organs.

In the author's experience over the past 17 years, the extrathecal or the transthecal route was employed between 5 and 10% of the time. I must emphasize that if repeated attempts at entry into the L5-S1 disc with the standard dorsolateral route fail, rather than cause further soft tissue damage, it is best to immediately switch to, first, the extrathecal route, and if this fails, to the transthecal route.

11

Complications of Percutaneous Laser Disc Decompression and Their Treatments

Daniel S.J. Choy

The author has experienced only three complications when the Neodymium:YAG (Nd:YAG) laser was used with a delivery system consisting of an 18-gauge needle, in a one-step access to the nucleus pulposus with a direct-firing fiber.

Paraspinal Muscle Spasm

Initially, the average patient's experience was total relief of back and sciatic pain immediately after the procedure, and as reported elsewhere in this text, 50% have return of absent reflexes, and nearly all have normalization of straight leg raising. On the third or fourth postprocedure day, approximately 10% of all patients develop right or left paraspinal muscle spasm that varies in severity from mild discomfort and stiffness responding well to mild analgesics to disabling pain. The onset can be gradual or abrupt. In the severe cases, physical examination discloses spinal curvature laterally with the concavity on the side of the spasm. Palpation reveals tender and very tight musculature with an area of maximal tenderness having a diameter of 1 to 2 cm.

It is my practice to prepare all patients for this possibility during the laser procedure. However, with the preoperative sedation with midazolam (Versed), and the stress of the percutaneous laser disc decompression (PLDD) procedure, some patients may not remember this cautionary note. I generally repeat this warning to the accompanying person. Both patient and spouse or companion are reassured that the muscle spasm usually disappears after 3 or 4 days, and in no way affects the outcome of the treatment.

Hence, reassurance is the first treatment. Diazepam is an excellent muscle relaxant, and this is prescribed in 5 to 10 mg doses, four times a day, depending on the size and weight of the patient. Patients are advised not to drink alcohol, make important decisions requiring judgment, perform acts requiring manual dexterity, or drive a car while on diazepam. They are advised to use local heat and/or soak in a hot tub three times a day. If a heating pad is used while supine, the setting should never be on "high" because if the patient falls asleep, a local burn can result. If heat is found to be ineffective, ice packs may be tried. A supine position is best during the phase of spasm. Walking for short periods is encouraged. Sitting still in one position, because it is associated with the highest intradiscal pressure, is discouraged.

Sacral–Iliac Joint Inflammation

In a private communication, Martin Knight of the Spinal Foundation (Manchester, U.K.) confirmed my own observation derived from over 17 years' experience with PLDD, that approximately 2% of patients show sacral–iliac (S-I) joint inflammation.

The symptoms consist of unilateral pain and tenderness over the S1 or S2 joints. The onset usually occurs several days after excellent relief of sciatic pain by the PLDD. The patient is usually unable to differentiate between the new pain, which may be referred down the leg, from the original pain. It is only on examination that one is able to find a sharply defined point of tenderness over the S-I joint. Pressure on this point aggravates the low back as well as the radicular pain. The remaining positive findings of sciatic involvement (e.g., reflex changes, straight leg raising, etc.) are absent. There may or may not be leukocytosis, elevated sedimentation rate, and a positive bone scan. With early onset of S-I joint inflammation and even later on, if the inflammation is not severe, these signs may continue to be normal. Diagnosis is made by thinking of it, and demonstrating sharply localized point tenderness over the S-I joint. In a personal communication, Dr. Arpad Fejos, a physiatrist at the Columbia University College of Physicians & Surgeons, provided a reasonable mechanism to explain this complication. During the pretreatment period of low back and sciatic pain, some patients defensively *lock* a right or left S-I joint to minimize pain on locomotion. After the sciatic pain has been abolished by PLDD, the defensive locking is no longer needed. The S-I joint then opens and the resulting friction on walking leads to local inflammation.

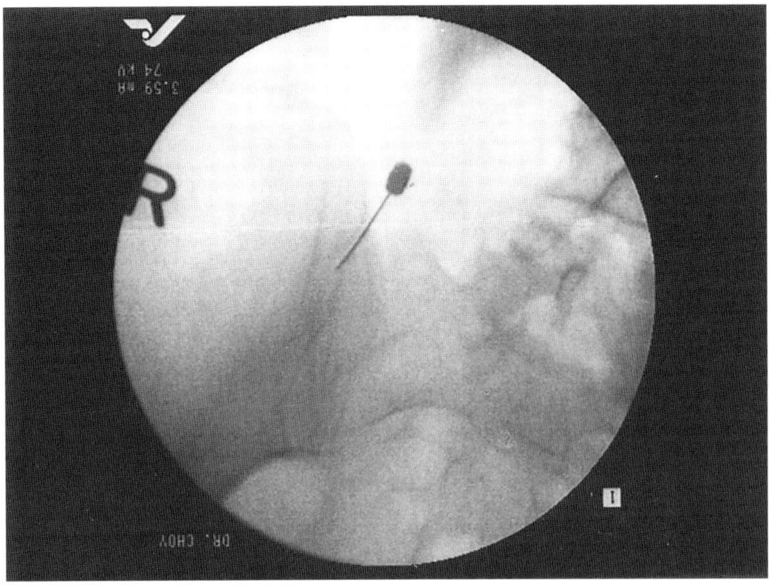

Figure 11.1. Under fluoroscopy and local anesthesia, a spinal tap needle is inserted into the affected sacroiliac joint. Infiltration is performed with 1 mL of lidocaine (Xylocaine) in the distal portion of the syringe and 3 mL of dexamethasone (Decadron) in the proximal portion into the joint. If the diagnosis is correct, relief is experienced within 1 to 2 hours and may last a few days. Oral nonsteroidal anti-inflammatory agents are then prescribed.

This is explained to the patient with the aid of a model of the lumbosacral spine and pelvis. Local infiltration of 3 mL of dexamethasone after prepping and freezing with ethyl chloride spray is usually effective (Fig. 11.1). The usual sequence of events, if the diagnosis is correct, is onset of pain relief in approximately 2 hours, lasting anywhere from 12 hours to a week. Repeat steroid injections may be performed at appropriate times, but not more than a total of three times in 6 months. An oral anti-inflammatory agent may be prescribed such as a COX-A inhibitor.

Disciitis: Aseptic or Infectious

In my first 200 patients treated at St. Luke's–Roosevelt Hospital, there were two cases of infectious disciitis. Both were caused by *Staphylococcus aureus,* and both responded to curative vancomycin given intravenously for 6 weeks. The incidence was therefore 1%. In the next 1850 patients treated on an outpatient basis at the New York Laser Spine Center, I encountered seven with infectious disciitis, four with *S. aureus,* and one with *Streptococcus viridans,* for an incidence of 0.38%. There were an equal number of aseptic disciitis cases in both institutions, but these required only conservative, symptomatic treatment further described here.

The usual onset of infectious disciitis is from day 3 to 5 after PLDD. Fever and severe pain occurs over the affected disc. Early on, the white blood cell count (WBC) and erythrocyte sedimentation rate (ESR) may be normal. All fever, however, is not disciitis. After a cervical PLDD, one of my patients had fever that turned out to be due to a viral pneumonia, another had bronchitis, a third had a fever of unknown origin (F.U.O.). If disciitis is suspected, an magnetic resonance imaging (MRI) with gadolinium enhancement should be performed promptly. Signs of disciitis are readily appreciated by an experienced radiologist, with changes in the T2-weighted images and positive contrast enhancement. In doubtful cases a bone scan may be obtained, but usually this is not necessary. Thin-needle aspiration of the suspected disc should be performed under fluoroscopic control for identification of bacteria and sensitivity studies. Since the usual infective agent is *S. aureus*, an access port is inserted early on and intravenous (IV) vancomycin started pending receipt of the results of bacteriologic studies. This treatment is continued on an outpatient basis for 6 weeks after discharge from the hospital when the patient has defervesced.

Two patients required open drainage of epidural abscesses. All recovered with antibiotic therapy.

The lower incidence of infectious disciitis when the procedure site was changed from the hospital to a stand-alone surgical suite reflects the higher incidence of nosocomial infections in a hospital. It is hard to ascribe the 0.38% incidence of infectious disciitis to a break in aseptic technique, since the same standard of site preparation has been used and the same draping of patient and fluoroscopic C-arm practiced with exceptional care and precision. Despite careful preoperative studies for systemic infection, there may have existed, in the few patients who developed this complication, some hidden locus of infection such as a small dental absess, or even a low-grade skin infection. The poorly vascularized disc is then "seeded" from this source.

Aseptic Disciitis

Aseptic disciitis is a diagnosis of exclusion. The signs and symptoms are the same as for infectious disciitis. Fever, however, is absent, and the WBC and ESR remain normal. Disc aspiration is negative. These patients respond to 3 to 4 days of bed rest, anti-inflammatory agents, and analgesics appropriate to the pain perceived by the patient. Analgesia is important, since every patient has his or her own pain threshold. Every experienced physician is aware of this. The type of analgesic must therefore be tailored to the individual patient. A *cookbook* approach should be avoided.

A patient who has pain relief is a grateful patient. A patient in pain is an angry one.

Other Complications

Some other complications seen with multistep, side-firing laser systems such as the Holmium:YAG (Ho:YAG) laser and the potassium triphosphide (KTP) system. These are described briefly.

Thermal Endplate Necrosis

Extensive reports of thermal endplate necrosis have been published by Botsford and others, and I have seen it in litigation cases in which I have been called as an expert witness. The problem is caused by inadequate training of an operator, who has obeyed incorrect instruction manuals that advise firing the laser throughout a 360-degree fiber rotation. I have actually seen such a manual, apparently written by a committee with little or no experience in laser–tissue interaction. Obviously if one fires a side-firing fiber while the laser output is directed cephalad or caudad, the laser beam will damage the endplate. This thermal necrosis often extends beyond the end plate to cause necrosis in the vertebral body (Fig. 11.2).

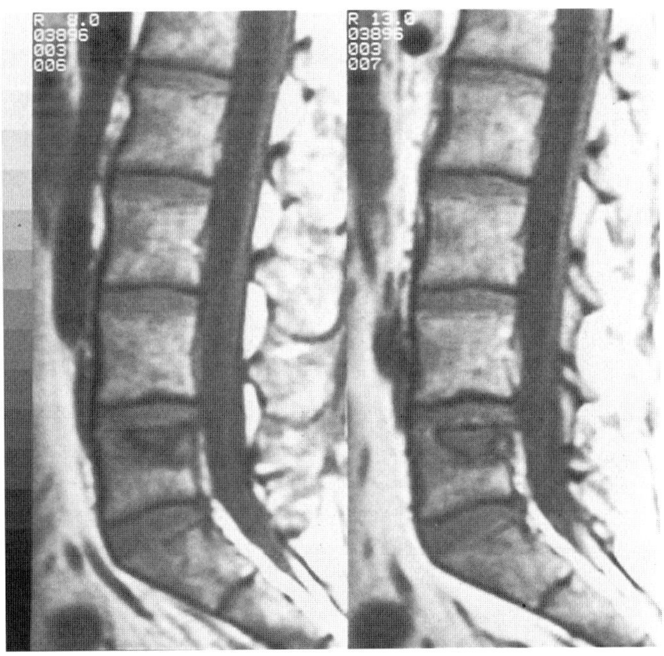

Figure 11.2. Necrosis of the cranial portion of the L5 vertebra has been caused by the side-firing fiber system of the potassium triphosphide (KTP) laser. I have also seen this effect with the Ho:YAG laser, but never with the direct-firing Neodymium:YAG (Nd:YAG) laser.

These patients have immediate exacerbation of local back pain that can last more than a year. The treatment, which consists of anti-inflammatories and/or steroids, is often ineffective.

Perianular or Epidural Ecchymosis and/or Hematoma

Ecchymoses and hematomas are a consequence of the larger bore trochars necessitated by the need for cooling the trochar and fiber with saline irrigation in the Ho:YAG laser. The multistep requirement, with dilatation and trephining of the annulus, also contributes to local soft tissue damage and blood vessel disruption. Diagnosis is dependent on radiology; the computed tomography (CT) scan is best in this application. Treatment consists of immobilization of the spine. Direct local pressure is of doubtful value, but correction of abnormal thrombotic cascade is essential.

Nerve Root Damage

I have seen, again as an expert witness, cases of permanent nerve root damage caused by incorrect placement of side-firing fibers. As Botsford likes to say, "Laser not in disc, laser cause much trouble."

There is no treatment for a damaged nerve root.

Cauda Equina Syndrome

Cauda equina syndrome in postprocedure PLDD patients results from excessive anesthesia. Patients being treated with PLDD may have mild sedation, but sedation should not be pushed to a point at which the patient is unable to feel nerve pain. Severe local and/or radicular pain is produced by direct contact of the needle or trochar with a nerve root, and by firing of a laser onto a nerve root. If the patient is overanesthetized, this "last defense" is gone and great damage can result. Again, there is no treatment for this complication except prevention.

Perforation of Viscus

Incorrect needle placement due to inadequate training of the operator is the only cause of perforation of the viscus. If the needle or trochar is precisely placed, with the terminal opening just past the annulus and the needle or trochar parallel to the disc axis, midway between the two endplates, the laser, if fired properly, can do no damage, since the laser beam interacts only with the nucleus pulposus. If, on the other hand, the needle is inserted too far, the laser beam may penetrate the opposite annulus and perforate intestine. Figure 11.3 shows two lateral views of the L5-S1 disc. In the upper one, the needle is inserted to the correct

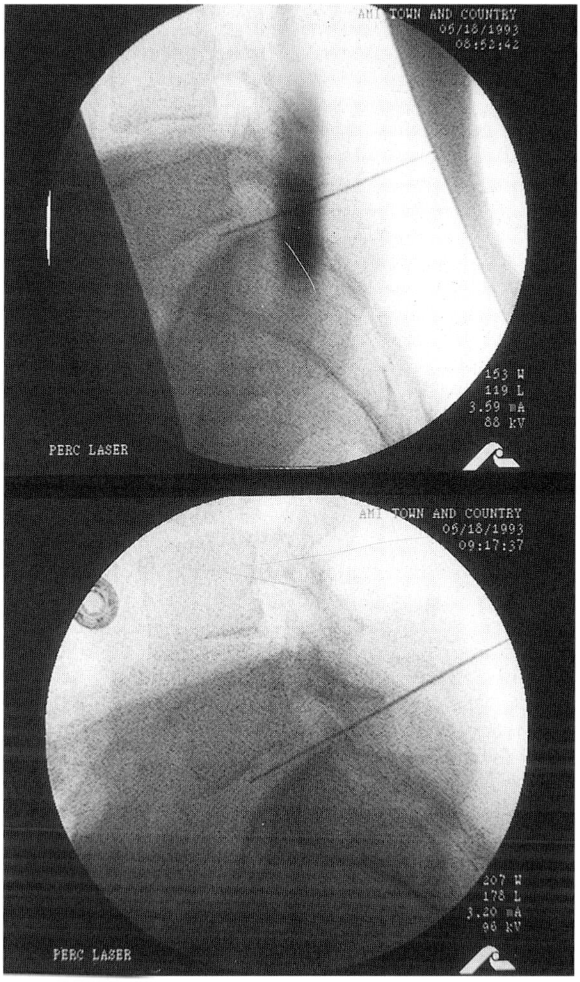

Figure 11.3. In the upper view of the L5-S1 disc, the needle has been inserted to the proper depth, just beyond the annulus, so that the laser tract will be entirely within the nucleus pulposus. In the lower view, the needle has been inserted too far into the disc, so that there is danger of laser perforation of the opposite annulus given the 2 cm length of the Neodymium:YAG (Nd:YAG) laser tract.

depth—the tip is just beyond the annulus. In the lower view, the needle is too far into the disc, and there is risk of laser perforation of the opposite annulus. The treatment is prevention; if perforation is suspected, an immediate laparotomy is indicated.

Needle Tract Heating

Rarely, a fiber tip in contact with nuclear material will "catch fire," become incandescent, and light up the entire proximal fiber.

If this "burnback" occurs, the operator should stop the laser, pull out the fiber, and measure its tip protrusion by inserting it into an identical needle. In the case of the Nd:YAG laser, the fiber tip should protrude 1.0 cm from the needle tip. If it is shorter, there is danger of the needle heating up when the laser is on, and there may be thermal injury along the needle tract. It is safer then to open another delivery set and use a new fiber. If heating of the needle tract occurs, the patient will experience sharp local pain every time the laser is fired.

It is my practice to pull the fiber at 500 joules, both to inspect the tip and to smell the needle opening for the odor of burning protein. One should use all one's senses to ensure that the lasing process is occurring and that one does not have a "dead" laser or a "dead" fiber.

Burnt Needle Tips and Burnt Fiber Tips

Botsford, again, has seen burnt needle and fiber tips in the course of PLDD with KTP and Holmium:YAG (Ho:YAG) lasers. Sometimes failure of the saline cooling irrigation system (blockage of inflow or outflow ports) in the case of the Ho:YAG laser has resulted in such burning. The *foreign bodies* have been left behind (Fig. 11.4) in the discs with unknown consequences.

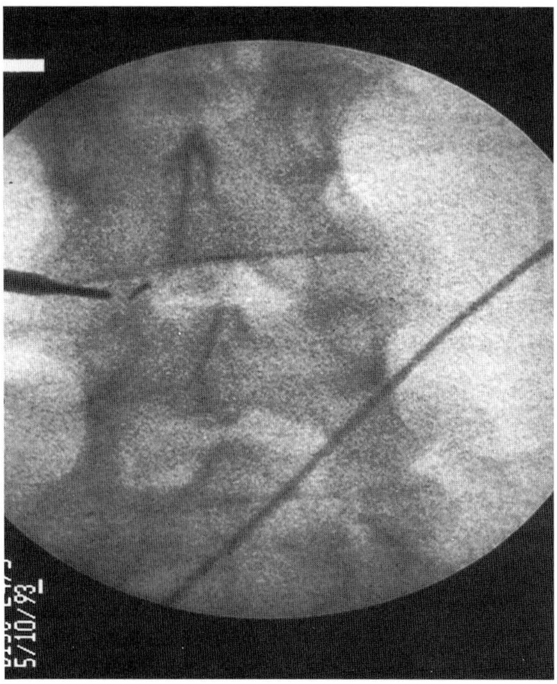

Figure 11.4. Burnt needle/fibertip left behind in a Ho:YAG-treated patient.

General Comments

A paraphrase of Occam's razor states that the simplest solution is the best solution. It is the author's strong convictiion that of the three available laser systems, the best and safest is the Nd:YAG. This requires the smallest trochar (1.0 mm), a one-step insertion into the disc, and only 800 to 1500 joules of total laser energy. There is no requirement for multiple steps to open the way for a 2.5 mm trochar, and no requirement to irrigate continuously to cool the trochar and fiber tip. The need for 18,000 to 19,000 joules (Ho:YAG) versus the 800 to 1500 joules (Nd:YAG) is like driving a car with one foot on the gas pedal and one foot on the brake. The more complicated a system, the more that can go wrong.

Witness the long list of complications of the more complex system. Worldwide, the Nd:YAG has the longest follow-up and the longest history of safe use.

12

Postprocedure Physical Therapy

Arpad S. Fejos

As mentioned in earlier chapters, the majority of patients undergoing percutaneous laser disc decompression (PLDD) experience relief of low back and leg pain immediately after the procedure. However, this immediate relief does not prescribe return to full activity. This chapter outlines postprocedural rehabilitation protocols for PLDD.

Unfortunately, the typical patient undergoing PLDD has had a long, protracted course of discogenic pain with radiculopathy caused by herniated discs. During this prolonged course, patients usually assume poor biomechanics as a result of the body's natural instinct to splint the painful lumbar segment. This coping attempt sequentially affects the kinetic chain above and below the initial injury, and to prevent reinjury or new injury to adjacent segments, the domino effect must be corrected. It is therefore important to correct the predisposing and the ensuing muscular disparity.

Basic Anatomy and Biomechanics

Before going further, it is important to review some basic anatomy and biomechanics of the lumbar spine. Lumbar spinal stability is influenced by activation of proper muscles, coordinated contractions, as well as sufficient strength and endurance of this muscular system. The components of this system, the lumbar extensors, are divided into the deep multifidi and superficial erector spinae. The deep multifidi insert and originate over one or many vertebral segments. They are believed to provide stability to individual motion segments and are most active during rotational motions. They are predominantly postural fibers that are able, because of their proximity to vertebral bodies, quickly and directly affect stability. The erector spinae muscles are much stronger and longer. They therefore provide counterbalance while a person is lifting and bending, and act to preserve lumbar lordosis.

The abdominal muscle, specifically the rectus abdominis, provides lumbar flexion and preserves lordosis. The transversus abdominis and oblique abdominal muscles stabilize the lumbar spine by inhibiting translation and rotation. The quadratus lumborum provides stability during lumbar bending and twisting and therefore acts as a dynamic stabilizer.

Weakness, decreased endurance, or alterations in agonist–antagonist muscle group contractions can cause increased, unbalanced stress to be exerted on the lumbar intervertebral discs. A sedentary lifestyle is one of the largest contributors to developing muscular fatigue and dysfunction. Overuse of stabilizing muscle, as in heavy or improper lifting, causes muscle imbalance secondary to injury. Postural muscles tend to become overused secondary to prolonged standing or sitting. These biomechanical imbalances can result in or be a result of a lumbar herniated disc. Also, new research has identified a common risk factor, confirming that genetics play a significant role in lumbar disc disease. It is therefore vital that proper biomechanics be taught through a comprehensive therapy program to minimize the risk of reinjury. Since there is little evidence to prove that one rehabilitation method is better than another, the most familiar method will be summarized. It has been established that bed rest and inactivity are detrimental to recovery.

Rehabilitation After Percutaneous Laser Disc Decompression

Activity guidelines after PLDD include rest for 24 hours, reclining or lying down with limited sitting or walking. After the first 24 hours, walking and sitting tolerance can be increased to 20 minutes. The patient should wear a corset for all activities to limit bending and twisting motions for the first 2 weeks. A small percentage of patients will experience paraspinal spasticity 3 to 4 days postprocedure. This can be controlled with warm packs for 30 minutes, four times per day, as well as cyclobenzaprine (Flexeril) if the symptoms are severe. Pain is well controlled with nonsteroidal anti-inflammatory drugs (NSAIDs); in the odd severe case, short-acting opioids can be used. Deep tissue massage is contraindicated in the first 2 weeks to allow for complete healing of the needle tract. Patients may return to work 3 days postprocedure, provided the work is in an office, with no bending or twisting and limited sitting as dictated by symptoms. Patient's who do physical labor can return to light duty in 7 to 10 days. Light housework can resume after 1 week, but again, no bending or twisting.

The level of the initial physical therapy program depends on the patient's functional staging prior to PLDD. Staging depends on the acuteness and severity of the symptoms. Patients in stage 1 before PLDD have difficulties performing basic daily activities such as sitting, standing, or walking. Patients in stage 2 can perform most activities of daily living but cannot perform heavier activities of lifting and vacuuming. Stage 2 patients usually have less severe symptoms that have lasted for a prolonged period of time. The goal of therapy is to progress the patient to a higher stage.

Physical therapy should be initiated one-week postprocedure, supervised by a therapist experienced in spine care. The patient should also carry out a home exercise program. These exercises should be initially taught to the patient by a physical therapist to insure precision. The home exercises include a core program of (1) supine hamstring stretch (Fig. 12.1), 5 reps, hold for 60 seconds on each side; (2) knee to chest, single (Fig. 12.2), 5 reps, hold for 60 seconds on each side; (3) piriformis stretch, 5 reps, hold for 60 seconds on each side; (4) buttock squeeze (Fig. 12.3), 10 reps, hold for 20 seconds; and (5) walking for 20 to 60 minutes daily. This program, which should continue for 4 to 6 weeks, will

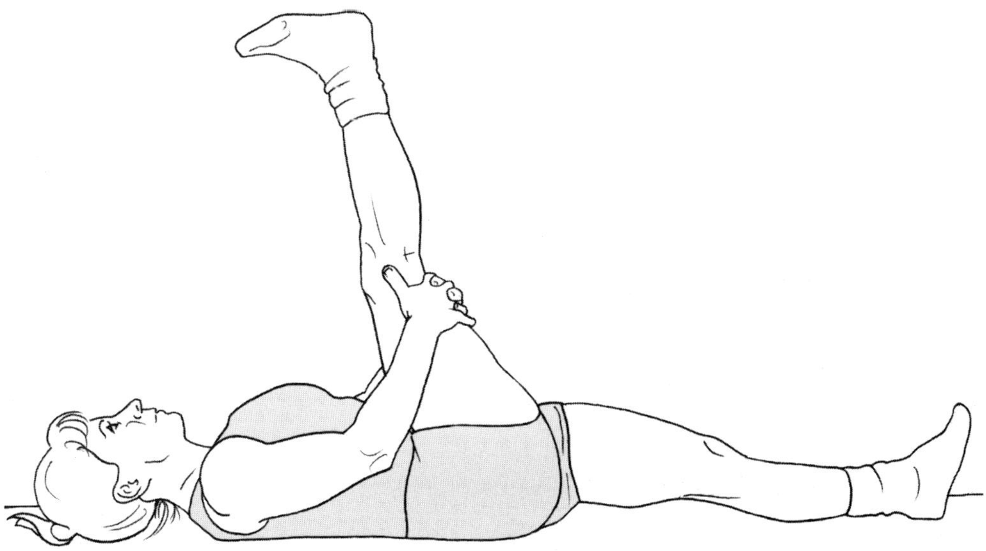

Figure 12.1. Supine hamstring stretch: hold for 60 seconds on each side; repeat 5 times.

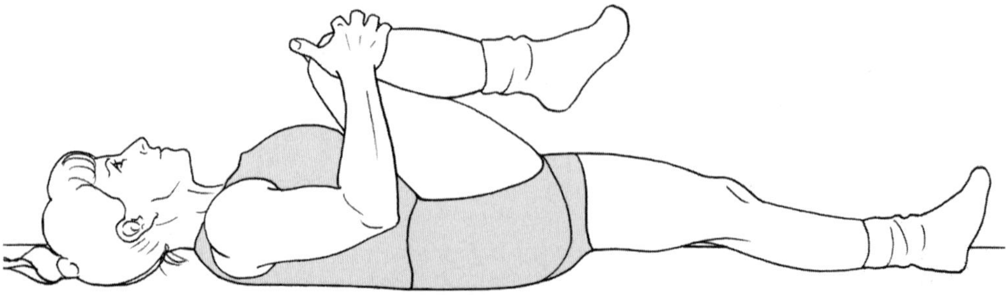

Figure 12.2. Knee to chest, single: hold for 60 seconds on each side; repeat 5 times.

supplement stage 1 exercises in therapy. Further home exercises are prescribed by the therapist and are based on the patient's progress in therapy.

Stage 1

Stage 1 of therapy can begin one week postprocedure and generally lasts 4 to 6 weeks. Patients who fall into stage 2 can bypass this level of therapy. Stage 1 focuses around flexion or extension exercises, depending on patient symptoms. That is, if symptoms are exacerbated by flexion, these exercises will be avoided, likewise for extension exercises. This stage is known as the centralization stage, in which the goal is to prevent pain from radiating peripherally.

In extension exercise programs, the patient assumes the quadruped position with gentle rocking back and forth (Fig. 12.4). This motion should be repeated 10 to 20 times, four times a session, with 5-minute rest intervals. In other exercises, the prone-on-elbows (Fig. 12.5A), and prone press-up exercises, the patient is lying prone with elbows used as a prop. This position is held for 30 seconds and repeated 8 to 10 times. This may progress to prone press-ups (Fig. 12.5B), holding for 30 seconds and repeating 10 to 20 times, depending on patient strength. As with all exercises, the response of patient symptoms dictates whether they will be continued.

In flexion exercise programs, the patient starts in the supine position (Fig. 12.6) bringing the knees to the chest, holding for 20 to 30 seconds, then repeating 10 to 20 times.

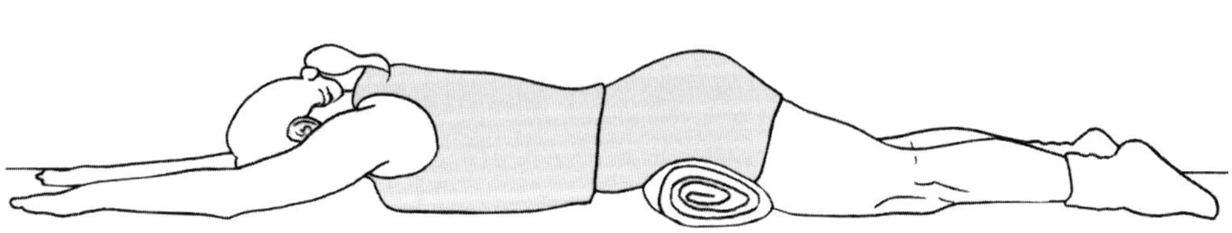

Figure 12.3. Buttock squeeze: hold for 20 seconds; repeat 10 times.

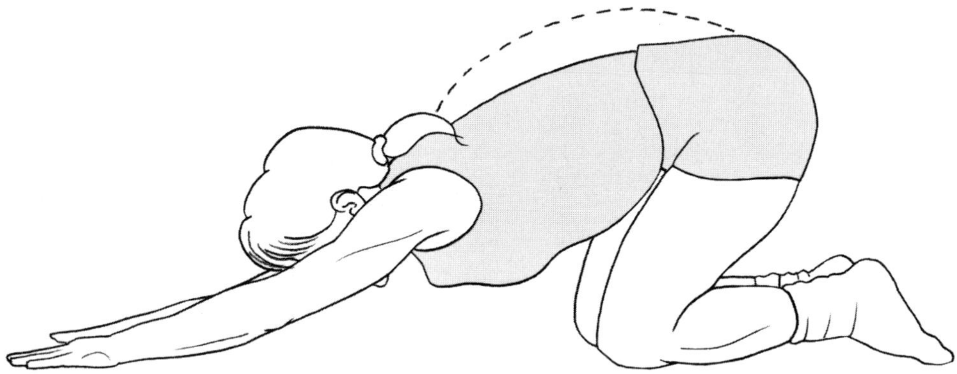

Figure 12.4. Quadruped position with gentle rocking back and forth: repeat 10 to 20 times, 4 times a session, with 5-minute rest intervals.

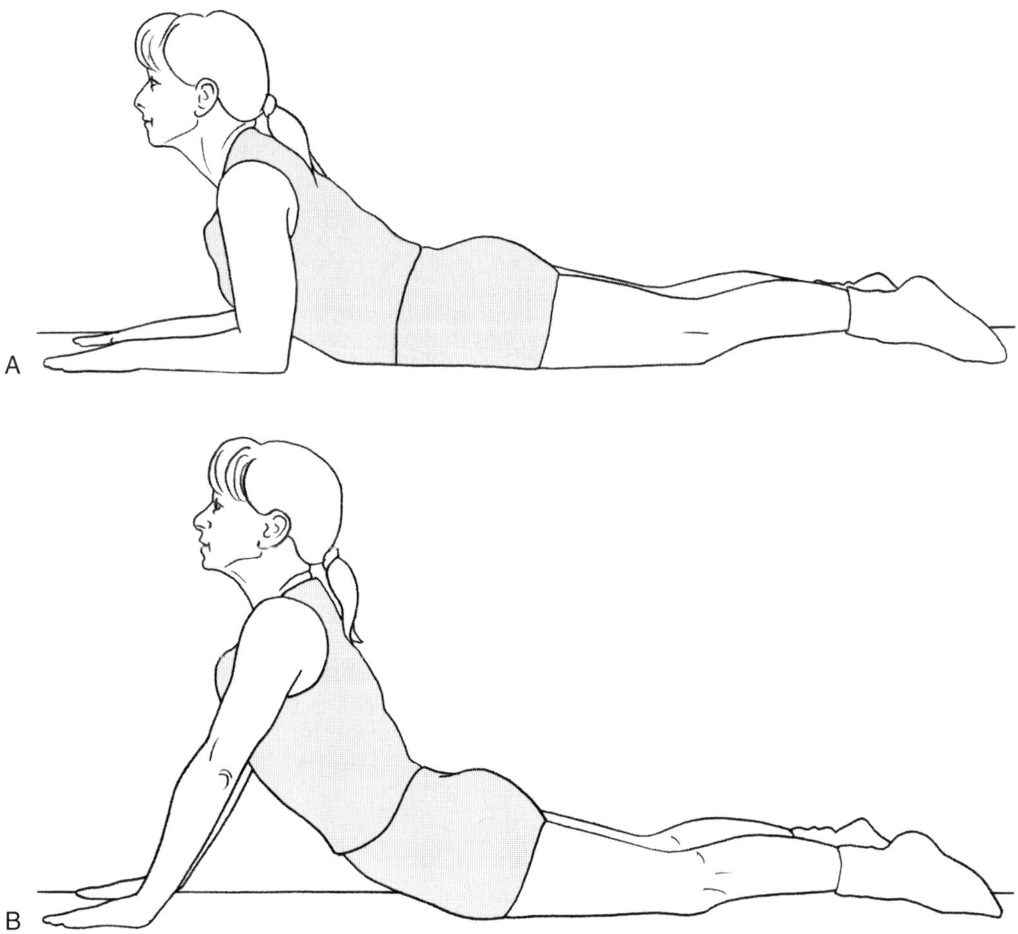

Figure 12.5. (A) Prone on elbows: hold for 30 seconds; repeat 8 to 10 times. (B) Prone press: hold for 30 seconds; repeat 8 to 10 times.

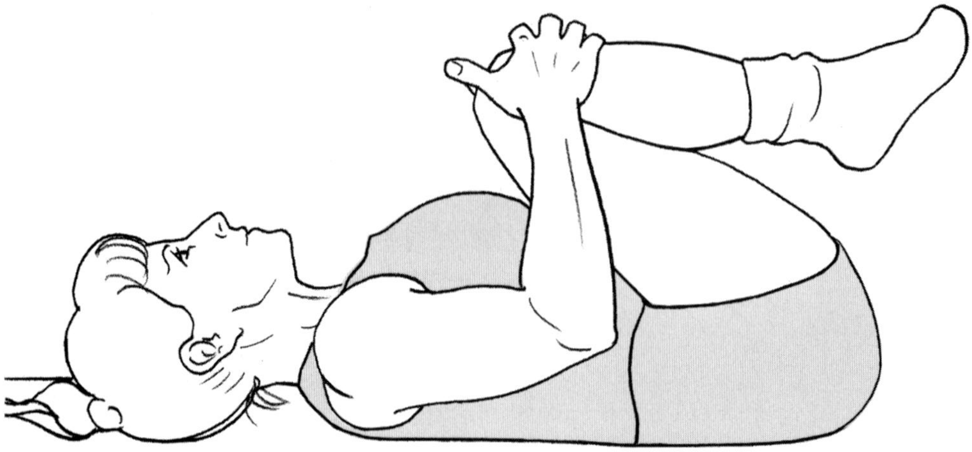

Figure 12.6. Knees to the chest: hold for 20 to 30 seconds; repeat 10 to 20 times.

Stage 2

Stage 2 will usually begin in 4 to 6 weeks or when the patient's pain becomes centralized. This stage is known as the lumbar stabilization stage and focuses on strengthening the static stabilization muscle groups. Strengthening of the transverse abdominis muscles is accomplished through the abdominal hollowing exercise (Fig. 12.7). This exercise, which isolates the deep abdominals without activating the rectus abdominis, is performed by drawing the abdomen toward the head and spine. This position is held for 20 seconds and the hollowing repeated 10 times. Once this has been mastered, more challenging exercises can be added. These include abdominal hollowing with repetitive leg movements (Fig. 12.8A) or bridging (Fig. 12.8B). The hollowing move-

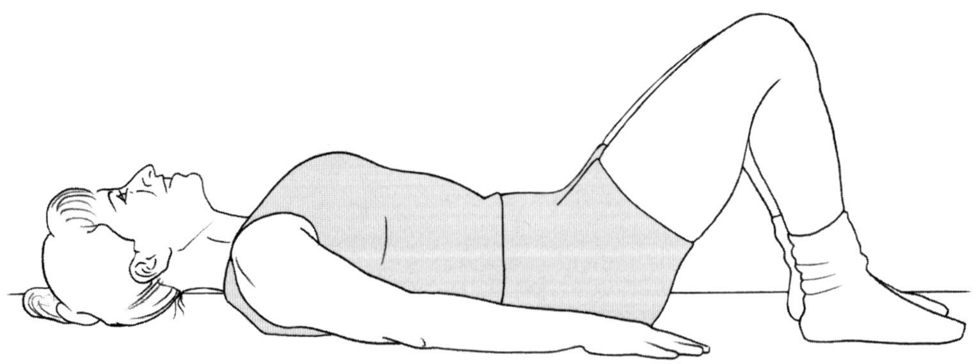

Figure 12.7. Abdominal hollowing: hold for 20 seconds; repeat 10 times.

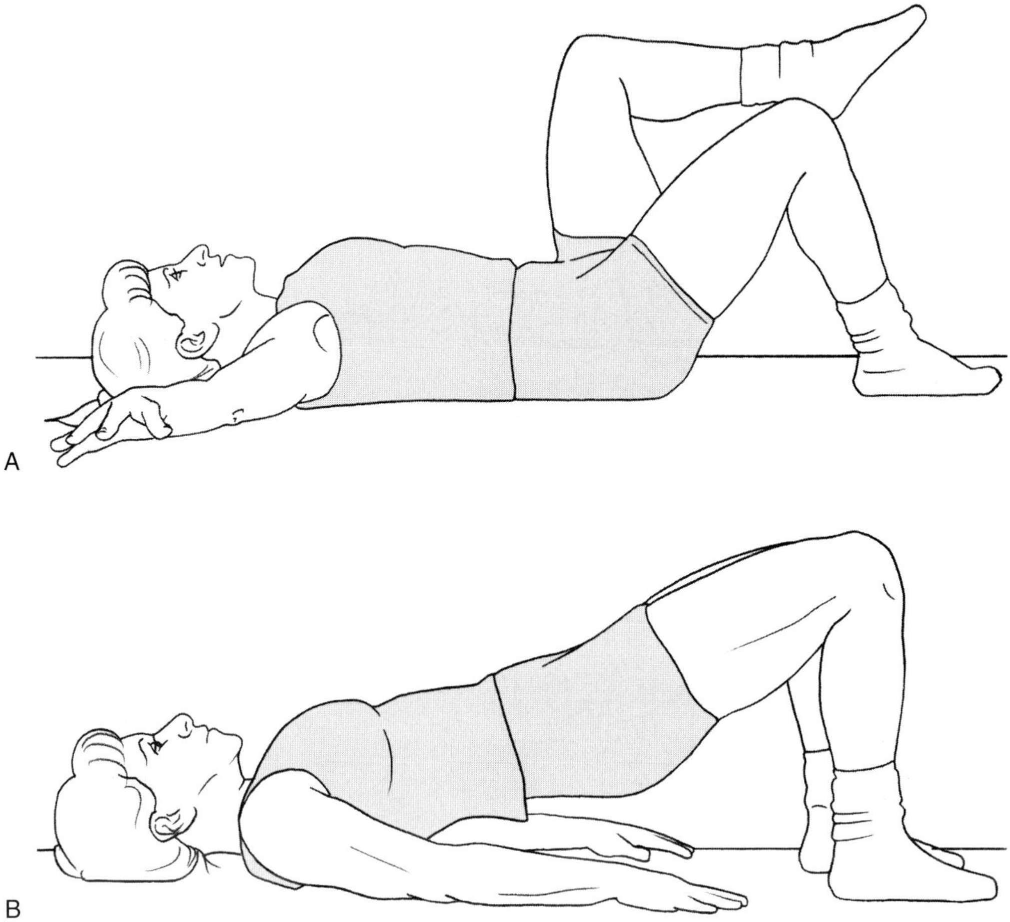

Figure 12.8. (A) Abdominal hollowing with repetitive leg movements. (B) Abdominal hollowing with bridging.

ment can then be incorporated into the patient's daily activities, such as sitting, standing, or bending.

Strengthening of the multifidi and erector spinae muscles is accomplished through single-leg/opposite-arm extensions performed in the quadruped position (Fig. 12.9). It is important that the patient maintain abdominal hollowing during these exercises. The position should be held for the count of 10 and repeated 10 times on each side. This exercise produces minimal compressive forces while activating the proper musculature.

Strengthening of the quadratus lumborum and oblique abdominal muscles is accomplished by performing the horizontal side support exercise with knees flexed (Fig. 12.10A) or extended (Fig. 12.10B). This position should be held for 10 seconds and the exercise repeated 10 times. The position can be sustained longer and repetitions increased as patient displays increased endurance.

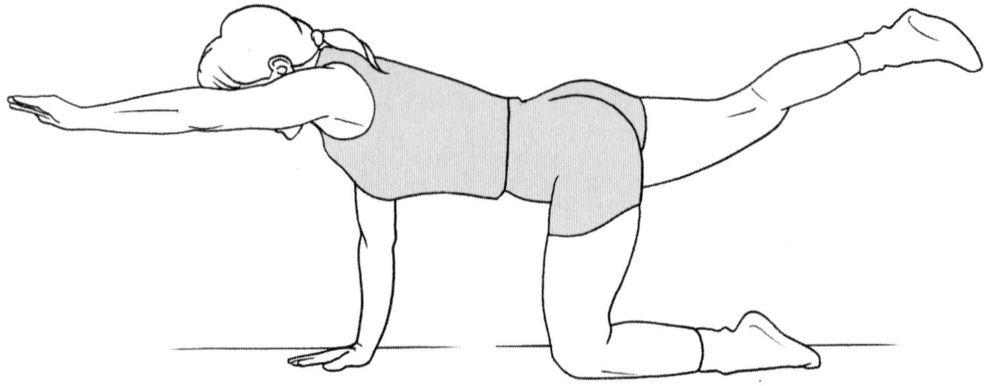

Figure 12.9. Single leg and opposite arm extension performed in the quadruped position, held for the count of 10 and repeated 10 times on each side.

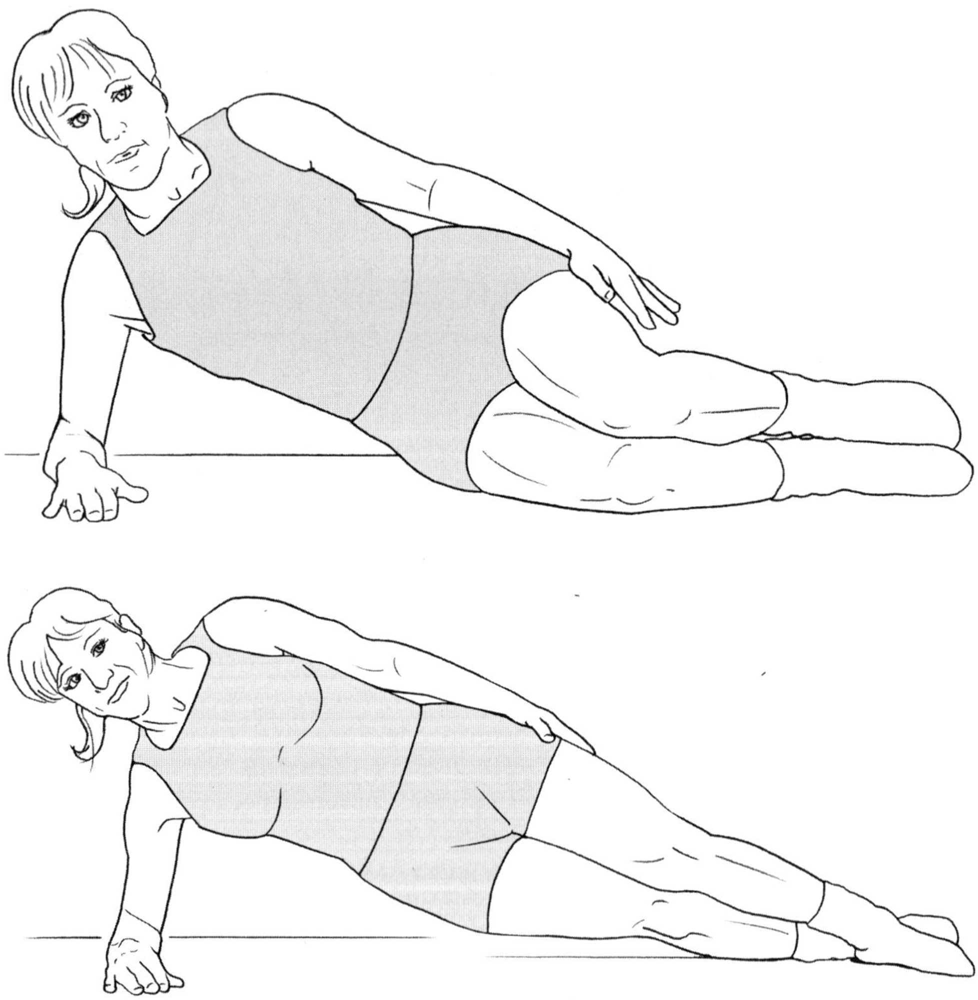

A

B

Figure 12.10. (A) Horizontal side support with knees flexed: hold for 10 seconds; repeat 10 times. (B) Horizontal side support with knees extended: hold for 10 seconds; repeat 10 times.

Stage 3

Stage 3 focuses on the dynamic stabilization of the lumbar spine. These exercises, which can be tailored to the patient's specific requirements by the therapist, can include work with the gym ball: bridging, Superman, and single-leg extensions (Fig. 12.11).

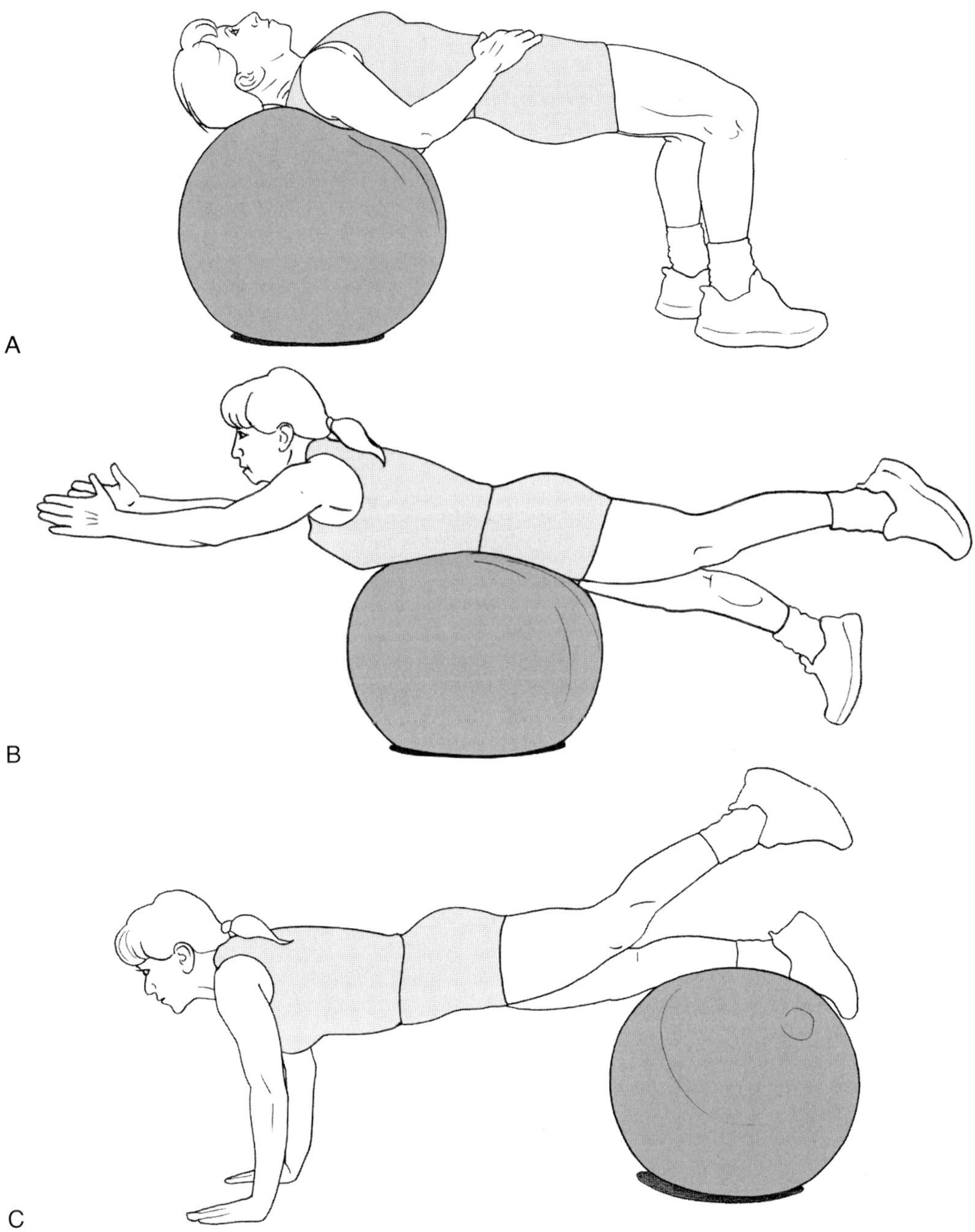

Figure 12.11. Gym ball exercises. In each case, hold for 60 seconds; repeat 5 times. (A) Bridging. (B) Superman. (C) Single-leg extensions.

The patient must maintain abdominal hollowing throughout all motions.

Once these stages have been mastered, the patient should be able to participate in all activities of daily living. Patients should adopt proper lifting and posture as taught in the therapy program. These safe back techniques emphasize neutral lumbar posture and lifting with the weight as close to the patient's center of gravity as possible.

Long-Term Maintenance

Patients should maintain a healthy exercise program, consisting of aerobic and anaerobic routines, three or four times per week. This helps maintain endurance and strength of the trunk musculature. Heavy weight training should be avoided.

Participation in sports should be gradual, to decrease the risk of reinjury. High-impact sports should be avoided. Activities such as golf or tennis that consist of twisting motions should be modified to decrease the amount of lumbar loading. These sport-specific modifications can be done with the guidance of someone with experience in a particular sport.

Again the goal is to prevent reinjury or new injury by maintaining trunk muscle tone and following safe back practices. By assuring patient compliance in the postprocedural protocols, outcome will be maximized.

Bibliography

Bogduk N. *Clinical Anatomy of the Lumbar Spine and Sacrum*. 3rd ed. New York: Churchill Livingstone; 1997.

Choy, DSJ. Rapid correction of neurological deficits by percutaneous laser disc decompression (PLDD). *Lasers Surg Med* 1996;14:13–15.

Cox J. *Low Back Pain Mechanism, Diagnosis and Treatment*. 6th ed. Philadelphia: Lippincott Williams & Wilkins; 1999.

Liemohn W. *Exercise Prescription and the Back*. New York: McGraw-Hill Medical Publishing Division; 2001.

Paassilta P, et al. Identification of a novel common genetic risk factor for lumbar disk disease. *JAMA* 2001;285:1843–1849.

Twomey L. *Physical Therapy of the Low Back*. 3rd ed. New York: Churchill Livingstone; 2000.

13

Complicated Disc Herniations Responding to Percutaneous Laser Disc Decompression

Daniel S.J. Choy

Extruded Herniated Discs

My early publications specifically excluded patients with herniated discs that were extruded, even if nonsequestered, as candidates for percutaneous laser disc decompression (PLDD). This policy was to ensure that the early clinical database for analysis would consist of information that was *clean* and susceptible to scientific analysis. Complicated clinical syndromes would have made analysis difficult if not impossible.

When a patient with a left foot drop and low back and sciatic pain appeared at the Laser Spine Center 6 years ago, magnetic resonance imaging confirmed the clinical diagnosis of an L4-5 disc lesion. There was extrusion of the disc, with a caudad component extending halfway down the L5 disc. I turned the patient down for PLDD. Visibly upset, he wanted to know the reason. I told him that it was against all I had ever written about PLDD, and that I had difficulty visualizing the vertical extruded portion of the disc shrinking in a cephalad direction and turning 90 degrees to retreat centrally into the parent disc.

"What is the alternative?" the patient wanted to know.

"Open surgery," I replied.

"I'd rather have an arm cut off than have open surgery," he said.

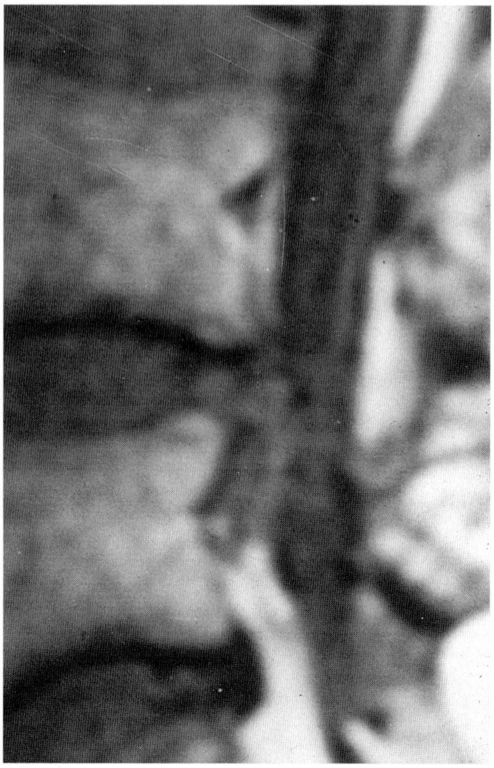

Figure 13.1. Disc herniation (L4-5) with a caudad extrusion.

I was adamant in my refusal to consider this patient for PLDD. He then asked me a very unfair question: " If our positions were exchanged, would you have open surgery?"

After a moment's thought I said, "No."

"Then," he responded, "you'll have to use the laser on me. I'll sign any kind of letter you write."

My lawyers drafted the most severe and restrictive consent form I have ever encountered: how the procedure was against my written advice, how the patient was determined to proceed at his own risk, and so on, and so forth. Both the patient and his wife signed the letter of informed consent, with witnesses.

In this patient's presurgery magnetic resonance imaging (MRI) (Fig. 13.1), the caudad extrusion is clearly seen. I performed PLDD on the L4-5 disc with 1500 joules. At the end of the procedure the patient's back and sciatic pain were gone. His foot drop was also gone.

The next two patients with extruded discs signed similar letters and also obtained good results from PLDD.

Subsequent patients have had extrusions of cephalad (Fig. 13.2), caudad, and mushroom-shaped (Figs. 13.3 and 13.4) lesions. They have occurred in the lumbar and cervical spines. De-

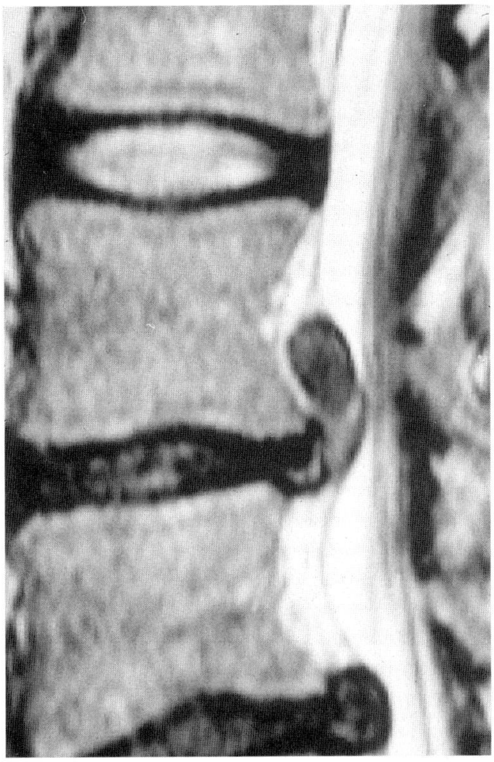

Figure 13.2. Disc herniation with cephalad extrusion.

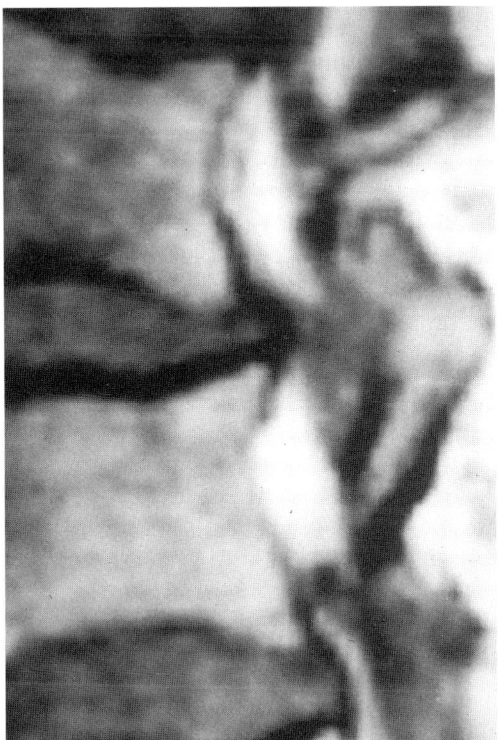

Figure 13.3. Disc herniation with a mushroom extrusion.

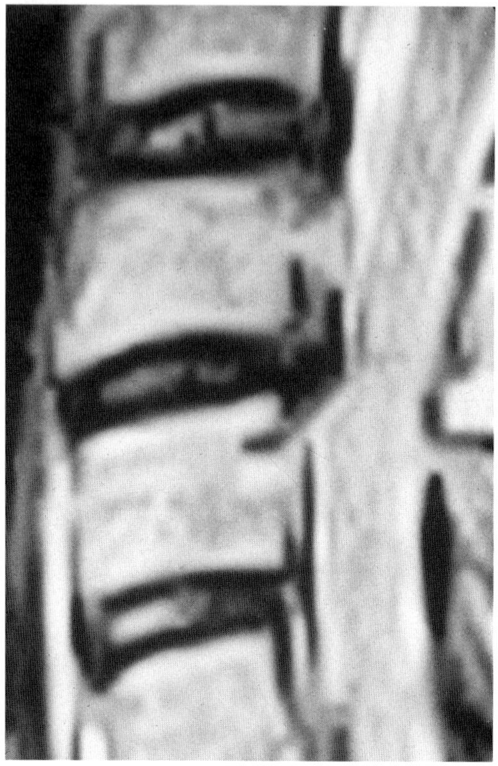

Figure 13.4. Another disc herniation with a mushroom-shaped extrusion.

tails of the first 21 such patients were reported in the *Journal of Clinical Laser Medicine & Surgery*.[1]

As of May 26, 2002, 36 patients with extruded discs had been treated with PLDD. Surprisingly, the results have not differed significantly from PLDD to the *normal* disc herniations, with success being achieved in 80 to 85% according to the MacNab criteria.

Extrusions per se are therefore no longer contraindications to PLDD, provided continuity with the parent disc is maintained.

Spinal Stenosis

In 1997 Dr. Jeffery Ngeow, an interventional anesthesiologist at the Hospital for Special Surgery in New York, asked if I had treated patients with spinal stenosis with PLDD. When the answer was in the affirmative, he took on himself the task of reviewing all the charts of my patients treated with PLDD from September 1988 to June 1997.

Spinal stenosis of pure bony origin would naturally not respond to PLDD. However, we thought that spinal stenosis contributed to by disc protrusion into the spinal canal might respond

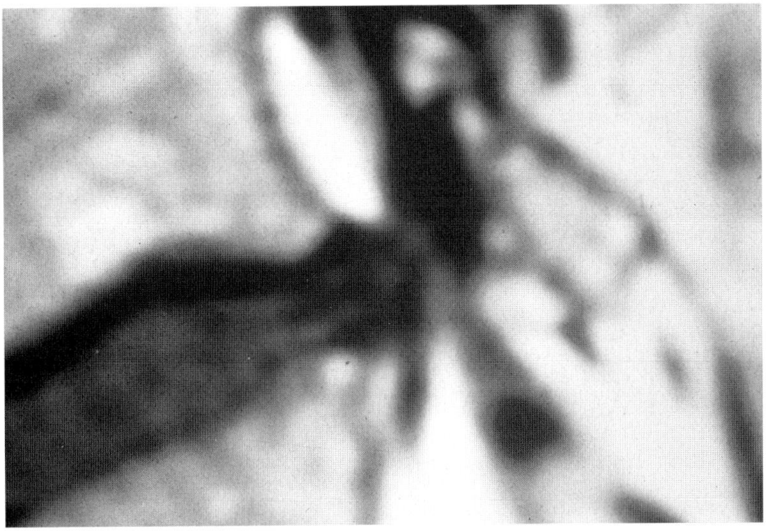

Figure 13.5. Spinal stenosis with disc protrusion contributing to the spinal canal narrowing.

well to PLDD, since the laser shrinks the disc, thereby relieving stenosis.

Dr. Ngeow found a total of 35 patients with radiologic documentation of spinal stenosis and disc herniation (Figs. 13.5 and 13.6). Again using the MacNab criteria and both chart and telephone follow-ups, he found a 69% response rate.[2]

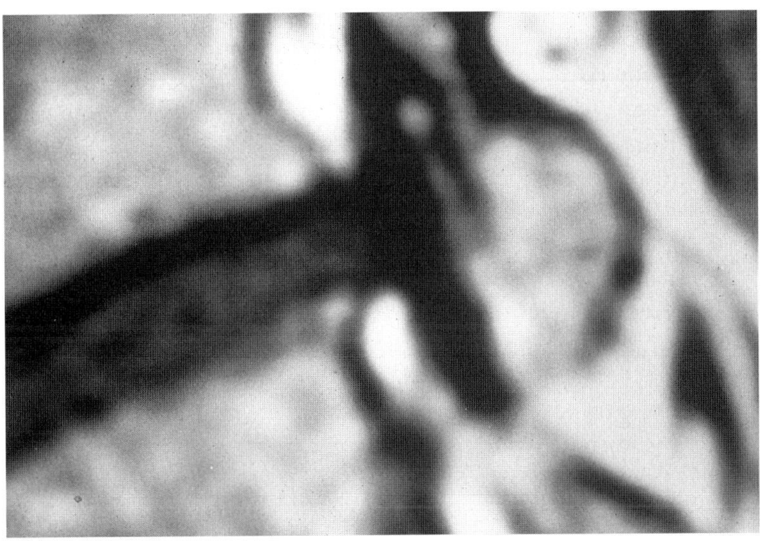

Figure 13.6. Another example of spinal stenosis with disc protrusion.

From June 1997 to the present (May 2002), the Laser Spine Center has accumulated another 61 patients with spinal stenosis and herniated discs. The response rate has remained unchanged. Thus, of 96 such patients, 66 have obtained good results, or 70%.

Spinal stenosis with associated disc herniation may now be added to the list of indications suitable for PLDD.

Discogenic Pain Without a Radicular Component

How does one approach a patient with an obvious disc herniation demonstrated by MRI if he or she has no pain radiation to the buttocks or legs? This is obviously a controversial issue, and many spine surgeons are entirely justified in not offering interventional therapy in the traditional manner, with laminectomy and discectomy. Open surgery carries with it the baggage of a low success rate, soft tissue damage, scaring, morbidity, and a relatively long recuperative period.

Percutaneous laser disc decompression (PLDD), on the other hand, is relatively noninvasive, has low morbidity, no scarring, a relatively high success rate, and a short recovery period. Most white collar workers are back at work within 4 to 6 days.

The strictures against interventional therapy, in my opinion, are not as rigid for PLDD as they are for open surgery.

I would still insist that the following criteria to be met:

1. Failure of adequate conservative treatment for 3 months.
2. Continued pain interfering with lifestyle and/or occupation.
3. Continued need for daily painkillers.
4. A positive Valsalva test result.
5. Local tenderness over the affected disc.
6. Local pain induced by forward, posterior, and lateral bending of the trunk.
7. Presence of paraspinal muscle pain or spasm that may cause scoliosis.
8. Although it can be seen from other chapters that I am not a great fan of discography, in extreme borderline cases I will accept a positive discogram. A negative discogram does not exclude a discogenic cause for back pain.
9. In lieu of discography, a positive pain response to disc compression using the lumbar disc compression frame described in Chapter 8.
10. Absence of severe osteoarthritis, facet joint syndrome, neural foraminal impingement by scar or osteophytes, severe disc degeneration and desiccation, osteoporotic vertebral collapse, greater than a grade 1 spondylolisthesis, pending litigation in which the patient may have secondary economic gain, and cancer.

11. The patient must be informed that the indications for use of PLDD in this clinical situation is not as clear-cut as when there is a radicular component to the pain.

Low back pain accompanied by peripheral numbness and/or neurologic deficits is acceptable as a definitive indication for PLDD without the constraints just enumerated.

In my experience, if the foregoing criteria are observed, PLDD has an excellent chance of producing a salutary effect in the patient with pure discogenic pain.

References

1. Choy DSJ. Response of extruded intervertebral herniated discs to percutaneous laser disc decompression. *J Clin Laser Med Surg* 2001;19(1): 15–20.
2. Choy DSJ, Ngeow J. Response of spinal stenosis to PLDD. *J Clin Laser Med Surg* 1998;16:123–125.

14

Unexpected Results in Patients Treated with Percutaneous Laser Disc Decompression

Daniel S.J. Choy

Rapid Correction of Neurologic Deficits after Percutaneous Laser Disc Decompression

Chapter 1 relates the story of the first patient treated with percutaneous laser disc decompression (PLDD) at the Neurosurgical Institute, University of Graz, Graz, Austria. The back and sciatic pain of a middle-aged Turkish man disappeared after application of 600 joules of laser energy in a procedure in which we had planned to deliver 1000 joules.

Since that first experience, it has become commonplace for laser surgeons performing PLDD around the world to observe disappearance of pain after, and sometimes, even during the procedure. From a physics point of view, this is not surprising, since disc shrinkage occurs concurrently with laser vaporization of water and proteoglycan in the nucleus pulposus. This shrinkage is documented by magnetic resonance imaging (MRI) in only one third of patients, since the best resolution of MRI is 2.0 cm or slightly less. A 100 Å movement of the herniation away from the nerve root relieves sciatic pain. In the first 100 patients treated at St. Luke's–Roosevelt Hospital who had complete resolution of back and sciatic pain, MRIs were performed at 6 weeks. Only one third of these images demonstrated measurable disc shrinkage.

What was unexpected was the rapid return of absent deep tendon reflexes, improvement of restricted straight leg raising (SLR), and the ability of patients to arise from a supine to a sitting position without progressing through the series of learned maneuvers termed the Choy sign by Dr. Robert April (i.e., by rolling over to one side, bending one knee, and assisting the upper body with an upper extremity while swinging the legs off the table).

One hundred eighty-two consecutive patients with MRI-documented herniated discs (lumbar, 251; cervical, 8; thoracic, 1), with corresponding clinical symptoms and an age distribution of 23 to 68 years, were studied. All 89 male and 93 female patients were examined both by the author and by an independent neurologist. No patient was receiving payments from an employer's workmen's compensation insurance. No control group was available for comparison. Deep tendon reflexes were rated at 0 when they were absent even with reinforcement, and at 1 plus and 2 plus without reinforcement. Straight leg raising less than 45 degrees was considered abnormal, and 80 degrees to be normal. Thus, a 10-degree change was not considered to be an improvement. The results cover the Achilles and patellar reflexes, as well as SLR, the Choy sign, and foot drop. The summary in Table 14.1 is amplified as follows.

1. There was absence of the Achilles reflex in 37%. Twenty-four percent became positive immediately after PLDD; 24% at day 1, 6% at one week, and 46% remained unchanged. At one week, therefore, 54% had returned to normal by one week.
2. Patellar reflex was absent in 38%. 32 percent became normal immediately; 26% at one day, and 6% at one week. It was unchanged in 36%. Thus, at one week, 64% had returned.
3. Seventy-four percent had an abnormality in SLR. Fifty-one percent returned to normal immediately, 28% on day one, and 2% at one week. Nineteen percent showed no improvement. Hence, 81% were normal by one week.

Table 14.1 Correction of Neurologic Deficits after Percutaneous Laser Disc Decompression

Procedure and Total Cases	Return to Normal			
	Immediate	1 Day	1 Week	No Change
Achilles reflex, 67 (37%)	16 (24%)	16 (24%)	4 (6%)	31(46%)
Patellar reflex, 69 (38%)	22 (32%)	18 (26%)	4 (6%)	25 (36%)
Straight leg raise, 134 (74%)	68 (51%)	37 (28%)	3 (2%)	26 (19%)
Choy sign 38 (15%)	22 (58%)	10 (26%)	6 (16%)	

4. The Choy sign was positive in 15%. Fifty-eight percent became negative immediately and 26% at one day, 16% at one week. Thus, 84% returned to normal by day 1.
5. Since 1988, of 28 patients with foot drop, 52% returned to normal immediately, 25% at one month, and 23% showed no change.

Discussion

When I first reported on these findings at a workshop on PLDD at the Deaconness Hospital, in Cincinnati, Ohio, in 1990, the presentation was greeted with expressions of disbelief. One year later, at the same institution, other laser spine surgeons reported similar observations. These results have been seen abroad as well. It is thought that these early returns of neurologic function are not seen with open operative procedures because of the associated increased soft tissue damage, local inflammation, and perhaps scar tissue formation.

The 81% improvement of SLR and the 84% change in the positive Choy sign correspond well to the published data on PLDD success rates ranging from 75 to 90%.[1–6]

The lower figures for improvement of Achilles and patellar reflexes perhaps indicate that relief of sciatic pain is not necessarily reflected by changes of the deep tendon reflexes. However, the rapid return of these absent reflexes make it necessary to reassess long-held concepts of neurophysiology. Sudden release of prolonged extrinsic pressure on nerve roots can allow immediate return of electrical transmission by those nerves. Hongell and Mattson, who found improvement in nerve conduction within 30 minutes of surgical decompression in 50 cases of carpal tunnel syndrome, further state, "it is a common clinical experience that patients with median nerve compression in the carpal tunnel are relieved of their pain and paresthesias the day after decompression."[7] Brown reported rapid return of nerve function following laminectomy and discectomy.[8] Rydevik et al. state "the rapid improvement of nerve function seen in these situations is consistent with a recovery of intraneural blood flow, which restores the supply of oxygen and other nutrients to the nerve tissue."[9] The rapid return of nerve function in these patients implies the absence of Wallerian degeneration. The existence of such degeneration would delay return of nerve function by some months, given the putative nerve regeneration velocity of 1.0 mm per day.

The position of the dorsal ganglion in the central part of the intervertebral foramen[10] makes this structure extremely vulnerable to compression by a disc herniation, with resultant radicular pain. By the same token, reversal of these compressive forces is likely to benefit the dorsal ganglion first, and pain relief is the earliest result of PLDD. The return to normal of SLR and the Choy sign indicate that it is possible in the successful cases to stretch the previously involved sciatic nerve. Thus, these last two signs have predictive value for continued success after PLDD.

Relief of Erectile Dysfunction

Shafer and Rosenblum[11] reported on an occult disc causing impotence, followed by Velcek's[12] report of 20 other cases of erectile dysfunction caused by spinal disc herniation.

In 1998 a 25-year-old white man with a 7-year history of low back pain and numbness of the posterior aspect of the right leg involving the foot and great toe, together with erectile dysfunction, despite stimulation for the past 2 years' duration, presented to the Laser Spine Center. Positive findings were absent right Achilles reflex, hypalgesia of the penis, and SLR 30 degrees on the right and 80 degrees on the left. There was a positive Valsalva sign. Magnetic resonance imaging for this patient (see earlier, Fig. 8.1) revealed a broad-based central/right paracentral herniation of the L4-5, and a mild annular bulge of the L5-S1 discs. Decompression of both discs with PLDD was performed in two stages, 3 weeks after the patient was first seen (L4-5) and 7 weeks later (L5-S1). Pain relief was essentially complete and the numbness was 90% improved after the first procedure.

Approximately 1 hour after PLDD, the patient experienced a spontaneous erection lasting 15 to 20 minutes. The patient was more excited by this phenomenon than by his pain relief. The second PLDD was performed 2 weeks later for residual leg pain. The pain disappeared at the end of the procedure, SLR increased from 30 to 80 degrees and the absent Achilles reflex became plus/minus. Seven years later we received an announcement that the patient had become a father.

A report on this and a second case was published in 1999.[13] Since then four additional patients with erectile dysfunction have been treated with PLDD. Three of the four achieved normal erectile function from 1 to 4 weeks after PLDD. There was no change in the fourth patient. Thus, of a total of six patients with erectile dysfunction, PLDD resulted in normal function in five. These numbers are too small to permit meaningful statistical analysis, but for the mathematically minded, these data represent an 83% response rate.

The lesson? Ask about erectile dysfunction during the history taking.

References

1. Choy DSJ, Case RB, Fielding W, et al. Percutaneous laser nucleolysis of lumbar disc. *N Engl J Med*. 1987;317:771–772.
2. Gottlob C, Kopchok G, Peng S, Tabbara M, Cavage D, White R. Holmium:YAG ablation of human intervertebral disc. Preliminary evaluation. *Lasers Surg Med* 1992;12:86–91.
3. Quigley M, Shih T, Elrifai A, Marron J, Lesiecki M. Percutaneous laser discectomy with the Ho:YAG laser. *Lasers Surg Med* 1992;12: 21–24.
4. Sherk H, Black J, Rhodes A, Lane G, Prodoehl J. Laser discectomy. *Clin Sports Med* 1993;12:569–577.
5. Choy DSJ, Ascher PW, Saddekni S, Alkaitis D, Liebler W, Hughes J, Diwan, S, Altman P. Percutaneous laser disc decompression—a new therapeutic modality. *Spine* 1992;17:949–956.
6. Casper D, Mullins LL, Hartman VH. Laser assisted disc decompression. A clinical trial of the Ho:YAG laser with side-firing fiber. *J Clin Laser Med Surg* 1995;13:27–31.
7. Hongell A, Mattshon HS. Neurographic studies before, after, and during operation for median nerve compression in the carpal tunnel. *Scand J Plast Reconstr Surg* 1971;5:103–109.
8. Brown MD. Intraoperative somatosensory evoked potentials in compressive lumbar root lesion. Presented to the International Society for the Study of the Lumbar Spine; April 1983; Cambridge, U.K.
9. Rydevik B, Brown MD, Lundberg G. Pathoanatomy and pathophysiology of nerve root compression. *Spine* 1984;9(1):7–14.
10. Goldstein TB, Mink JH, Dawson EG. Early experience with automated percutaneous lumbar discectomy in the treatment of lumbar disc herniation. *Clin Orthop* 1989;228:77–82.
11. Shafer N, Rosenblum J. Occult disc causing impotency. *N Y State J Med* 1969;69:2465–2470.
12. Velcek D. Discogenic impotence. *Int J Impotence Res* 1989;1:95–113.
13. Choy DSJ. Early relief of erectile dysfunction after laser decompression of herniated lumbar disc. *J Clin Laser Med Surg* 1999;17(1): 25–27.

15

Endoscopic Laser Foraminoplasty: A Treatment Concept and Two-Year Outcome Analysis

M.T.N. Knight and A.K.D. Goswami

The impact of back pain on modern industrial society has been well established.[1] Approximately 2 to 5% of people suffer from acute back pain every year.[2,3] Of those with acute pain, 0.5% have pain and neurology requiring surgery, while the rest slip into chronicity.

The available methods of treatment such as osseous decompression, removal of discs to decompress nerve roots, and spinal fusion provide the standard armamentarium of the spinal surgeon. Widely varying claims of success are attributed to these techniques.[3] The realization of the shortcomings of conventional techniques has led to the development of minimalist midline foraminal decompression, with improved results.[4] The recent deployment of endoscopic techniques to the spine has allowed visual inspection of the disc to be carried out through the *keyhole*, with the patient in the aware state and intradiscal decompression to be effected.[5] However, these techniques could not address abnormalities in the foramen, the epidural space, or the posterior disc wall.

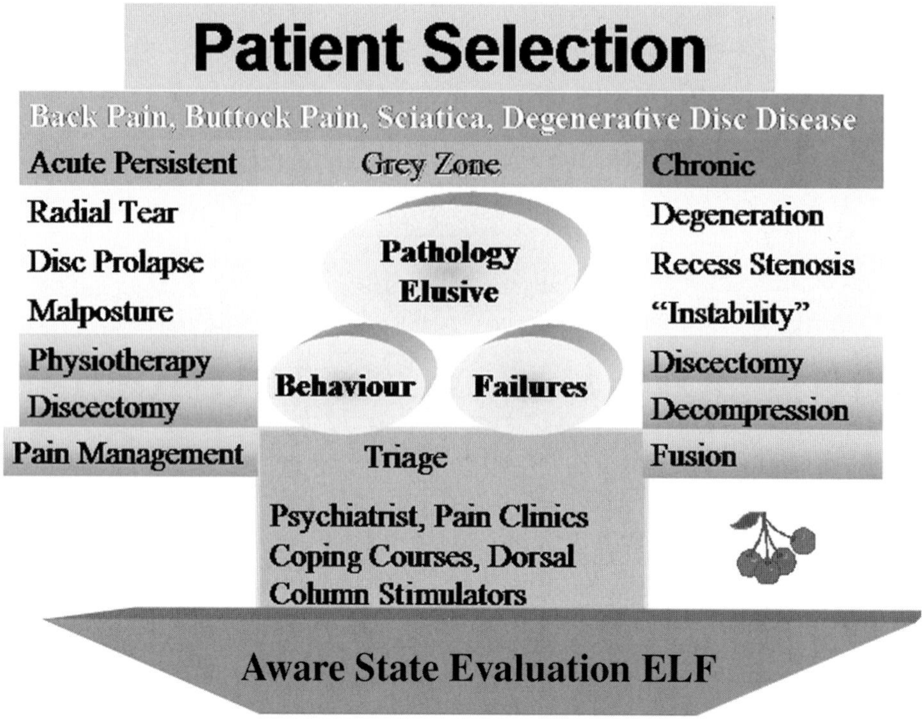

Figure 15.1. Shortcomings and limitations of conventional indications for spinal surgery focus on chronic manifestations but are limited to careful *cherry picking* of patients with overt symptoms. Those with significant symptoms but less clear pathology are denied surgery, and surgery is limited in the treatment of failed back surgery syndrome. These patients fall into the gray zone category, poorly served by current techniques. Endoscopic laser foraminoplasty has been used to address the conventional indications, the gray zone category of patients, as well as those with shorter lived but progressive symptoms.

Laser as a tool for tissue ablation has been tried in several surgical specialties with encouraging results. Not only has it been effective in *precision surgery*, but it has also been shown to reduce morbidity associated with conventional surgery.[6] In 1986 the laser disc decompression procedure was introduced by Choy and others[7]; recently, it has been combined with endoscopy to effect intradiscal clearance.[8,9] Its wider application as a surgical tool in spinal surgery remained underestimated until it was used to ablate bone and scar tissue (Fig. 15.1).[10]

Recent appreciation of neural mechanisms of pain, pain mediators in and around the spinal canal, and pain modulation in the peripheral and central nervous systems have cautioned us against excessive dependence on purely mechanical concepts of back pain (Fig. 15.2).[12,13] Importantly, the sensitivity, reliability,

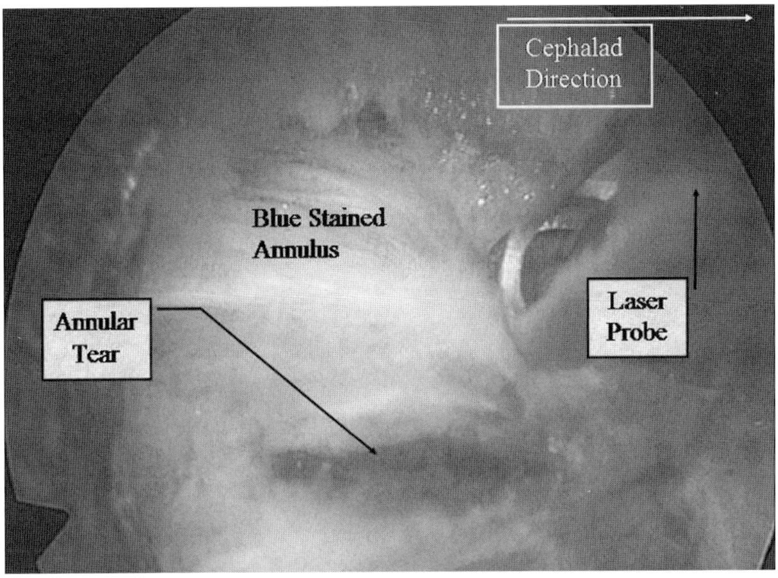

Figure 15.2. Endoscopic view of a leaking radial tear that may breach the annulus either under the posterior longitudinal ligament (PLL) (subligamentous) or through the PLL (transligamentous), causing symptoms according to the point of liberation of breakdown products. The most symptomatic are those releasing breakdown products directly onto the nerve in the foramen. Their effect is amplified where the nerve is tethered adjacent to the exit portal of the tear. The fibrous response may cause encapsulation of the leakage, resulting in containment and concentration of the breakdown products around the nerve.

and predictive value of diagnostic tools such as magnetic resonance (MR) scans, computer-assisted tomography, myelography, and discography, singly or in combination, cannot reliably establish the source and cause of back pain.[14]

The function of the foramen is a delicate balance between the size of the foraminal boundaries and the status of their contents. Pathology, irritation, or sensitization of tethered tissues and abnormal motion easily compromises this balance. In this prospective study, we present the results of the management of back pain using the *Viviprudence* system of aware-state spinal probing and discography (SP&D) and endoscopic diagnosis of the causes of pain, followed by pain source ablation in the epidural, foraminal, and extraforaminal zones combined with lateral recess and intradiscal decompression achieved by endoscopic laser foraminoplasty (ELF) (Fig. 15.3).

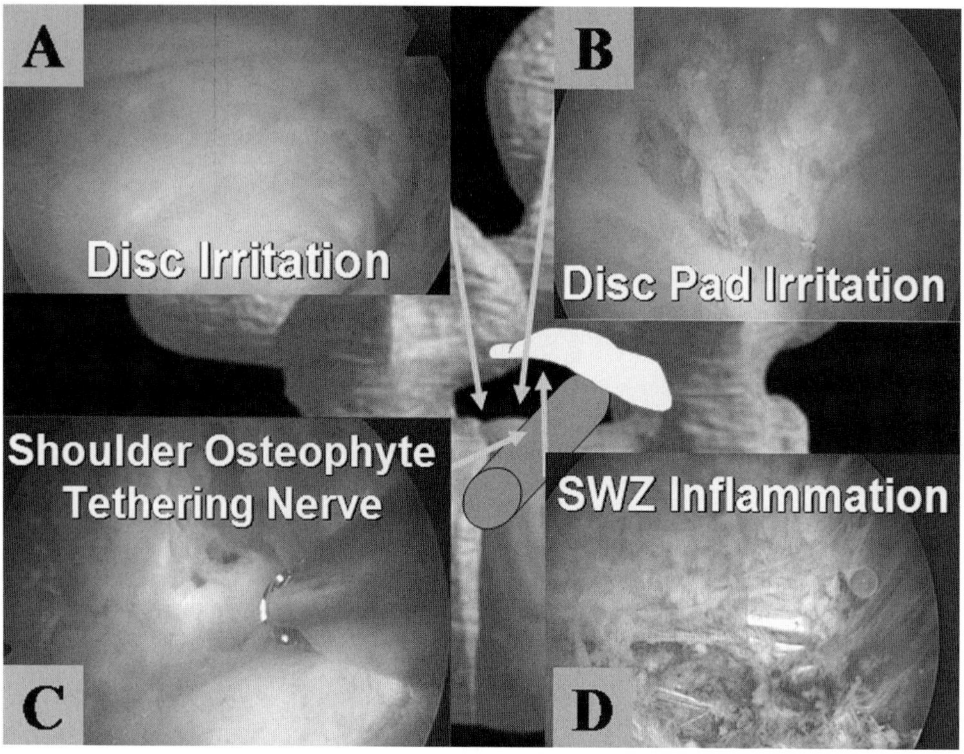

Figure 15.3. A collage of pain sources (right-sided view). (A) The annulus is injected and tender on probing. (B) The disc (stained blue) tissues are hyperemic, appear irritated, and are tender to probing. (C) An exposed shoulder osteophyte that will be ablated by a side-firing laser probe. The nerve then rolls back, free of impingement. (D) The exposed safe working zone (SWZ) reveals a leaking radial tear, as well as an irritated nerve root that was tender, hyperemic and injected.

Materials and Methods

Study Construct

The study was designed prospectively and consisted of 250 consecutive patients treated between March 1994 and June 1997.

Data Acquisition

Full details of history and symptoms were recorded in a questionnaire including a pain manikin, a visual analogue pain (VAP) scale, Oswestry Disability scores, patient satisfaction scores, patient target achievement scores, and psychological indices. Patients were evaluated at 6 and 12 weeks and 6 months following surgery and were reviewed at yearly intervals unless clinical symptoms required closer supervision.

Clinical Evaluation

Full clinical neurologic and postural analysis was performed together with plain anteroposterior and neutral weight-bearing radiographs and a dynamic series of digitized *instability* radiographs in flexion and extension, both sitting and standing. Patients were prescribed muscle balance physiotherapy for a period of 3 months. If the pain intensity remained high, and the response to physiotherapy remained inadequate, patients were referred for a magnetic resonance imaging (MRI) scan. Gadolinium enhancement was added when prior spinal surgery had been involved or perineural scarring was suspected.

Definitions

If the MRI scan clearly identified loss of perineural fat and a foraminal dimension of less than 5 mm, patients were deemed to have lateral recess stenosis.

Surgical Protocol

Spinal probing and discography were done at those suspected levels, which demonstrated degenerative changes and clinically reproduced the site of back pain and neurologic radiation.

Symptom reproduction by probing indicated ELF with flexible endoscopic intradiscal discectomy, neurolysis, undercutting, and osteophytectomy as required.

Where probing reproduced symptoms at several levels, differential discography was performed. Differential discography consists of instillation of depomedrol (Depomedrone, Pharmacia Ltd, Milton Keynes, Bedfordshire, U.K.) after discography and observation of the effect of the symptoms over a number of weeks. At an adjacent level with concordant symptoms, Marcaine (Astra Pharmaceuticals, Kings Langley, Hertfordshire, U.K.) anesthetic agent was inserted. Symptom amelioration over the initial 5 to 8 hours indicated the Marcaine-instilled level as the index level, and longer term symptom modification indicated that the methylprednisolone (Depo-Medrol)-instilled level should be addressed.

Independent Evaluation

Patients were selected from the study series database on a blinded randomized basis by using a computer random number generator linked to the research unit (Spinal Foundation) number. These patients were evaluated by the independent observer (a neurosurgeon). A total of 58 (23%) patients were randomly selected to assess the accuracy of outcome and data recording. Patients were interviewed by telephone, and their questionnaires were checked against the computer database record. Forty-eight (19%) could be directly contacted. Only one inaccuracy was detected (a transcription of a postoperative VAP score of 4 on the questionnaire was marked as 6 in the computer).

Operative Technique

The patients were operated under neuroleptic (aware-state) analgesia. The skin and subcutis were infiltrated with local anesthetic. The procedures were done under image intensifier control. The evoked sensations were recorded both in distribution and intensity on a data sheet describing the patient response to facet joint probing and annulus probing, and during discography.

Lasing Technique

During the entire procedure, an image intensifier is used to ensure the correct position of the endoscope and the laser probe. A Richard Wolfe endoscope with an eccentrically placed 2.5 mm working channel and two irrigation channels was inserted. A side-firing 2.1 mm diameter laser probe with internal irrigation was inserted through the endoscope. The facet joint was displayed, defined, and undercut, providing access to the disc and the epidural space. The exiting and transiting nerve roots were mobilized and decompressed medially and laterally until the axilla of the root at the apex of the safe working zone was displayed. The nerve was cleared of perineural fibrosis. Clearance was extended to the bone margin of the superior notch and the superior foraminal ligament was resected. Osteophytes along the

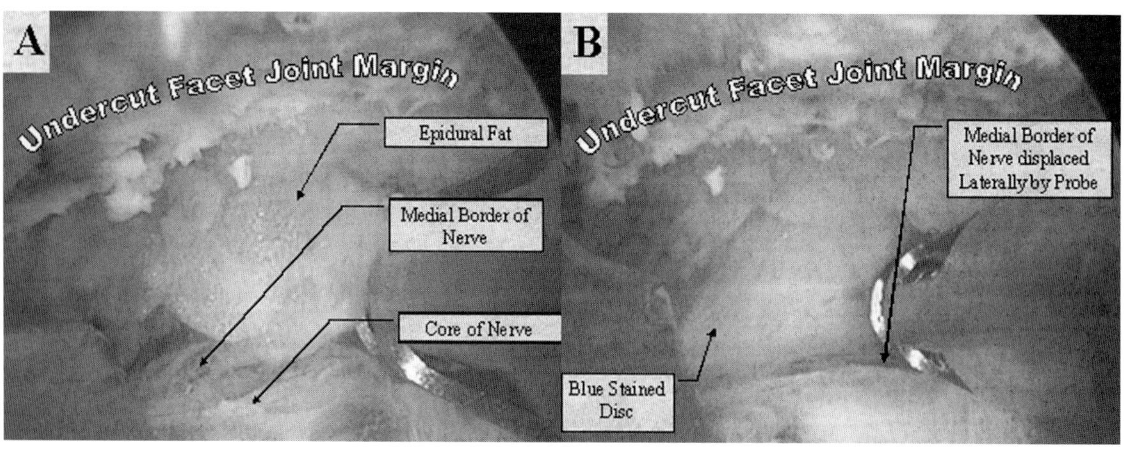

Figure 15.4. Endoscopic view of exiting nerve before and after displacement. (A) The core of the nerve has been decompressed of the impacting facet joint. The nerve is partially covered by mobilized epidural fat. (B) Lateral displacement has occurred. Endoscopy allows discrete areas of the nerve to be gently probed and the elicited response recorded.

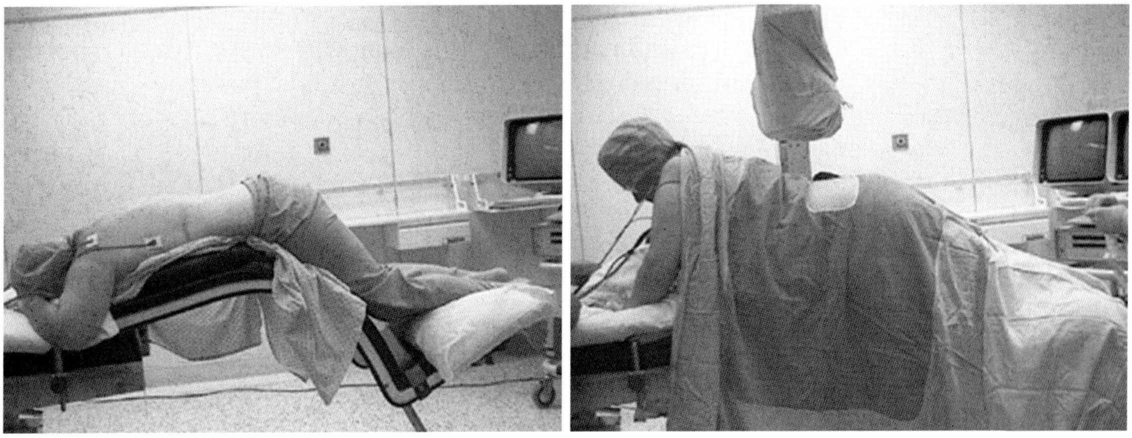

Figure 15.5. The push-up test with the patient flexed and prone (left) and extended prone (right). The test attempts to reproduce the patient's predominant symptoms before surgery by effecting a push-up test on the operating table by pushing the shoulders upward to their maximal extent by extending the arms while leaving the hips on the operating table, hyperextending the spine, and encouraging the abdomen to sag. If the test reproduced leg pain before the procedure but does not do so at the end, then sufficient clearance has usually been effected. This test is valuable in evaluating efficacy of clearance of leg pain but less so for buttock and back pain.

ascending facet joint, the superior notch, the dorsum of the vertebral margin, and the vertebral shoulder (shoulder osteophytes) were ablated under endoscopic vision (Fig. 15.4). The absence of pain at the end of the surgical procedure during the push-up test and leg extension test denoted sufficient clearance of the cause of pain (Fig. 15.5).

Follow-up

Patients were discharged the day following surgery. The muscle balance physiotherapy regime was recommenced on the first day following surgery and amplified with neural mobilization drills.

Results

The cohort consisted of 121 male and 129 female subjects. The average age of the patients was 48 years (range, 21 to 86 years). The average follow-up period was 30 months. A cohort integrity of 97% was maintained at 2 years' follow-up. The overall duration of symptoms was 6.1 years (range, 5 to 21 years; SD, 2.4).

Oswestry Disability Index

An Oswestry Disability Index score of 50 or more was used to designate good and excellent outcome: 61% of patients exceeded this score for back pain, 66% for buttock pain, and 65% for leg pain. The global improvement was 74, 77, and 75%, respectively (fair, good, and excellent). In patients with one prior operation, the corresponding figures were 49, 46, and 51%. Sixty-four percent of patients with one to three open operations improved with Oswestry Disability Index scores of 20 or more.

Satisfaction Scores

Seventy-two percent of patients were satisfied with the outcome of the procedure.

Visual Analogue Pain Score

On the VAP scale, 57% of patients had more than a 50% improvement, while 5% of patients had deterioration of pain symptoms following surgery.

Patient Target Achievement Score

Sixty-two percent of patients were satisfied with the targets achieved specific to their needs, chosen before surgery.

Revision Endoscopic Surgery

Five percent of patients (n = 13) required revision surgery (Table 15.1). Two patients underwent a revision ELF at the index level on the same side. Six required ELF at an adjacent or contralateral level with success. Five underwent conventional open exploration and fusion at other centers. Ninety-five percent of patients did not require any further surgical intervention. Only 2.5% required conventional intervention; 3% required adjacent or contralateral ELF.

If all the patients in this study were taken as a group, the Oswestry Disability Index on a global scale demonstrated that 61% had excellent or good result (19% excellent results and 42% had good results) for their back pain, 66% for their buttock pain, and 65% for their leg pain. For patients who had had no previous operations, the corresponding figures were 76, 72, and 71%. At the 2-year follow-up review, 17 patients (7%) evidenced continuing degeneration and were worse on the Oswestry Disability Index, but only 5% of patients described their pain as worse than before.

Table 15.1. Incidence and Type of Revision in 250 Patients

Technique	Level and Side	Number
Revision endoscopic laser foraminoplasty	Index level same side	2
	Adjacent level	3
	Contralateral side	3
Conventional fusion	Index level	5

Prior Open Operations

Seventy-five patients had had between one and four conventional open operations on the spine. Perineural fibrosis with or without epidural fibrosis was identified in all patients. In the 62 patients who had undergone one previous operation, ELF resulted in an excellent or good Oswestry Disability Index score of 49% for back pain, 46% for buttock pain, and 51% for leg pain. However, when overall results are assessed for all the patients who had had open operations, 50% improved to the good-and-excellent category and an additional 14% of patients demonstrated appreciable clinical improvement.

Spondylolytic Spondylolisthesis

Twenty-three patients had spondylolytic spondylolisthesis (16 grade I, 7 grade II) involving L4-5 and at L5-S1 levels. Seventeen patients achieved excellent or good results according to the Oswestry Disability Index. Five patients had a poor outcome because of bilateral perineural and epidural scarring from previous open surgery and fusion.

Preoperative Foot Drop

There were 10 patients who had foot drop grade 1–2 before surgery. All these patients had had the foot drop for more than 3 years, and all except one demonstrated improvement in the dorsiflexion power at the ankle at the end of 2 years (grade 4–5), although none reached normal power.

Morphine Sulfate Usage

Nineteen patients were on morphine sulfate therapy (MST) before surgery. Only two patients were still on MST at the end of 2 years. Fifty percent of the patients achieved excellent to good results, while another 15% had clinically appreciable change on the Oswestry Disability Index (ODI).

Multiple Sclerosis

Four patients had multiple sclerosis diagnosed before surgery. All four patients were wheelchair bound. All improved their VAP index by more than 80%, but their function remained impaired by the underlying condition.

Discussion

Sciatica and back and buttock pain have been attributed to many sources, but these have not been examined by using aware-state patient feedback combined with posterolateral endoscopy as a means of true verification.[11]

Viviprudence System

Spinal probing and discography followed by ELF represents part of a treatment algorithm termed *Viviprudence*. The Viviprudence system is based on detailed analysis of the clinical presentations, clinical and postural examination, and dynamic weight-bearing radiographs, followed by advanced spinal physiotherapy using the muscle balance approach. Failure of the symptoms to respond sufficiently to specific dynamic postural restabilization and correction of segmental loading leads to MRI scanning. Spinal probing and discography, with differential discography led by concordant response, provided the final arbiter for the indication of the index level for surgery.

Magnetic Resonance Imaging and Its Shortcomings

Endoscopy reveals that static MRI fails to demonstrate the tethering and impaction of the superior facet joint, the infolded ligamentum flavum, the facet joint capsule, the inferior foraminal ligament and the superior foraminal ligament onto the nerve and local structures. The presence of disc protrusions may be directly misleading compared with the side and site of the true pathology subsequently located by means of aware-state spinal probing and endoscopy. A number of patients who were thought to have no compression of the nerves on the basis of MRI scans because of preserved *fat lucency* around the nerve were found to have significant edema of the nerve sheath, which was causing compression of the nerve within the exit foramen. The latter condition arose in the presence of a dynamically impacting ascending facet joint and tethering of the nerve to the posterolaterally weakened annulus. Endoscopy also revealed that the MRI scan underestimates the degree of local scarring and the vascular hyperemia and thrombosis occurring within.

Outcome and Systemic Status

Endoscopic laser foraminoplasty (ELF) has proved beneficial in the management of back pain in patients with multiple sclerosis, rheumatoid arthritis and seronegative arthritis, and recent vascular and coronary heart disease, as well as in patients on anticoagulants, patients with bleeding disorders, and the infirm and the elderly.

Dynamic and Adynamic Lateral Recess Stenosis

The extent of bony excision needed to bring about adequate conventional decompression is not defined.[15,16] However, many patients who have conventional lateral recess decompression undergo spinal fusion to forestall the hypothetical, incompletely understood concept of spinal instability. By undercutting the facet and mobilizing the nerve, ELF achieves the same net effect while maintaining segmental mobility and avoiding aggravated domino degeneration or spondylolisthesis.

Postoperative Flares

In this early series postoperative flares occurred in 28% of patients and were significant in 12%. A flare may result from the swelling associated with the postoperative inflammatory response or revascularization and remodeling of the laser-ablated bone. Timely caudal epidural steroid infiltration, with manipulation under anesthesia, has helped to quench such symptoms. That these patients responded to the steroid infiltration supports the inflammatory hypotheses of the cause of the flare. The flare may last up to 3 weeks. The incidence has decreased with greater experience and foraminal undercutting and clearance.

Complications

One patient suffered neurologic deficit following surgery (grade II) owing to residual protrusion. However, 2 years later her power had recovered considerably (grade IV). Another patient had an aseptic disciitis.

Scarring

Scarring noted endoscopically was almost always associated with vascular bands. The exiting or traversing nerve was often hyperemic and particularly tender at discrete points along its course, with these points located at the areas of entrapment. Swelling and engorgement of veins and thrombosis therein were noted endoscopically in the foramen and the perineural region. These features have been suggested as a cause of lateral recess stenotic symptoms by compromise of the available space in the spinal exit foramen or compromise of neural drainage.[17] Endoscopic laser foraminoplasty (ELF) provides a means of excision of the scar from the nerve using the side-firing probe as well as resection of the engorged veins and inflammatory tissue masses that occur in the safe working zone and on the disc and posterior longitudinal ligament.

Sequestration

Ten of 14 patients who had sequestration of disc material had excellent to good results. Four patients had a poor outcome. Failures were long-term sequestra with advanced degeneration and extensive displacement predominantly at the L5-S1 level in male subjects. These patients underwent surgery elsewhere for sequestrectomy by fusion.

Conclusions

This series of endoscopic laser foraminoplasties represents the initial attempt to address degenerative disc disease of the spine, lateral recess syndrome, and failed back surgery as a complex of multiple sources of pain production. That so little tissue handling could do so much to so many who had no alternatives available brings into focus once again our lack of understanding of back pain and our persistent overkill, relying on major potentially damaging surgical procedures such as instrumented or noninstrumented fusions to treat such pathology. The principal cause for the failure of conventional spinal surgery is attributed to "operating on the wrong level."[18] Viviprudence and endoscopy indicate that the cause of failure is in reality a failure to identify not only the level, but the pain site in the level.

Endoscopic laser foraminoplasty (ELF) provides a day case means of treating the effect of disc protrusion, chronic lumbar spondylosis, lateral recess stenosis, spondylolytic spondylolisthesis, and failed back syndrome that will widen the beneficial role of minimal invasive spine surgery for the treatment of back pain and referred pain.

References

1. Nettelbladt E. Antalet reumatikerinvalder I Sverige under en 30-arsperiod. *OPMEAR* 1985;30:54–56.
2. Report of the Commission on the Evaluation of Pain. *Soc Security Bull* 1987;50:13–44.
3. Nachemson A. Recent advances in the treatment of low back pain. *Orthopaedics* 1985;9:1–10.
4. Hijikata S, Yamagishi M, Nakayama T, et al. Percutaneous discectomy: a new treatment method for lumbar disc herniation. *J Toden Hosp* 1975;5:5–13.
5. Kambin P, Casey K, O'Brien E, Zhou L. Transforminal arthroscopic foraminal decompression of lateral recess stenosis. *J Neurosurg* 1996;84:462–467.
6. Simpson JM. Indications for laser surgery in the treatment of degenerative disk disease of the lumbar spine. *J South Orthop Assoc* 1996;5:174–180.
7. Choy DS, Michelsen J, Getrajdman G, Diwan S. Percutaneous laser disc decompression: an update—spring 1992. *J Clin Laser Med Surg* 1992;10:177–184.
8. Knight MTN. Laser-assisted percutaneous and endoscopic lumbar discectomy. In: Ramini PS, ed. *Textbook of Spinal Surgery*. Mumbai, India: Department of Neurology and Spinal Surgery; 1996:449–454.

9. Knight MTN, Pantoja S. KTP/532. Percutaneous laser disc decompression for lumbar disc prolapse. *Clin Neurosci* 1996;49:330–336.
10. Knight MTN, Vajda A, Jakab GV, Awan S. Endoscopic laser foraminoplasty on the lumbar spine—early experience. *Minimally Invasive Neurosurg* 1998;41:5–9.
11. Kushlick SD, Ijlstron CL, Michael CJ. The tissue origin of low back pain: a report of pain response to tissue stimulation during operations on lumbar spine using local anesthesia. *Orthop Clin North Am* 1991;22:181–187.
12. Almay BGL, Johansson F, Von Knorring L, et al. Substance P in CSF of patients with chronic pain syndromes. *Pain* 1988;33:3–9.
13. Rydevik B, Brown MD, Lundborg G. Pathoanatomy and pathophysiology of nerve root compression. *Spine* 1984;9:7–15.
14. Spitzer WO, LeBlank FE, Dupuis M, et al. Scientific approach to the assessment and management of activity-related disorders: a monograph for clinicians. Report at Quebec Task Force on Spinal Disorders. *Spine* 1987;12(suppl):S1–S59.
15. Johnsson K, Willner S. Postoperative instability after decompression of lumbar spinal stenosis. *Spine* 1986;11:107–110.
16. Goswami A. *Laminotomy versus Laminectomy: Is There a Difference in Stability? A Biomechanical Study on Cadaveric Spines.* Thesis: MCh (Orth) Liverpool, UK: University of Liverpool; 1994.
17. Parke WW, Watnabe R. The intrinsic vasculature of the lumbosacral spine nerve roots. *Spine* 1985;10:508–515.
18. McCulloch J. Complications of lumbar microdiscectomy. *Acta Orthop Belg* 1987;53:272–275.

16

Role of Percutaneous Laser Disc Decompression in the Treatment of Discogenic Back Pain

William Black, Arpad S. Fejos, and Daniel S.J. Choy

Discogenic back pain is a syndrome of nonradicular pain in the absence of spinal deformity, instability, and neural tension signs.[1] Pain generators from discogenic pain are believed to be produced from the nociceptive fibers through the sinuvertebral nerve, which is stimulated by fissures or tears in the posterior longitudinal ligament and annulus fibrosus.[2–4] More specifically, the outer posteriolateral part of the annulus has a rich sensory innervation.[5] It has been documented that the outer annulus is the tissue of origin in most cases of low back pain.[6] It is conceivable, then, that increased discal pressure can cause stretching of the annulus and firing of these nerve endings. It is also believed that provocative discograms will reproduce this pain. Discograms had previously been used exclusively in determining the anatomic segment thought to be responsible for the patient's pain. This use has been controversial, and many published studies have supported[7–9] or refuted it.[10–12]

Studies that accepted discography as a valid diagnostic tool treated patients with positive discograms. Surgical treatment outcomes for percutaneous discotomy, discectomy, interbody fusion, posterior lumbar interbody fusion, and global fusion revealed success rates from 30 to 96%.[13] Donelson et al. reported that the McKenzie assessment reliably differentiated discogenic pain from nondiscogenic pain as well as competent from an incompetent annulus in symptomatic discs and was superior to magnetic resonance imaging (MRI) in distinguishing painful from nonpainful discs.[14]

In 1986, Choy and Ascher first employed laser technology to decompress discs.[15] This procedure is based on the concept that the intervertebral disc, when contained by the annulus and the dorsal longitudinal ligaments, is a closed hydraulic space, subject to pressure and volume relationships. Choy and others have demonstrated that a small decrease in intradiscal volume results in a substantial reduction on intradiscal pressure.[16,17] Despite refinements in technique and the recognition that discogenic pain can cause low back pain, percutaneous laser disc decompression (PLDD) has been recommended only for cases of lumbar radiculopathy and not for low back pain alone. However, over the course of time and aided by the work of Botsford, with discography, low back pain caused by central herniation or disc degeneration (discogenic pain) seemed to be treatable with PLDD. It can be theorized that the decompressive affects of PLDD reduce the activity of the sensory fibers of the outer annulus, decreasing pain sensation.

The objective of this retrospective study is, to evaluate patients (see Table 1.2), using the McNab criteria who were treated with PLDD for discogenic pain. Until now, no long-term follow-up on this patient population has been performed.

A total of 37 patients were selected. The majority of the patients (32) were selected from the Laser Spine Center (D.S.J. Choy) based solely on their clinical symptoms of low back pain with absence of radicular symptoms on initial evaluation. The other five, from Northeastern Neurological Associates (W.A. Black), were selected based on clinical findings as well as a concordant provocative discogram. Patients who underwent PLDD from December 14, 1993 to June 19, 2001, were selected for attempted interview via telephone to evaluate their response to PLDD as outlined by the McNab criteria. One patient was deceased, and three could not be contacted. This left 32 patients participating in the survey.

Case Studies

Case JB

This patient was first seen in November 1993 with a 3-year history of low back pain, which was progressive. JB had been treated with reduction of activity (quit playing tennis) and chiropractic manipulations. Low back pain occurred with sitting, bending, lifting, or standing in one position. Only changes in activity gave relief. He became intolerant.

Discography performed on July 18, 1994, showed central disc herniation of L2-3 and L3-4 with reproduction of low back pain. The L3-4 pain was more pronounced than L2-3; L1-2 showed no herniation and no reproduction of back pain. JB underwent PLDD on July 20, 1994, at L2-3 and L3-4. He experienced a post-operative facet syndrome, which was treated with exercise and methylprednisolone (Medrol) dose pack. During an interview in December 2001 the patient stated, "The surgery changed my life." He reported that he is able to play golf and engage in other activities that had not been possible before. At times JB still at times experiences low back pain, which is relieved with massage, but he acknowledged being out of shape and having dropped his exercise program.

Case TG

This patient was a 29-year-old auto mechanic who twisted while crouching and lifting. He had transient pain in the calf. He was treated with physical therapy for 3 months while working in a light-duty position and did well. However, he experienced chronic, recurrent back pain with bending and lifting and could not return to his profession. His MRI scans of June 1992 and 1993 demonstrated Schmorl's node in the superior end plate of L3. He was seen in June 1994 because of 8 months of inability to work secondary to back pain. A discogram of L2-3 reproduced his back pain, and the contrast medium entered the Schmorl's node. PLDD, performed on November 19, 1994, resulted in relief of back pain and TG's return to employment as an auto mechanic. During an interview on December 12, 2001, the patient reported that he continues to work as an auto mechanic. His work includes bending over into engines. He does note occasional back pain, which can be relieved by ibuprofen (Motrin).

Case Summaries

More specifically, 23 male and 9 female patients were contacted. PLDD was performed on 59 separate disc levels: one each at T8-9, T12-13, and L1-2; 4 at L2-3, 11 at L3-4; 20 at L4-5; and 21 at L5-S1 (Table 16.1).

Survey results revealed that 14 patients (44%) reported a good response, 14 (44%) reported a fair response, and 4 (12.5%) reported a poor response. The 28 patients (88%) who reported good or fair responses were considered to represent successful cases. Those 4 patients (12.5%) who reported a poor response were considered to be treatment failures. Of these 4 failures, 2 reported reinjury as the cause of pain in the treated discs. The remaining 2 patients reported having relief postprocedure for a few days before their preprocedure pain levels returned.

Table 16.1 Case Summaries and Patient-Reported Responses for Percutaneous Laser Disc Decompression for Discogenic Back Pain from December 14, 1993 to June 19, 2001

Total number of patients	32
Female	9
Male	23
Disc levels operated	
T8-9	1
T12-13	1
L1-2	1
L2-3	4
L3-4	11
L4-5	20
L5-S1	21
Patient response	
Good	14 (44%)
Fair	14 (44%)
Poor	4 (12.5%)

Conclusions

These results indicate that discogenic back pain, whether diagnosed clinically or via discogram, is amenable to PLDD. In the future, more comprehensive studies must be performed to support these findings. Based on this small study population, it can be concluded that PLDD may be an effective treatment for discogenic back pain with minimal natural recurrence.

References

1. Rhyne AL, et al. Outcome of enumerated discogram-positive low back pain. *Spine* 1995;20:1997–2001.
2. Fischgrund JS, et al. Diagnosis and treatment of discogenic low back pain. *Orthop Rev* 1993;22:311–318.
3. Groen G, et al. The nerves and nerve plexus of the human vertebral column. *Am J Anat* 1990;188:282–296.
4. Mooney V, et al. Position statement on discography, the Executive Committee of the North American Spine Society. *Spine* 1988;13:1343.
5. Yoshizawa H, et al. The neuropathology of intervertebral disc removed for low back pain. *J Pathol* 1980;132:95–104.
6. Kuslich SD, et al. The tissue origin of low back pain and sciatica. *Orthop Clin North Am* 1991;22:181–187.
7. Birney TJ, et al. Comparison of MRI and discography in the diag-

nosis of lumbar degenerative disc disease. *J Spinal Disord* 1992;5:417–423.
8. Colhoun E, et al. Provocative discography as a guide to planning operations on the spine. *J Bone Joint Surg Br* 1988;70:267–271.
9. Hudgins WR. Diagnostic accuracy of lumbar discography. *Spine* 1977;2:305–309.
10. Holt E. The question of lumbar discography. *J Bone Joint Surg Am* 1968;50:720–726.
11. Maezawa S, et al. Pain provocation at lumbar discography as analyzed by computed tomography/discography. *Spine* 1992;17:1309–1315.
12. Nachemson A. Lumbar discography—where are we today? *Spine* 1989;14:555–557.
13. Zdeblick TA. The treatment of degenerative lumbar disorders—a critical review. *Spine* 1995;20(suppl):126S–137S.
14. Donelson R, et al. A prospective study of centralization of lumbar and referred pain—a predictor of symptomatic discs and anular competence. *Spine* 1997;22:1115–1122.
15. Ascher PW. Application of the laser in neurosurgery. *Lasers Surg Med* 1986;2:91–97.
16. Choy D, et al. Percutaneous laser disc decompression: an update. *J Clin Laser Med Surg* 1992;10:177–184.
17. Nachemson A, et al. In vivo measurements of intradiscal pressure discometry, a method for the determination of pressure in the lower lumbar discs. *J Bone Joint Surg Am* 1964;40(5):1077–1092.

17

Clinical Experience in 2088 Percutaneous Laser Disc Decompression Procedures

Daniel S.J. Choy

Present Status (February 13, 2003)

Since the first patient treated with Professor Peter Wolf Ascher at the Neurosurgical Institute, University of Graz, Graz, Austria, in February 1986, percutaneous laser disc decompression (PLDD) has spread throughout the world. The best current estimate is that approximately 35,000 PLDD procedures have been performed to date. They are being done in most countries in western Europe, the United Kingdom, the United States, Cuba, Colombia, Argentina, Japan, Korea, and India. This chapter deals only with the author's experience.

Laboratory Investigations

Two years of laboratory investigations at the Laser Laboratory, an outgrowth of Professor Robert B. Case's Investigative Cardiology Laboratory at St. Luke's–Roosevelt Hospital, Columbia University, preceded the first clinical case in Graz. The author is heavily indebted to Dr. Case's scientific insights, active encouragement, and generous collaboration. Without the unlimited use of the fine laboratory facilities made available to me, the elaboration of the basic science precepts underlying PLDD described

Table 17.1 Summary of Percutaneous Laser Disc Decompression (PLDD) from February 15, 1986 to February 13, 2003

Number of procedures:	2088
Number of patients:	1109
Age range:	17–92 years
Male:	682
Female:	427
Discs:	
C3-4	15
C4-5	29
C5-6	70
C6-7	44
T4-5	1
T5-6	5
T6-7	4
T7-8	5
T8-9	4
T9-10	1
T10-11	1
T11-12	4
T12-L1	6
L1-2	29
L2-3	98
L3-4	249
L4-5	799
L5-S1	724
Success rate past 17 years:	89%
Complication rate:	0.38%

in this book would not have been possible. Fresh human autopsy specimens and bovine discs were used in in vitro experiments. The initial PLDDs were performed in anesthetized mongrel dogs. The animals were killed in a humane way and autopsied.

Professor Peter Wolf Ascher possesses the vision and boldness that combined to make him one of the first pioneers in the use of lasers in neurosurgery. Without his active collaboration, the first human patient could not have been treated only two short years after I started my laboratory experiments.

Table 17.1 summarizes the author's experience. It can be seen that the most commonly involved discs in the lumbar area are at L4-5 and L5-S1. The frequency of involvement of these two discs may be related to two factors: (1) the posterior longitudinal ligament is thinnest and narrowest at these two levels, and (2) these two discs are at the spinal location bearing the maximum weight of the body. Taken together, the lumbar discs account for 91% of all intervertebral disc protrusions. The cervical discs are involved in 7.5%, and the thoracic discs in 1.5%. It may be that the cervical disc is involved more often than the thoracic discs because the cervical spine is a collection of relatively delicate vertebral bodies that must support the entire weight of the head and also must serve flexion, extension, and rotatory functions. The thoracic spine, on the other hand, is composed of larger, stronger vertebrae with limited rotatory function, and it is supported by a relatively rigid rib cage. For anatomic reasons it is not possible to enter the thoracic discs from TI to T5 from the usual dorsolateral direction.

The first 200 cases were performed in the angioplasty x-ray suite at St. Luke's–Roosevelt Hospital. The common complications are discussed in Chapter 11. There were two cases of infectious disciitis in this group, for a rate of 1%. 1%. Laser surgeons from around the world report a complication rate of 1 to 20%. Scheduling conflicts and the disadvantage of using a fixed operating table led me to move the procedure to a stand-alone surgical facility, the Laser Spine Center. In the 1888 procedures performed at this facility between infectious disciitis was encountered 7 times, for an incidence rate of 0.38%. Why was there a threefold decrease in incidence? Hospitals are *dirty* places, and the infections called nosocomial are not uncommon. Also, the use of a movable radiolucent table (see earlier: Fig. 10.1) improved imaging during the procedure. A fixed table mandates a motor-driven C-arm. With the inertia to be overcome, the C-arm does not move immediately when the button is pressed, and also does not stop as soon as the finger is lifted from the button. The imaging is therefore just slightly off. With a movable table the imaging is precise and accurate. Was this responsible for the improvement of success rate from 75% to the present 89%? Since the learning curve had been achieved before the first 100 cases, this speculation may indeed have merit.

I am often asked by patients if there is need to repeat the magnetic resonance imaging (MRI) scan after PLDD. In the first 100 patients who had 100% pain relief from PLDD, we were able to convince third-party payers to approve a second MRI 6 weeks after PLDD. In only 33 patients was there demonstrable retraction of the disc protrusion. Since the best resolution of the MRI is of the order of 2.0 mm, any dimensional change less than 2.0 mm will not appear. One needs to move the disc only 100 Å away from the nerve root to achieve a pain-free state.

A repeat MRI is needed in only two situations: (1) if disciitis is suspected and (2) if, because of reinjury, there is a cause to suspect a reherniation.

As clinical experience was gained, it was possible to *expand the envelope*. First, previously operated patients were accepted for

PLDD if a gadolinium-enhanced MRI did not demonstrate nerve entrapment by scar tissue. Second, it was found that spinal stenosis to which a bulging disc had contributed could be treated (see Chapter 13). Third, we began to accept patients with low back pain without a radicular component, but with MRI positive for disc protrusion, who might or might not have tenderness over the affected disc or to one side of the disc, especially if aggravated by trunk flexion (see Chapter 13). Finally, patients with extruded discs that were not sequestered and maintained physical contact (or a *bridge*) with the *parent* disc who were unsuccessfully treated (see Chapter 13). This last group now numbers 33, with success in 85%. The success rate in the lumbar, cervical, and thoracic discs has been 89, 85, and 100%, respectively. I have not encountered pneumothorax in PLDD of the thoracic discs. Professor Johannes Hellinger, in a personal communication, reported one instance of pneumothorax in 42 thoracic discs treated with PLDD.

The recurrence rate at 5% compares favorably with the reported 5 to 37% recurrences after open surgery.[1–4] The PLDD patients with recurrences generally report instances of reinjury. These have included lifting a heavy weight, playing golf, falling during sports, a severe coughing episode in an HIV-positive patient with pneumocystis pneumonia, and in one case, a mugging.

If there is initial improvement followed by recurrence of all symptoms at the same level of severity within 3 months, a new MRI with gadolinium enhancement is ordered. If there are root compression signs in the neurologic examination, a repeat PLDD can be offered to the patient. In my long experience, second and third procedures are infrequent events, and when performed, have generally been successful approximately 75% of the time. One patient required four PLDDs. He was an electrician working on commercial buildings and had to pull on heavy cables. When he finally took my advice and became a supervisor, his need for repeat PLDDs ceased.

Why is there a 11% failure rate? Approximately half of PLDD-failed patients who proceed to open surgery have been found to have free disc fragments. Free, sequestered disc fragments are missed 20% of the time by the best MRIs.[5–7] My theory is that free fragments, missed by the MRI, are the principal cause of PLDD failure. Botsford champions the use of preprocedure discography to identify such patients. My objection to routine discsography is based on (1) the need for another procedure that is invasive, (2) the extra pain, (3) the extra expense, and (4) the low yield.

Vacuum phenomena, best imaged by computed tomography, are another possible cause of PLDD failure. A disc with a large gas bubble is no longer a homogeneous hydraulic entity, and vaporization of a small volume of water will not result in a pressure decrease.

The usual single disc can be treated in 15 to 30 minutes, unless needle entry is impeded by osteoarthritic changes. It is not uncommon to treat two discs at one sitting. The usual time for two discs can be 30 to 60 minutes. On rare occasions, as with a patient from out of town who wishes a minimum hotel stay, I have treated as many as five discs at one sitting. It is unusual to have five discs all causing symptoms, but I have seen this two or three times.

Sometimes a high iliac crest prevents satisfactory needle placement in the L5-S1 disc. In this case the extrathecal, and sometimes a transthecal route (see Chapter 10) can be used. In over 125 such procedures I have encountered post–spinal tap headache only two or three times. No adverse neurologic sequelae have occurred.

The last six male patients between 80 and 92 years of age all failed, probably because their discs had a low water content. Because of this I no longer accept male patients over 80 as PLDD candidates. There appears to be no age limit for women.

I started with the Neodymium:YAG (Nd:YAG) laser and, for reasons discussed in Chapter 18, have continued to favor this over the Potassium Triphosphide (KTP) system and Holmium:YAG (Ho:YAG).

References

1. Delamarter RB, Bohlman HH. Failed lumber microdiscectomies. American Association of Orthopedic Surgeons; 1990;515.
2. Malter AD, McNeney B, Loeser JD, Deyo RN. Five year reoperation rates after different types of lumbar spine surgery. *Spine* 1998;23: 814–820.
3. Matsunaga S, Kabayama S, Yamamoro T, Yone K, Sakou T, Nakanishi K. Strain on intervertebral discs after anterior cervical decompression and fusion. *Spine* 1999;24:670–675.
4. Weir BKA, Jacobs GA. Reoperation rate following lumbar discectomy. *Spine* 1980;5:366–370.
5. Thornbury SR, Fryback DG, Turski PA, et al. Disk-caused nerve compression in patients with acute low back pain. Diagnosis with MR, CT myelography, and plain CT. *Radiology* 1993;186:731–738.
6. Greenspan A. CT discography vs MRI in intervertebral disc herniation. *Appl Radiol* March 1993:34–40.
7. Joubert JM, Laredo JD, Ziza JM, et al. Gadolinium-enhanced MRI imaging in the preoperative evaluation of lumbar disc herniations. Presented at the 78th Scientific Assembly and Meeting of the Radiological Society of North America; November 29–December 4, 1992; Chicago. Abstract 304.

18

Percutaneous Laser Disc Decompression: A 10-Year Follow-Up of Clinical Data

Daniel S.J. Choy and Arpad S. Fejos

In today's world of fad diets and miracle cures, one might be skeptical when first finding out about percutaneous laser disc decompression (PLDD). How effective and long lasting could this seemingly painless and instantaneous procedure be? After seeing the results of the PLDD firsthand, one could still query what the long-term outcomes might be. After further research, a study was devised to follow-up on patients who underwent this procedure 10 years ago.

Low back pain is one of the major causes of lost work time and disability in the United States. For pain due to herniated discs, a variety of treatment modalities have been prescribed, including open discectomy, microdiscectomy, and automated nucleotome discectomy. The disadvantages of these treatment options are general anesthesia, greater risks, the requirement for hospitalization and the longer recovery times associated with the procedures. By contrast, PLDD is an enticing alternative given the low risk, immediate relief, and long-lasting benefits. Percutaneous laser disc decompression is indicated for nonsequestered herniated discs, failed back syndrome, repeat procedures on reinjured discs and most recently, extruded nonsequestered discs.[1]

Since Choy and Ascher first introduced PLDD in Austria in February 1986, over 35,000 procedures have been performed worldwide.[2] With a growing need came Food and Drug Administration (FDA) premarket approval of the delivery system in 1991, and the American Medical Association granting a Current Procedural Terminology (CPT) code in January 2000.[3] The procedure is innovative and ingenious. Under local anesthesia and fluoroscopic guidance, an optical fiber is introduced from a posterolateral approach into the disc through an 18-gauge needle. Applying Neodymium:YAG (Nd:YAG) laser energy via an optical fiber causes a small volume of the nucleus pulposus to be vaporized, with a corresponding marked decrease in disc pressure. The effect is immediate, with patients walking out of the office virtually pain free.[4]

Objective

Until now, there has not been a documented study that demonstrates the long-term benefits of PLDD. The objective of this retrospective, nonrandomized, nonblinded study is to show the outcomes 10 years post-PLDD.

Design

Patients were selected from among those seen at the Laser Spine Center who had undergone lumbar PLDD from September 9, 1989, to March 20, 1991. The selection criteria included having herniated discs documented by magnetic resonance imaging or computed tomography, and corresponding clinical symptoms. In addition, patients had to have failed 3 months of conservative management, including anti-inflammatory medications, rest, muscle relaxants, physical therapy, and/or epidural steroid injections. Also, a second concurring opinion was sought from a neurologist, neurosurgeon, or orthopedic surgeon. Exclusion criteria included ongoing litigation, cancer, vertebral fracture, myositis, lateral recess syndrome, severe osteoarthritis, myositis, bone spur impingement on nerve roots, previous surgery with scar tissue nerve root entrapment, severe spondylolisthesis, or pure bony spinal stenosis.[2]

Patient Selection

A total of 61 patients met the entrance criteria and were surveyed by telephone. Despite several attempts to reach everyone, 31 could not be contacted. Of the remaining 30 patients, 2 were deceased, and 9 advised that they had undergone unspecified back surgery. A total of 19 participants were able to participate in the study (15 men, 4 women). Of these 19 eligible participants, 2 had PLDD done at the L3-L4 level, 11 at L4-L5, and 6 at L5-S1. Patients participating in the survey were asked questions allowing them to be categorized as having had good, fair, or poor response to therapy as indicated by the MacNab criteria[5] (see Table 1.2). This classification was further divided into good (MacNab good and fair) and poor (MacNab poor). Statistical analysis was performed using a logistic regression.

Methods

The procedure was performed in an outpatient setting with the patient lying in the left lateral decubitus position and an 18-gauge needle entering with a posterior lateral approach under C-arm fluoroscopic guidance. For the L5-S1 level on patients with a high iliac crest, the needle is guided 2 to 3 cm from the midline at a 5-degree angle from the sagittal plane in a posterior extrathecal approach[6] (Fig. 18.1). Once the skin and deep fascia have been anesthetized, the needle is inserted into the disc, midway through and parallel to the endplates with the tip just past the annulus (Fig. 18.2). After needle placement has been confirmed from both the anterior–posterior and lateral views, an optical fiber is guided through the needle. This fiber has a metal stopper that prevents the tip from being advanced further than 1 cm past the needle

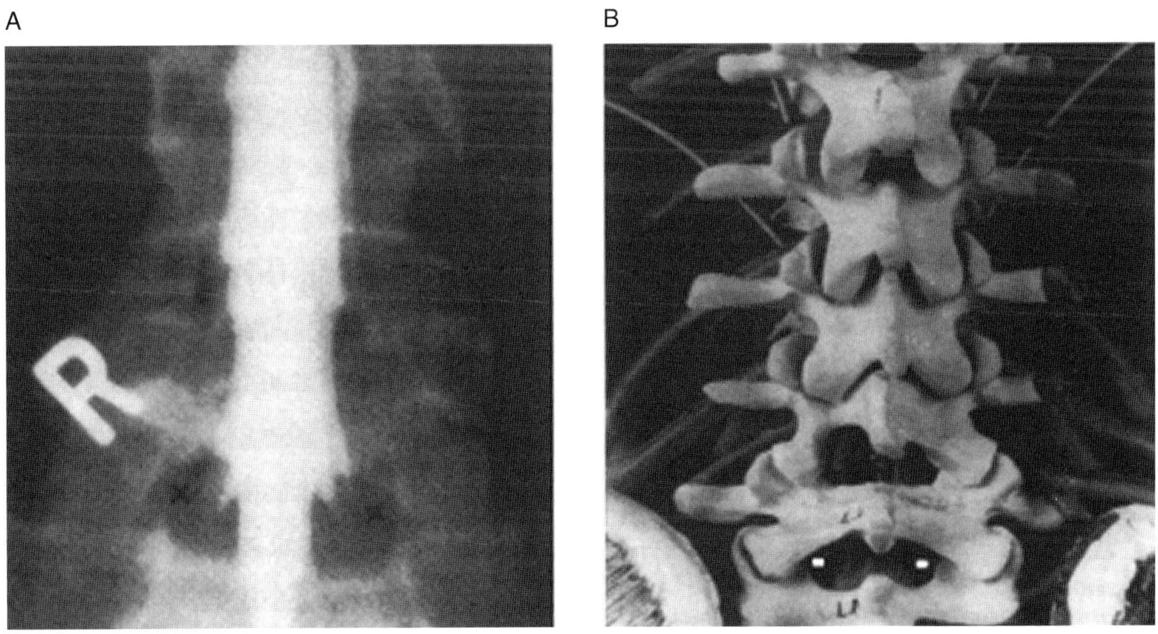

Figure 18.1. The extrathecal route is marked by Xs on a model (A) and on white dots on a routine myelogram (B). (Reprinted with permission from Choy DSJ. Percutaneous laser disc decompression (PLDD): 352 cases with an 8½-year follow-up. *J Clin Laser Med Surg* 1995;13:17–21.)

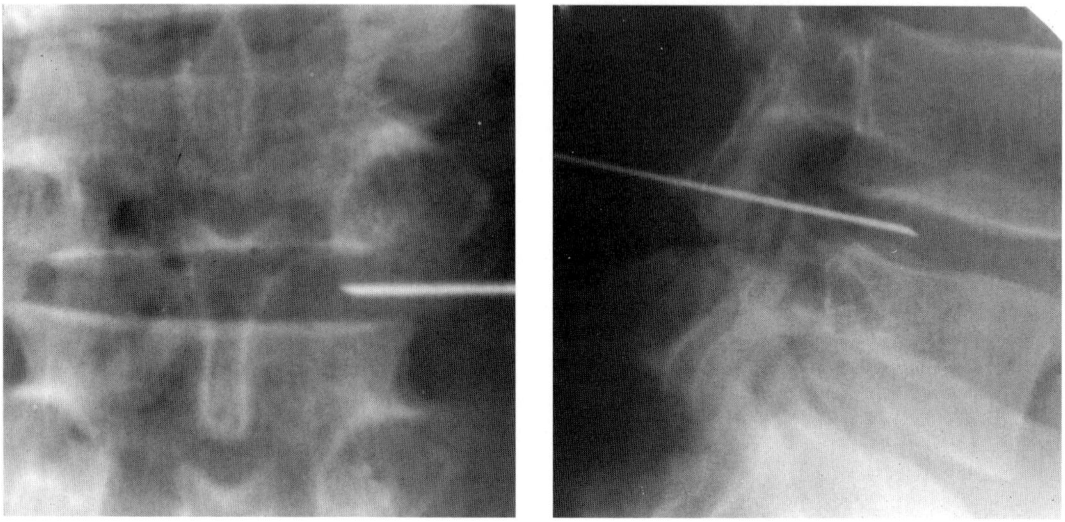

A B

Figure 18.2. The posterior view (A) shows the needle just past the annulus, while the same needle in the lateral view (B) is parallel to the disc axis and between the two end plates. (Reprinted with permission from Choy DSJ. Percutaneous laser disc decompression (PLDD): 352 cases with an 8½-year follow-up. *J Clin Laser Med Surg* 1995;13:17–21.)

tip. When the fiber is in place, calibrated 20-watt pulses of 1-second durations (20 joules) are delivered with 5-second pauses to allow for thermal dissipation,[6] for a total of 1000 to 2000 joules applied to the disc. With the application of the laser energy, a 50% decrease in intradiscal pressure occurs,[7] causing the herniation to retract away from the affected nerve root toward the center of the disc.[8,9]

Results

A two-tailed *t*-test was performed on the MacNab outcomes demonstrating statistical significance ($p < 0.0001$). This indicated that the MacNab outcome observed was not a chance occurrence. Specifically, 10 years post-PLDD 16 (84%) patients reported a good response and 3 (16%) reported a poor response to PLDD. When gender, age, and disc level are compared, there was no statistically significant correlation of the MacNab criteria with respect to the PLDD outcomes for the study population. This indicates that outcome is independent of gender, age, or disc level. Also when gender, age, disc level, and MacNab criteria were compared, a chi-squared analysis did not show statistical significance with the patients in the study group that had postprocedure back surgery. Of the 9 patients eventually undergoing discectomy and/or fusion, 7 surgeries are attributed to reinjury. The remaining 2 patients had no pain relief postprocedure and went on to surgical decompression 3 years later. Of the 7 patients who were reinjured, 4 had greater than 50% pain relief for 2 to 4 years, while the remaining 3 patients reported less than 6 months of pain relief. Of the 7 patients reporting pain relief, all stated greater pain after surgical decompression than after PLDD.

Discussion

The success of PLDD is based on a simple pathophysiologic phenomenon. The disc can be compared with a closed hydraulic space.[5,10,11] When approximately 98 mg of disc tissue is removed from a 1.0 cm × 3.5 mm diameter laser tract,[9] a 50% decrease in intradiscal pressure[7] occurs (see Fig. 1.5).[2] The pressure gradient between the tissue adjacent to the herniation and the disc results in movement of the herniation away from the affected nerve root.[4] As a result, this provides relief to the previously encroached-upon nerve root. In addition, there is clinical evidence that the disc continues to shrink for as long as 11 months after PLDD. In the past, approximately 5% of patients who did not experience immediate pain relief did so 2 to 12 weeks after the procedure.

Worldwide there has been reported a complication rate of 1% and a recurrence rate of 5%. The majority of complications have been due to infectious disciitis; less common are cauda equina syndrome and bowel perforation. Infectious disciitis responds well to appropriate antibiotics; bowel perforation is due to poor needle placement or use of side-firing tips.[2] All patients in this study underwent PLDD with the Nd:YAG laser at 1.06 μm. This laser has the greatest use worldwide.[2] As stated throughout this book, PLDD is a simple, safe, and effective procedure providing long-lasting pain relief to patients with herniated discs. It is performed in an outpatient setting under local anesthesia; it has a short recovery time; and it is relatively painless. There is no scar formation, and no spinal instability, which means that segment mobility is preserved. This allows patients to return to work relatively quickly with minimal rehabilitation (depending on previous functioning) required. Considering PLDD's strong merits, segment mobility preservation and long-lasting outcome, why does a 69-year-old operation precede it as a first-line treatment in herniated disc disease? In the age of new percutaneous disc interventions, PLDD with its 17-year track record should precede all other surgeries and interventions as a treatment option when indicated.

References

1. Choy DSJ. Response of extruded intervertebral herniated discs to percutaneous laser disc decompression. *Lasers Surg Med* 2001;19:15–20.
2. Choy DSJ. Percutaneous laser disc decompression (PLDD): a first line treatment for herniated discs. *Lasers Surg Med* 1995;19:1–2.
3. Choy DSJ. New CPT code for percutaneous laser disc decompression awarded by the American Medical Association. *Lasers Surg Med* 2000;17:239.
4. Choy DSJ. Rapid correction of neurological deficits by percutaneous laser disc decompression (PLDD). *Lasers Surg Med* 1996;14:13–15.
5. MacNab I. Negative disc exploration: an analysis of the causes of nerve root involvement in 68 patients. *J Bone Joint Surg Am* 1971;53: 891–903.
6. Choy DSJ. Percutaneous laser disc decompression (PLDD): 352 cases with an $8\frac{1}{2}$-year follow-up. *Lasers Surg Med* 1995;13:17–21.
7. Choy DSJ. Percutaneous laser disc decompression using the 1.06- and 1.32-μm Nd:YAG lasers. *Spine* 1993;7(1)(state-of-the-art review: laser discectomy):41–47.
8. Choy DSJ. Percutaneous laser disc decompression (PLDD): twelve years' experience with 752 procedures in 518 patients. *Lasers Surg Med* 1998;16:325–331.
9. Choy DSJ, Ngeow J. Fall of intradiscal pressure with laser ablation. *Spine* 1993;7(1):23–29.
10. Nachemson A. The effects of forward leaning on lumbar intradiscal pressure. *Acta Orthop Scand* 1965;35:314–328.
11. Nachemson A. The lumbar spine: an orthopaedic challenge. *Spine* 1976;1:59–71.
12. Choy DSJ, Ascher PW, Saddekni S, et al. Percutaneous laser disc decompression—a new therapeutic modality. *Spine* 1992;17(8):949–956.

Index